Corneal Infection and Inflammation

Corneal Infection and Inflammation

A Colour Atlas

Edited by

Noopur Gupta

Ritika Mukhija

Radhika Tandon

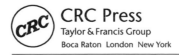

CRC Press
Taylor & Francis Group
Boca Raton London New York

CRC Press is an imprint of the
Taylor & Francis Group, an **informa** business

First edition published 2021
by CRC Press
6000 Broken Sound Parkway NW, Suite 300, Boca Raton, FL 33487-2742
and by CRC Press
2 Park Square, Milton Park, Abingdon, Oxon, OX14 4RN

© 2021 Taylor & Francis Group, LLC
CRC Press is an imprint of Taylor & Francis Group, LLC

Library of Congress Cataloging-in-Publication Data
Names: Gupta, Noopur, editor. | Mukhija, Ritika, editor. | Tandon, Radhika, editor.
Title: Corneal infection and inflammation : a colour atlas / edited by
Noopur Gupta, Ritika Mukhija, Radhika Tandon.
Description: First edition. | Boca Raton, FL : CRC Press, 2021. | Includes
bibliographical references and index. | Summary: "This book is a comprehensive treatise on slit lamp illustrations of infective and inflammatory pathologies of the cornea. Both infectious (bacterial, fungal, viral, and protozoan) and non-infectious keratitis that cause corneal vascularization, scarring and vision loss, have been extensively covered, supported by illustrated case scenarios"— Provided by publisher.
Identifiers: LCCN 2020049633 (print) | LCCN 2020049634 (ebook) | ISBN
9780367457129 (hbk) | ISBN 9780367761561 (pbk) | ISBN 9781003024897 (ebk)
Subjects: MESH: Keratitis—pathology | Cornea—pathology | Atlas | Case Reports
Classification: LCC RE336 (print) | LCC RE336 (ebook) | NLM WW 17 | DDC
617.7/1900222—dc23
LC record available at https://lccn.loc.gov/2020049633
LC ebook record available at https://lccn.loc.gov/2020049634

ISBN: 9780367457129 (hbk)
ISBN: 9780367761561 (pbk)
ISBN: 9781003024897 (ebk)

Typeset in Palatino
by KnowledgeWorks Global Ltd.

eResources available at: www.routledge.com/9780367761561

To my parents
Mrs Annapurna Gupta and Mr Gopal Sharan Gupta
Mrs Sushila Parakh and Mr Keshri Chand Parakh

Noopur Gupta

To my parents, Mrs Sushma Mukhija and Mr Suresh Mukhija, and my
husband, Dr Mayur Nayak, for always being my pillars of strength.

Ritika Mukhija

To my family, teachers, students and patients.

Radhika Tandon

Table of Contents

Foreword

Henry David Thoreau (1817–1862): *'We cannot see anything until we are possessed with the idea of it, take it into our heads, – and then we can hardly see anything else.'*[1]

D.H. Lawrence (1885–1930): *'What the eye doesn't see and the mind doesn't know, doesn't exist.'*[2]

Robertson Davies (1913–1995): *'… the eye sees only what the mind is prepared to comprehend.'*[3]

The medical atlas is often one of the very first textbooks purchased by beginning medical students, and thus holds a special place in the libraries of physicians and surgeons long after the rigours of their training have passed. The great medical atlases are broad compendiums of medical knowledge, providing invaluable visual examples and descriptions of health and disease. Medical atlases are often also great works of art. This is true particularly for atlases of ophthalmology, for the eye's beauty even in illness is every ophthalmologist's secret joy.

It is my great pleasure and high honour to introduce this wonderful new atlas, authored exclusively by the magnificent clinicians and senior trainees on the Cornea, Cataract and Refractive Surgery Service of the Dr Rajendra Prasad Centre for Ophthalmic Sciences, All India Institute of Medical Sciences, in New Delhi. The editors of the atlas, Drs Noopur Gupta, Ritika Mukhija and Radhika Tandon, have assembled an exhaustive and fully comprehensive tome, encompassing the broad array of corneal infectious and inflammatory disorders, replete with useful and representative clinical photographs, diagrams, case descriptions and teaching videos. The atlas will serve as a single resource for residents-in-training, corneal fellows, and comprehensive ophthalmologists. Academic cornea specialists will find it a welcome addition to their library, as the book includes disorders both rare and common.

The All India Institute of Medical Sciences was established in 1965 through an Act of the Parliament of India and is the largest government hospital in the country. Its Dr Rajendra Prasad Centre for Ophthalmic Sciences, named after the first President of India and known affectionately as the RP Centre, was established in 1967 and quickly became the leading centre in India for training young ophthalmologists. Over one-half million patients are seen at the RP Centre every year, and their ophthalmologists have the privilege of seeing, and the attendant responsibility of caring for, the entire spectrum of corneal disorders. This book will serve well any budding ophthalmologist seeking to learn to recognise corneal disorders and is fully consistent with the motto of the RP Centre: "Tamso Ma Jyotirgamaya" (from darkness to light).

Enjoy!

James Chodosh, MD MPH
Edith Ives Cogan Professor of Ophthalmology
Massachusetts Eye and Ear
Harvard Medical School
Boston, Massachusetts, USA

NOTES

1 Henry David Thoreau, Autumnal Tints. First published, 1862.
2 D.H Lawrence, Lady Chatterley's Lover. 1928.
3 Robertson Davies, Tempest-Tost. 1951.

Preface

Ophthalmology is a very visual specialty. The field is blessed among the other medical domains as having a very clear view of most of what is happening, both literally and figuratively. Of the various clinical aspects of ophthalmology, the diagnosis and management of corneal disorders has a distinctive edge of greater accessibility clinically for assessment and evaluation. Because the cornea is an essential component of the visual apparatus of the eye, playing a crucial role as the protective front layer of the globe and being richly innervated, diseases of the cornea have a high morbidity and far-reaching consequences due to their sequelae, particularly those related to infections and inflammations. Timely recognition and suitable intervention can go a long way in stemming the tide of blindness or permanent visual loss. Though there is an abundance of excellent textbooks on corneal disorders and their medical and surgical treatment, few cover a wide range of samples conveying the true spectrum of pathologies related to the topics of corneal infections and inflammations. Corneal infections are a major cause of blindness in developing countries and a significant contributor to ocular morbidity worldwide. The thought processes and motivation behind the landmark herpetic eye disease studies are key indicators of how the extreme discomfort and debilitating effects of corneal disorders can be a major driving force for actions to induce change.

The wealth of information available in textbooks and journal articles is supplemented by practical aspects gained by seeing and working up patients with the disorders. Theoretical knowledge is given a boost by actual clinical experience to provide the required know-how for best patient care and, also teaching. Clinical practice and acumen are skills honed by an inquisitive mind, supported by a systematic approach with logical reasoning and analytical thought processes that distil the known knowledge and combine it with the current case scenario to arrive at a suitable diagnosis and plan appropriate management. In most situations, a complex interplay of one's higher mental processes, retrieving past examples from the storehouse of one's brain to cogently combine them with the situation at hand and arrive at the 'what to do now' eureka moment, actually takes place at lightning speed and with remarkable accuracy. One can also rely on consulting one's peers or superiors or even consulting one's books or journals, various online platforms, chat groups and other professional social media platforms to get help and guidance when needed. There do arise situations, though, when one wishes one knew more ... be it at the stage of recognising a crucial clinical sign, learning the trick of what critical clues to look for or having an idea of what to expect over the clinical course, outcome of intervention and final prognosis.

On the other side of the fence, clinicians also face situations where the condition unravels itself over the course of investigations and treatment, the hidden truths being laid bare as the disease unfolds until finally they experience the eureka moment of seeing the secret revealed in all its splendour. In yesteryear these examples could be shared for posterity via case reports and short articles, but as the medical profession has raced ahead, the journals have kept pace, and there is consequently limited space for sharing such vignettes with a wider audience and documenting the clinical tips for future generations. In this context, a medical atlas plays a useful role. Having a plethora of interesting and unique cases to document and share was the inspiration, and our 'academic DNA' was the main motivation for writing this book.

We consulted our colleagues, including the residents with an interest in cornea, and explored the level of interest in a book of this nature. We were pleased to find a high level of enthusiasm and realised that there was indeed a wealth of resources in terms of case studies, clinical material and enthusiastic authors with a fresh perspective on what the end user would be looking for or likely to benefit from. In researching the topic, we were emboldened to find that we had substantial new information to add by using the clinical material available with our inputs of real-world experience and were confident of having plenty of useful stories to tell and create a good, practical resource for both students or ophthalmologists early in their career and experienced professionals. A plethora of knowledge can be unravelled with hands-on experience through a variety of clinical presentations, both common and new; the highlights being the crisply drawn schematic corneal diagrams, teaching videos and useful, pertinent tips related to management of clinical case scenarios.

We brainstormed with potential authors and enlisted interested residents who had contributed and actively participated in the patient care process. One realises how many people are involved in a busy tertiary care referral academic institution such as ours and how each person at every level has a critical role to play. In recognition of the individual clinicians and their contributions, we compiled their various skill sets for each chapter, harnessing their unique capacities efficiently and effectively. The strategy worked out extremely well and despite the COVID-19 pandemic throwing life out of gear we were able to use the various online platforms and virtual arenas to continue to work together on our project and meet our deadline.

In the completion of this book, we have many to thank. First, the academic ethos of All India Institute of Medical Sciences (AIIMS) and tradition of excellence of the Dr Rajendra Prasad Centre for Ophthalmic Sciences, the clinical platform afforded by the Centre with state-of-the-art facilities and the abundance of rare and exquisite cases we get to see. We are also indebted to our teachers, who have always been a guiding force and our students, a constant source of motivation to always exceed in our endeavours and excel. No words can describe the gratitude we feel for our patients, who come to our centre not only from different parts of the country, but also the world. We are thankful to them for the faith they place in us and their patience and understanding in the time-consuming process of data collection, clinical photography and treatment. And last but not the least, we are extremely grateful to Professor James Chodosh for being a source of great inspiration in the field and for taking the time to contribute a brilliant forward for this special book.

Noopur Gupta
Ritika Mukhija
Radhika Tandon

Editors

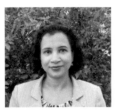

Noopur Gupta, MS (Gold Medal), DNB, PhD, is an eminent member of the Cornea, Cataract and Refractive Surgery Services at Dr RP Centre for Ophthalmic Sciences, All India Institute of Medical Sciences, New Delhi, India. With nearly 20 years of teaching and research experience, she has actively participated as chairperson, instructor, judge and faculty at various regional, national and international conferences. She has received numerous awards at national and international platforms for robust cornea research including the Excellence in Ophthalmic Research & AIIMS Excellence award. She received the ORBIS International Medal for best paper contributing to prevention of blindness in the developing world for her work on keratomalacia. Her contributions in the field of dry eye have been lauded both nationally and globally. With more than 200 publications to her credit, she is reviewer and editor of many national and international journals and has contributed immensely to national health policies and advocacy. She serves as an international expert to the World Health Organization, Geneva, and has actively contributed to developing recommendations for global elimination of neglected tropical diseases.

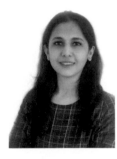

Ritika Mukhija, MD, MRCSEd, FICO, FAICO (Cornea), has been working as a Senior Resident in the Cornea, Cataract and Refractive Surgery Services at the Dr Rajendra Prasad Centre for Ophthalmic Sciences, AIIMS, New Delhi, India. She completed her undergraduate degree from Maulana Azad Medical College, New Delhi, in 2012 and postgraduate degree in Ophthalmology from the All India Institute of Medical Sciences, New Delhi, in 2017. She has over 30 publications in peer-reviewed indexed journals and seven book chapters to her credit. She received the 'best senior resident award' in 2019 and has many other awards and presentations to her name. She has been actively involved in academic, clinical and research work in the field of cornea for the last three years.

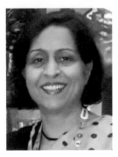

Radhika Tandon, MD, DNB, FRCSEd, FRCOphth, MNASI, is a Professor of Ophthalmology at the Dr Rajendra Prasad Centre for Ophthalmic Sciences, AIIMS, New Delhi, India. She is a leading expert in cornea, refractive and cataract surgery with nearly three decades of ophthalmic surgical and medical teaching experience. She has been accorded several national and international honours and fellowships and has been appointed as an expert to several task forces and high-powered committees. She served as the President of the Eye Bank Association of India (EBAI) 2016–2018 in which she has pioneered shaping and guiding eye banking standards and practices in India, combated corneal blindness and imparting training in cornea and keratoplasty.

Contributors

Sneha Aggarwal
Optometrist
Dr Rajendra Prasad Centre for Ophthalmic
  Sciences
All India Institute of Medical Sciences
New Delhi, India

Suresh Azimeera
Senior Resident
Cornea, Cataract and Refractive Surgery
  Services
Dr Rajendra Prasad Centre for Ophthalmic
  Sciences
All India Institute of Medical Sciences
New Delhi, India

Amit K Das
Senior Resident
Cornea, Cataract and Refractive Surgery
  Services
Dr Rajendra Prasad Centre for Ophthalmic
  Sciences
All India Institute of Medical Sciences
New Delhi, India

Noopur Gupta
Associate Professor of Ophthalmology
Cornea, Cataract and Refractive Surgery
  Services
Dr Rajendra Prasad Centre for Ophthalmic
  Sciences
All India Institute of Medical Sciences
New Delhi, India

Shikha Gupta
Assistant Professor of Ophthalmology
Dr Rajendra Prasad Centre for Ophthalmic
  Sciences
All India Institute of Medical Sciences
New Delhi, India

Yogita Gupta
Senior Resident
Cornea, Cataract and Refractive Surgery
  Services
Dr Rajendra Prasad Centre for Ophthalmic
  Sciences
All India Institute of Medical Sciences
New Delhi, India

Shubhi Jain
Research Optometrist
Dr Rajendra Prasad Centre for Ophthalmic
  Sciences
All India Institute of Medical Sciences
New Delhi, India

Alisha Kishore
Senior Resident
Cornea, Cataract and Refractive Surgery
  Services
Dr Rajendra Prasad Centre for Ophthalmic
  Sciences
All India Institute of Medical Sciences
New Delhi, India

Pooja Kumari
Senior Resident
Cornea, Cataract and Refractive Surgery
  Services
Dr Rajendra Prasad Centre for Ophthalmic
  Sciences
All India Institute of Medical Sciences
New Delhi, India

Neiwete Lomi
Assistant Professor of Ophthalmology
Cornea, Cataract and Refractive Surgery
  Services
Dr Rajendra Prasad Centre for Ophthalmic
  Sciences
All India Institute of Medical Sciences
New Delhi, India

Rachna Meel
Associate Professor of Ophthalmology
Dr Rajendra Prasad Centre for Ophthalmic
    Sciences
All India Institute of Medical Sciences
New Delhi, India

Ritika Mukhija
Senior Resident
Cornea, Cataract and Refractive Surgery
    Services
Dr Rajendra Prasad Centre for Ophthalmic
    Sciences
All India Institute of Medical Sciences
New Delhi, India

Nimmy Raj
Senior Resident
Cornea, Cataract and Refractive Surgery
    Services
Dr Rajendra Prasad Centre for Ophthalmic
    Sciences
All India Institute of Medical Sciences
New Delhi, India

Deeksha Rani
Junior Resident
Dr Rajendra Prasad Centre for Ophthalmic
    Sciences
All India Institute of Medical Sciences
New Delhi, India

Aishwarya Rathod
Junior Resident
Dr Rajendra Prasad Centre for Ophthalmic
    Sciences
All India Institute of Medical Sciences
New Delhi, India

Akash D Saha
Junior Resident
Dr Rajendra Prasad Centre for Ophthalmic
    Sciences
All India Institute of Medical Sciences
New Delhi, India

Nikita Sharma
Senior Resident
Cornea, Cataract and Refractive Surgery
    Services
Dr Rajendra Prasad Centre for Ophthalmic
    Sciences
All India Institute of Medical Sciences
New Delhi, India

Rashmi Singh
Ex-Senior Resident
Cornea, Cataract and Refractive Surgery
    Services
Dr Rajendra Prasad Centre for Ophthalmic
    Sciences
All India Institute of Medical Sciences
New Delhi, India

Vipul Singh
Junior Resident
Dr Rajendra Prasad Centre for Ophthalmic
    Sciences
All India Institute of Medical Sciences
New Delhi, India

T Monikha
Junior Resident
Dr Rajendra Prasad Centre for Ophthalmic
    Sciences
All India Institute of Medical Sciences
New Delhi, India

Radhika Tandon
Professor of Ophthalmology
Cornea, Cataract and Refractive Surgery
    Services
Dr Rajendra Prasad Centre for Ophthalmic
    Sciences
All India Institute of Medical Sciences
New Delhi, India

M Vanathi
Professor of Ophthalmology
Cornea, Cataract and Refractive Surgery Services
Dr Rajendra Prasad Centre for Ophthalmic
    Sciences
All India Institute of Medical Sciences
New Delhi, India

Praveen Vashist
Professor of Community Ophthalmology
Dr Rajendra Prasad Centre for Ophthalmic
    Sciences
All India Institute of Medical Sciences
New Delhi, India

Saumya Yadav
Senior Resident
Cornea, Cataract and Refractive Surgery Services
Dr Rajendra Prasad Centre for Ophthalmic
    Sciences
All India Institute of Medical Sciences
    New Delhi, India

SECTION A
OVERVIEW

1 Applied Anatomy and Pathophysiology

Nimmy Raj, Saumya Yadav, T Monikha, Akash D Saha, Noopur Gupta

INTRODUCTION

The cornea is an avascular, transparent tissue that forms a major structural barrier between the intraocular structures and the external environment. As the most exposed part of the eye, the cornea is particularly prone to environmental insults including microbial invasion. The transparency of the cornea is maintained by various structural and functional mechanisms. Due to its avascular nature, the process of wound healing after corneal injury is different from other parts of the body. This chapter gives a brief overview of the relevant anatomy and pathophysiology in corneal infection and inflammation.

ANATOMY AND PHYSIOLOGY OF THE CORNEA

The cornea is an aspheric, biconvex, avascular structure which forms the outer covering of the eye with an anterior curvature of 7.8 mm and posterior curvature of 6.5 mm. The refractive index of the cornea is 1.376. The corneal thickness in the centre ranges from 551 µm to 565 µm[1] and increases from the centre to the periphery.[2] It is composed of five layers: the epithelium, Bowman's membrane, the stroma, Descemet's membrane and the endothelium, along with a recently described, acellular layer in the pre-Descemet's region known as Dua's layer (Figure 1.1).

Each corneal layer serves a purpose to maintain the transparency of the cornea and hence helps in formation of a clear image at the fovea. The stratified squamous non-keratinised corneal epithelium is composed of relatively uniform five to seven layers of cells that are arranged regularly along with tight junctions. It not only helps to maintain the corneal transparency but also prevents fluid ingress and egress of pathological agents into the eye. The epithelium and the tear film form a symbiotic relationship that maintains a uniform surface over the eye. The peripheral cornea, owing to its unique anatomical and physiological characteristics, is more prone to local and systemic infectious diseases and inflammatory disorders.[3] Bowman's membrane lies just anterior to the stroma and is composed of type I and V collagen with a thickness of approximately 12 µm. This layer helps the cornea maintain its shape. As it has no ability to regenerate, injury can result in scar formation.

The corneal stroma constitutes approximately 80–85% of the total corneal thickness and forms the major bulk of the corneal tissue with extracellular matrix (predominantly type I collagen along with type III, V, VI and glycosaminoglycans) and keratocytes as the predominant components. Glycosaminoglycans are keratan sulphate (predominantly), chondroitin sulphate and dermatan sulphate. The regular and closely packed arrangement of the collagen fibrils and their smaller size play an important role in preventing diffraction of light and maintaining transparency. Descemet's membrane is made up of type IV collagen and laminin, is secreted continuously by the endothelium and makes an important surgical landmark in corneal lamellar procedures. The endothelium, which is a single layer of orderly arranged cuboidal cells of approximately 5 µm thickness, have a Na+ K+ ATPase pump on the lateral membrane which causes a net flux of ions from stroma to aqueous humour and thus helps in keeping the cornea in a dehydrated state. The endothelial cell density continues to change throughout one's lifetime, ranging from 3000 to 4000 cells/mm² at birth to around 2500 cells/mm² in adulthood and reduces at a rate of 0.6% per year.[4]

OCULAR SURFACE IMMUNE DEFENCE SYSTEM

The cornea is normally protected from microbial invasion by the natural ocular surface defence mechanisms present in the precorneal tear film (mucin, IgA, lysozyme,

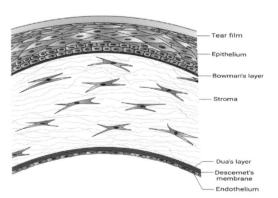

Tear film
Epithelium
Bowman's layer
Stroma
Dua's layer
Descemet's membrane
Endothelium

Figure 1.1 Schematic diagram illustrating the anatomical layers of the cornea.

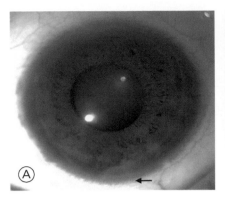
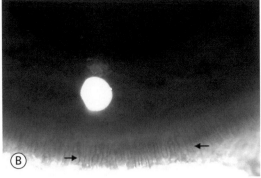

Figure 1.2 Slit lamp photograph of the cornea depicting (A) the limbal palisades of Vogt (black arrow). A magnified view of the inferior limbus shows (B) the same in greater detail with the pigmented linear structures at the limbus arranged in parallel rows (black arrows).

β lysin, lactoferrin, complement factors), conjunctiva (conjunctiva-associated lymphoid tissue) and the corneal epithelium. Derived from the surface ectoderm, an intact corneal epithelium acts as a mechanical barrier to invading organisms. Corneal epithelial cells are also capable of secreting cytokines to activate the immune defence mechanisms whenever there is deeper involvement from an injury. The cytokine interleukin (IL)-1 is stored in the corneal epithelial cells and is released when the cell membrane is ruptured by infectious agents or trauma leading to an enhanced immune response.[5]

In normal and diseased states, the ageing corneal epithelium is continuously replaced by the regular migration, proliferation and differentiation of corneal epithelial cells. These epithelial cells are derived from multipotent limbal stem cells located in the undulating folds of the palisades of Vogt and are usually replaced every 7–10 days. The palisades of Vogt (Figure 1.2) are a series of radially oriented fibrovascular ridges commonly located in the superior and inferior corneoscleral limbus. The palisades are more discrete in younger and more heavily pigmented individuals. The X, Y, Z hypothesis of corneal epithelial maintenance states that the sum of X (proliferation and anterior migration of cells) and Y (centripetal migration of cells) must equal Z (desquamation of superficial cells). This process gets accelerated if any epithelial injury occurs and hence those injuries that involves just the epithelium heal rapidly.

When corneal injury occurs, the earliest response that occurs is that of apoptosis of keratocytes and necrosis of corneal stromal tissue. Inflammatory biomarkers like transforming growth factor beta (TGF β) and IL-1 lead to accumulation and migration of inflammatory cells at the site of injury. This eventually leads to stromal remodelling and may result in either formation of a disorganised extracellular matrix leading to corneal scarring or apoptosis of keratocytes (Figure 1.3).

Microbial keratitis is a spectrum of ocular infectious diseases affecting the cornea caused by the proliferation of microorganisms (bacteria, fungi or other protozoal organisms) with resulting inflammation and tissue destruction (Figure 1.4). The severity of the condition may vary in each person depending on the pathogenicity of the organism involved, the susceptibility of the individual and the immunological state of the individual. The healing of an infectious corneal ulcer proceeds in three stages, namely, the initial progressive followed by the regressive and healing stages. The progressive stage is marked by a grey zone of infiltration, necrosis and ulceration, which, if it penetrates deeper, may lead to formation of a descemetocele. The regressive stage is seen as a demarcation line around the ulcer along with leucocytosis and macrophages that engulf the organisms and the neutrophils. Lastly, the healing phase takes over to promote epithelisation with a decrease in the size of infiltrates and the appearance of vascularisation and formation of ghost vessels. Herpes simplex keratitis has peculiarities as it results in activation of both innate and adaptive immune response and the latency of the infection resulting from the latter leads to recurrent attacks of herpes keratitis in the individual.[6] The innate response is mediated by the dendritic cells, macrophages and natural killer cells while the adaptive response is mediated by the antigen expressed memory T cells and B lymphocytes (Figure 1.5).

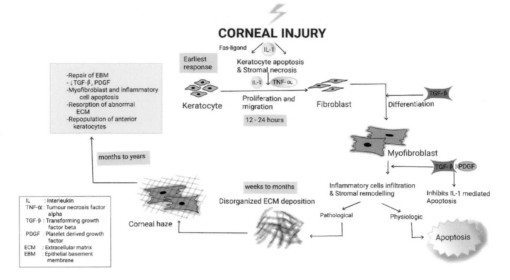

Figure 1.3 Immunological response to corneal injury and repair mechanisms.

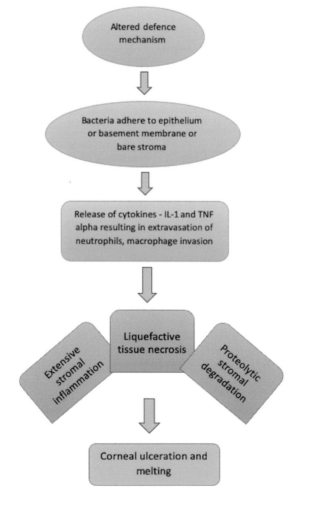

Figure 1.4 Pathogenesis of microbial keratitis and ulceration.

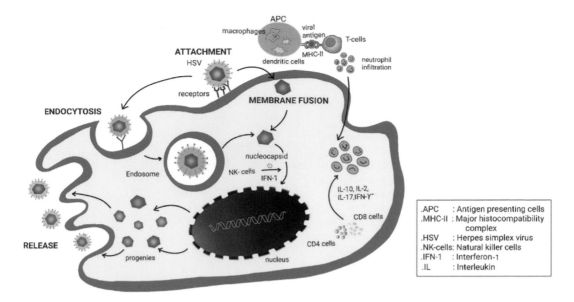

Figure 1.5   Innate and adaptive immune response to herpetic corneal infection.

CONCLUSION

A lucid understanding of the anatomical and physiological aspects of the cornea is important for the proper management of corneal infective and inflammatory disorders. A basic knowledge of the complex cellular and biochemical pathways involved in corneal wound healing can help modify treatment for each case and hence result in better anatomical and functional outcomes.

REFERENCES

1. Feizi S, Jafarinasab MR, Karimian F, Hasanpour H, Masudi A. Central and peripheral corneal thickness measurement in normal and keratoconic eyes using three corneal pachymeters. *J Ophthalmic Vis Res*. 2014; 9:296–304.
2. Fares U, Otri AM, Al-Aqaba MA, Dua HS. Correlation of central and peripheral corneal thickness in healthy corneas. *Cont Lens Anterior Eye*. 2012; 35:39–45.
3. Thoft RA, Friend J. The X, Y, Z hypothesis of corneal epithelial maintenance. *Invest Ophthalmol Vis Sci*. 1983 Oct; 24(10):1442–3.
4. Bourne WM, Nelson LR, Hodge DO. Central corneal endothelial cell changes over a ten-year period. *Invest Ophthalmol Vis Sci*. 1997; 38:779–82.
5. Niederkorn JY, Peeler JS, Mellon J. Phagocytosis of particulate antigens by corneal epithelial cells stimulates interleukin-1 secretion and migration of Langerhans cells into the central cornea. *Reg Immunol*. 1989; 2: 83–90.
6. Wang L, Wang R, Xu C, Zhou H. Pathogenesis of herpes stromal keratitis: immune inflammatory response mediated by inflammatory regulators. *Front Immunol*. 2020;11:766.

2 Clinical Evaluation

Saumya Yadav, Nimmy Raj, Aishwarya Rathod, Noopur Gupta

INTRODUCTION

The spectrum of microbial keratitis is dependent on a complex interplay between a diverse group of microorganisms and the host. A corneal ulcer may be defined as a discontinuation in the normal epithelial surface of the cornea associated with necrosis of the surrounding tissue and is pathologically characterised by oedema and cellular infiltration. Ulceration of the cornea, especially if severe and involving the visual axis or with extreme corneal thinning and impending perforation or if already perforated, is an ophthalmic emergency that needs immediate attention and, if not effectively managed, can lead to sight-threatening complications and in extreme situations irreversible loss of vision. This chapter gives a brief overview of the natural ocular defence mechanisms followed by the technique to approach the workup of a case of microbial keratitis.

CLINICAL ASSESSMENT

1. History

- Symptoms: pain, redness, foreign body sensation, burning, itching, photophobia, blurred vision, excessive tearing, purulent/mucopurulent/mucoid/watery discharge, swelling of the eyelids

- Mode and duration of onset

- Risk factors:

  - *Ocular*: trauma, contact lens wear, a recent history of chickenpox or shingles, history of ocular surgery, use of steroid eye drops/ointments, compromised ocular surface (Figure 2.1), adnexal infections, chemical/thermal injury, eyelid disorders

  - *Systemic diseases*: diabetes mellitus; immunocompromised states; connective tissue and autoimmune disorders (rheumatoid arthritis, Sjögren's syndrome); Stevens-Johnson syndrome; chronic infections like tuberculosis, leprosy and syphilis; dermatological diseases, generalised malnutrition in children

  - *Occupational*: farmers, animal handlers, chemical industry workers

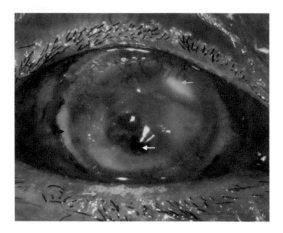

Figure 2.1 Slit lamp photograph of right eye of a patient with post-chemical injury corneal melt with secondary bacterial infection demonstrating diffuse congestion with superficial vascularisation (blue arrow) and a patch of limbal ischaemia (black arrow), central corneal melt with iris prolapse (white arrow), corneal infiltrates (yellow arrow) and frothy meibomian discharge (green arrow).

2. General Examination

- Face lesions (Herpes zoster/simplex)

- Facial palsy

- Blink rate

3. Ocular Examination

- Visual acuity

- External examination (diffuse light)

  - Lid oedema

  - Entropion, ectropion, trichiasis, lagophthalmos, lid margin

  - Dacryocystitis, nasolacrimal duct obstruction (regurgitation test)

  - Bell's phenomenon

  - Corneal/conjunctival exposure

- Slit lamp examination of the cornea (Figure 2.2)

  - Meibomian gland dysfunction

  - Conjunctival congestion – circumcorneal/diffuse

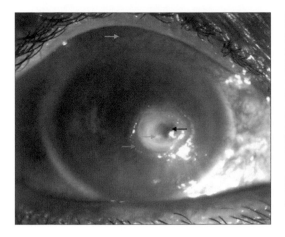

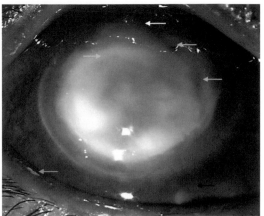

Figure 2.2 Slit lamp photograph of a case of infective keratitis depicting ciliary congestion (blue arrow), corneal epithelial defect (grey arrow), small infiltrate (green arrow) and corneal thinning (black arrow).

Figure 2.3 Slit lamp photograph of a case of corneal abscess (yellow arrow) with corneal (green arrows) and scleral (black arrow) thinning. Associated mucopurulent discharge (white arrow) and meibomian gland dysfunction (blue arrow) can also be seen.

- Purulent/mucopurulent discharge
- Corneal sensations
- Corneal ulcer (Figure 2.3)
  - Site, size, surface, margin, slough, depth of involvement, satellite lesions
- Anterior chamber
  - Cells, flare, hypopyon, endothelial pigments/exudates
- Fluorescein staining (1% sodium fluorescein) (Figure 2.4)
  - Size of the epithelial defect
  - Size of corneal infiltrate

- Seidel test (Video 2.1)
- Iris and pupil
- Lens
- Fundus evaluation/ultrasound B-scan for status of the posterior segment
- Schematic corneal diagram: a scaled, coloured corneal diagram should be drawn at the initial presentation and at follow-up visits as representative images of the ulcer and associated corneal features (Figure 2.5). They should follow the standard colour-coding guidelines

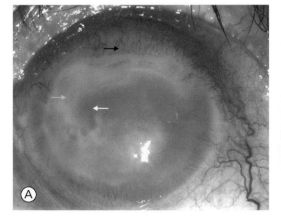

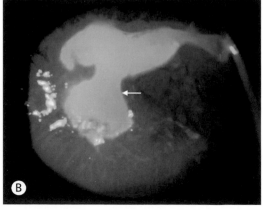

Figure 2.4 Slit lamp photograph of a case of bacterial corneal ulcer showing (A) epithelial defect (white arrow), superficial corneal vascularisation (black arrow) and corneal infiltrates (yellow arrow). Staining with 1% sodium fluorescein highlights (B) the epithelial defect delineating its margins (white arrow).

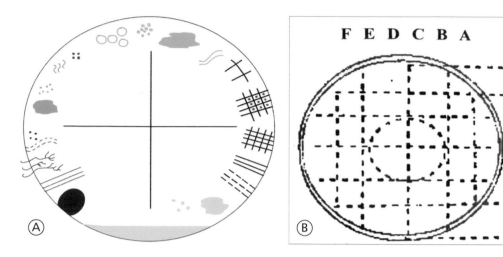

Figure 2.5 Schematic coloured diagram (A) and grid diagram (B) for documenting corneal pathologies. Each square on the grid diagram represents an area of 2×2 mm² on the cornea.

(Table 2.1).[1,2] The schematic diagrams help in assessing the course of the disease and response to therapy. This method of recording corneal pathologies should be practised for all corneal diseases as it provides simplified, standardised graphic documentation and serves as a universal language among ophthalmologists (Figure 2.6).

- Examination under anaesthesia (EUA): An ocular examination under general anaesthesia (GA) is sometimes necessary in cases of corneal ulcers when an external and/or slit lamp examination is not possible (paediatric/uncooperative/elderly patients). A comprehensive preoperative evaluation by the anaesthetist assessing fitness of the patient for GA is mandatory before scheduling an EUA. Associated risks with GA should be explained to the patient/relative/guardian and written informed consent should be obtained.

A complete eye examination, including measurement of epithelial defect/infiltrate size and measurement of intraocular pressure (IOP), and collection of corneal scraping samples should be done during the initial EUA, which can be repeated, if necessary, for monitoring response to treatment.

4. **Systemic Examination**

- General health
- Anaemia
- Lymph nodes palpation
- Protein energy malnutrition, vitamin A deficiency and immunisation status in children

Videos for Chapter 2 can be accessed at: www.routledge.com/9780367761561

Video 2.1: Positive Seidel test in a case of viral keratitis

Video 2.2: Technique of corneal scraping in a case of microbial keratitis.

Table 2.1: Colour Coding for Documenting Corneal Pathologies

Black	Blue	Yellow	Green	Red	Brown
• Scars • Degenerations • Guttae • Deposits • Contact lens (broken line) • Foreign body • Corneal nerves • Tissue adhesive	• Epithelial oedema • Epithelial bullae • Stromal oedema • Descemet's membrane folds	• Infiltrate • Hypopyon • Keratic precipitates	• Epithelial defects • Fluorescein stained areas • Superficial punctate keratitis • Filament • Vitreous	• Deep and superficial vascularisation • Ghost vessels (dotted line) • Hyphaema • Rose bengal stained areas	• Pigments (iron lines, epithelial melanosis, Krukenberg's spindles) • Iris • Peripheral anterior synechiae

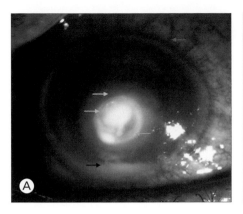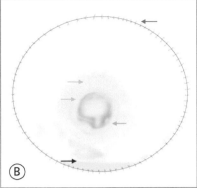

Figure 2.6 Slit lamp photograph (A) and corresponding coloured schematic diagram (B) of a case of fungal (*Aspergillus flavus*) corneal ulcer showing ciliary congestion (blue arrow), epithelial defect (green arrow), deep stromal infiltrates with feathery edges (yellow arrows) and hypopyon (black arrow).

INVESTIGATIONS

1. Routine Laboratory Investigations

- Complete hemogram including blood haemoglobin, total leucocyte count, differential leucocyte count, erythrocyte sedimentation rate, blood sugar levels and urine and stool examination

2. Microbiological Investigations

- Scraping from the base and margins of the ulcer (Video 2.2)

  - Smear: Gram stain, Giemsa stain, potassium hydroxide (KOH) mount

  - Culture: bacterial, fungal, *Acanthamoeba*, *Mycobacteria*

3. Ocular Investigations

- *In Vivo Confocal Microscopy (IVCM)*: a non-invasive imaging modality that allows direct visualisation of causative pathogens in real time and has proved to be a very useful aid in establishing a diagnosis of microbial keratitis especially those caused by fungi and *Acanthamoeba*. The Heidelberg Retinal Tomograph 3/Rostock Cornea Module (HRT3/RCM) provides high-resolution imaging and has been shown to have good sensitivity and specificity in detecting *Acanthamoeba* cysts (Figure 2.7) and fungal hyphae (Figure 2.8).[3,4] Recent studies have also demonstrated good sensitivity and specificity of HRT3/RCM in detecting atypical infectious keratitis and simultaneous infections by multiple organisms.[5]

- *Spectral Domain Anterior Segment Optical Coherence Tomography (ASOCT)*: a non-contact imaging modality that provides high-resolution cross-sectional images of the cornea and thus can be used to evaluate and serially monitor cases of infectious keratitis. The calliper tool of ASOCT can be used to measure corneal thickness at the site of infection, infiltrate depth (Figure 2.9), stromal oedema and width of the endothelial plaque, and serial standardised scans from the same area can be used to objectively assess the disease course and monitor response to therapy.[6]

- *B-scan Ultrasonography*: for posterior segment examination should be done in all cases of corneal ulcer as a dilated fundus examination is not possible in most of these cases. Endophthalmitis (Figure 2.10), serous choroidal detachment and suprachoroidal haemorrhage should be looked for and managed accordingly. These are important for guiding treatment in specific circumstances.

- *Corneal biopsy*: performed in cases where repeated smear examinations and microbial cultures of specimens obtained from standard corneal scraping technique reveal negative results such as deep stromal abscess and fungal ulcer.

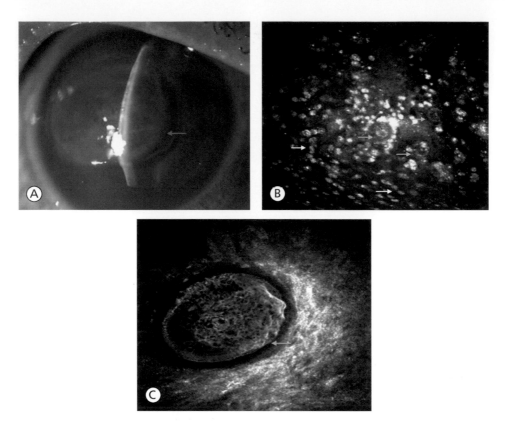

Figure 2.7 Slit lamp photograph of (A) a suspected case of *Acanthamoeba* keratitis in a patient with a history of exposure to contaminated water showing well-delineated, central ulcer (blue arrow). In vivo confocal microscopy (HRT3 with Rostock Corneal Module, Heidelberg Engineering, Heidelberg, Germany) image of the eye shows (B) multiple hyper-reflective, round to ovoid shaped, double-walled *Acanthamoeba* cysts (yellow arrows) in the corneal stroma with few cysts arranged linearly (white arrows). The magnified view (C) of an *Acanthamoeba* cyst highlights the cyst wall (green arrow) and the organism.

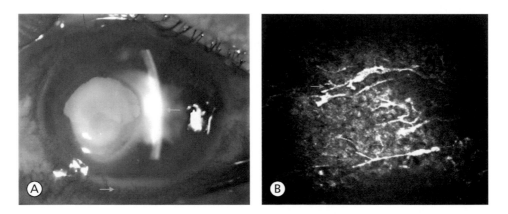

Figure 2.8 Slit lamp photograph of a patient with fungal keratitis shows (A) corneal infiltrate with feathery margins and elevated appearance (yellow arrow) associated with hypopyon (green arrow). In vivo confocal microscopy shows (B) hyper-reflective, branched, septate, linear structures with acute angle branching (blue arrows) typical of fungal hyphae (*Aspergillus* species).

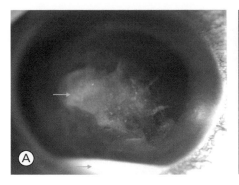
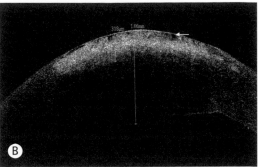

Figure 2.9 Slit lamp photograph (A) of a case of fungal keratitis showing corneal infiltrates (yellow arrow) and hypopyon (green arrow). The corresponding anterior segment optical coherence tomography image shows (B) hyper-reflective infiltrates in anterior corneal stroma with posterior shadowing, corneal oedema and necrotic/cystic spaces (white arrow).

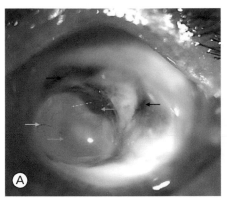
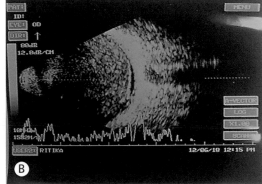

Figure 2.10 Slit lamp photograph of a diabetic male patient with bacterial (*Pseudomonas aeruginosa*) keratitis shows (A) total corneal melt (black arrows) with extrusion of lens (blue arrow) and vitreous (green arrow). Neovascularisation of the pseudo-membrane (yellow arrow) can also be seen. Ultrasonography B-scan of posterior segment shows (B) mild-moderate amplitude spikes suggestive of vitreous exudates.

REFERENCES

1. Waring GO, Laibson PR. A systematic method of drawing corneal pathologic conditions. Arch Ophthalmol. 1977; 95:1540–2.
2. Waring GO. Slit beam ruler. Am J Ophthalmol. 1976; 82:802–3.
3. Hau SC, Dart JKG, Vesaluoma M et al. Diagnostic accuracy of microbial keratitis with in vivo scanning laser confocal microscopy. Br J Ophthalmol. 2010; 94(8):982–7.
4. Vaddavalli PK, Garg P, Sharma S, Sangwan VS, Rao GN, Thomas R. Role of confocal microscopy in the diagnosis of fungal and *Acanthamoeba* keratitis. Ophthalmology. 2011; 118(1):29–35.
5. Wang YE, Tepelus TC, Vickers LA, Baghdasaryan E, Gui W, Huang P, Irvine JA, Sadda S, Hsu HY, Lee OL. Role of in vivo confocal microscopy in the diagnosis of infectious keratitis. Int Ophthalmol. 2019 Dec; 39(12):2865–74.
6. Sharma N, Singhal D, Maharana PK, Agarwal T, Sinha R, Satpathy G, Singh Bageshwar LM, Titiyal JS. Spectral domain anterior segment optical coherence tomography in fungal keratitis. Cornea. 2018 Nov; 37(11):1388–94.

SECTION B
CORNEAL INFECTION

3 Viral Keratitis

Ritika Mukhija, Vipul Singh, Aishwarya Rathod, Noopur Gupta, Radhika Tandon

INTRODUCTION

Infectious keratitis is an important cause of ocular morbidity across the globe and can affect people of all ages. Viruses, bacteria and fungi are responsible for the majority of the cases, while protozoa and other parasites are amongst the less commonly implicated micro-organisms. The various viral infections that can affect the cornea can be broadly grouped under the following categories: herpes simplex keratitis; varicella zoster induced keratitis and adenoviral keratitis; cytomegalovirus keratitis; measles and rubella infection.[1–3] Viral infections can have classical presentations, where the diagnosis is quite straightforward, but can also have variations in clinical features that are often confusing. The management of herpetic keratitis is largely guided by the Herpetic Eye Disease Study.[4,5] This chapter presents a variety of clinical scenarios to illustrate the various practical aspects of diagnosis and management.

CASE 3.1

CLINICAL FEATURES

A 30-year-old female presented with symptoms of photophobia, watering and mild diminution of vision in her left eye of three days duration. She did not give any prior history of such episodes or any other ocular or systemic disease. Examination findings and slit lamp appearance are illustrated in Figure 3.1.

KEY POINTS

Diagnosis:
- The above clinical scenario describes a case of dendritic ulcer, the classic herpetic corneal epithelial lesion, caused by a replicating virus.

Investigations:
- In most of the cases, the diagnosis is straightforward and based on clinical features; polymerase chain reaction (PCR), immunofluorescence (IF) and viral culture can be done if needed.

Treatment:
- The patient was treated with topical acyclovir ointment (3%) five times a day, topical antibiotic (moxifloxacin hydrochloride 0.5% four times a day), cycloplegic (homatropine hydrobromide 2% three times a day) and lubricants (preservative-free carboxymethylcellulose 0.5% six times a day).

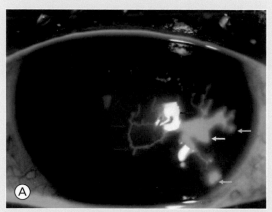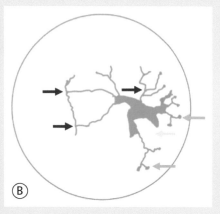

Figure 3.1 Slit lamp photograph of the left eye (A) with corresponding corneal diagram (B) showing herpetic dendritic ulcer (grey arrow) with dichotomous branching (red arrows) as visualised with fluorescein staining under cobalt blue filter. Note the terminal bulbs (yellow arrows), which also appear to be slightly raised.

Outcome:

- The lesion responded to treatment and healed without a scar in around ten days.

Supplementary Information and Additional Tips

- Debridement of the infected loose epithelium from the edge of the dendrite may also be useful in such cases.
- Classic dendritic ulcers in herpes simplex virus (HSV) keratitis stain positively for fluorescein along the length of the lesion, and negatively along the swollen and raised epithelial borders.
- In contrast, rose bengal stain, that is taken up by the devitalised cells, delineates the border of the ulcer (Figure 3.2). However, as it is toxic to HSV, it should not be used prior to viral cultures.

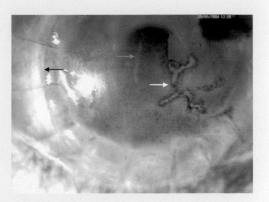

Figure 3.2 Slit lamp photograph of a patient with recurrent viral keratitis post penetrating keratoplasty showing HSV dendritic ulcer with its margins stained with rose bengal (white arrow). Note the central graft oedema with few Descemet's folds (grey arrow) and the graft-host junction (black arrow) with sutures in situ.

CASE 3.2

CLINICAL FEATURES

A 32-year-old male presented with symptoms of mild photophobia, pain, watering and diminution of vision in his left eye for three days. He gave a history of one similar episode in the past which resolved completely with topical medications. Examination findings and slit lamp appearance are illustrated in Figure 3.3.

KEY POINTS

Diagnosis:

- The above clinical scenario describes a case of recurrent dendritic ulcer, possibly evolving into a geographical ulcer.

Treatment:

- The patient was managed with similar treatment as the above case.

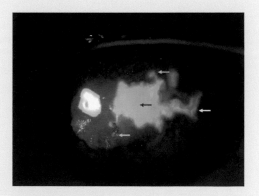

Figure 3.3 Slit lamp photograph of the right eye showing a large dendritic ulcer (white arrow) with terminal bulbs (yellow arrows) as visualised with fluorescein staining under cobalt blue filter. The ulcer seems to have taken up a partial amoeboid pattern (red arrow), indicating possible evolution into a geographical ulcer.

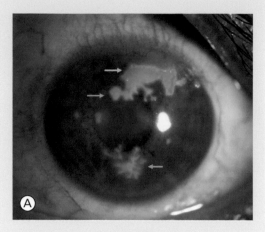 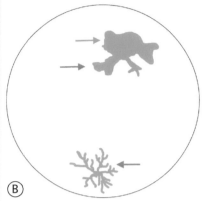

Figure 3.4 Slit lamp photograph (A) and corresponding corneal diagram (B) showing two herpetic dendritic ulcers (grey arrows), one of which has almost converted into a geographical ulcer (yellow arrow).

Outcome:
- The lesion responded to treatment and healed with a faint nebular corneal scar in around two weeks.

Supplementary Information and Additional Tips
- Multiple herpetic epithelial lesions in different stages may be present in the same eye (Figure 3.4).
- Possible sequelae of viral epithelial keratitis include healing without any scar formation or persistence of ghost dendrites (Figure 3.5), or progression to stromal keratitis.

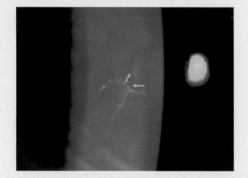

Figure 3.5 Slit lamp photograph showing ghost dendrite (yellow arrow) in a patient with previous epithelial keratitis.

CASE 3.3

CLINICAL FEATURES

A 55-year-old male presented to our outpatient department with symptoms of pain, redness, watering and diminution of vision in his right eye for the past ten days. Previous treatment records from elsewhere revealed that the patient had received topical steroids along with topical acyclovir ointment for viral keratouveitis. He also gave a history of two similar episodes in the past. Examination findings and slit lamp appearance are illustrated in Figure 3.6.

KEY POINTS

Diagnosis:
- The above clinical scenario describes a case of herpes simplex viral keratouveitis with both epithelial and endothelial involvement.

Treatment:
- This patient was managed with topical acyclovir (3% ointment) and oral acyclovir (400 mg five times a day) and was also kept on oral acyclovir prophylaxis (400 mg twice a day) to reduce the incidence of recurrence.

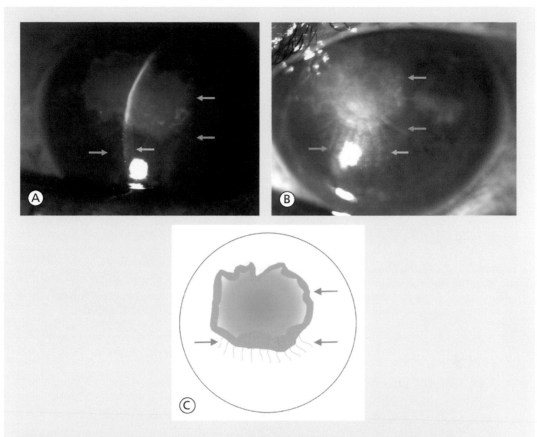

Figure 3.6 Slit lamp photographs (A, B) and corresponding corneal diagram (C) showing herpetic viral keratouveitis with localised stromal oedema (yellow arrows) with Descemet's folds (green arrows) and endothelial pigments along with a geographical ulcer (grey arrow).

Topical prednisolone acetate 1% was started in a tapering dose after the epithelial defect healed.

Outcome:

- The lesion responded to treatment and healed with a nebulo-macular corneal scar along with mild Descemet's scarring in around one month.

Supplementary Information and Additional Tips

- It is important to note that in such cases, topical steroids should only be started after the dendritic ulcer has healed, otherwise it can progress to a geographical ulcer, as happened in this case.

CASE 3.4

CLINICAL FEATURES

A 38-year-old male presented with blurred vision, mild pain and watering in his left eye for the past five days. There was no history of similar episodes in the past. Examination findings and slit lamp appearance are illustrated in Figure 3.7.

KEY POINTS

Diagnosis:

- The above clinical scenario describes a case of herpes simplex viral immune stromal keratitis with a classical immune ring.

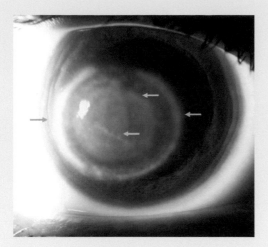

Treatment:
- The patient was managed with topical steroids (prednisolone phosphate 1% four times a day), cycloplegic (homatropine hydrobromide 2% three times a day) and lubricants (preservative-free carboxymethylcellulose 0.5% four times a day) along with a two-week course of oral acyclovir (400 mg five times a day).

Outcome:
- The lesion responded to treatment and healed with formation of a nebulo-macular corneal scar in around two months.

Figure 3.7 Slit lamp photograph of the left eye showing ring shaped stromal infiltrates (yellow arrows) along with an immune ring (grey arrows) suggestive of immune stromal keratitis. There was no overlying epithelial defect or associated epithelial keratitis.

Supplementary Information and Additional Tips

- A long tapering course of topical steroids of at least 10 weeks is recommended in stromal keratitis.
- In cases where there is associated epithelial keratitis (Figure 3.8),

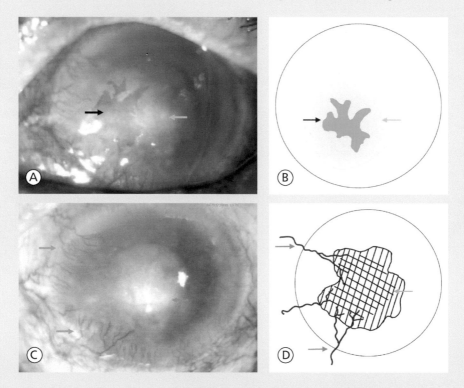

Figure 3.8 Slit lamp photograph (A) and corresponding corneal diagram (B) showing stromal infiltrates (yellow arrow) along with epithelial defect (black arrow) suggesting a combination of epithelial and stromal keratitis. Clinical picture of the same patient at a three-month follow-up (C) and corresponding corneal diagram (D) revealing healed lesion with scarring (green arrow) and vascularisation (grey arrows).

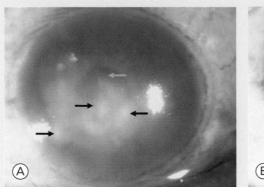
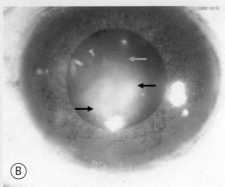

Figure 3.9 Slit lamp photographs showing two different clinical scenarios (A, B) with multifocal stromal infiltrates (black arrows) with mild oedema (grey arrows).

acyclovir ointment can be added and topical steroids withheld till the epithelial defect heals.

- Immune-mediated stromal keratitis can also manifest as punctate stromal lesions (Figure 3.9), Wessely immune ring or stromal neovascularisation (Figure 3.10).

- Necrotising stromal keratitis is a less common presentation and is characterised by severe corneal necrosis and ulceration (Figure 3.11) and/or dense infiltration of stroma (Figure 3.12) with frank perforation in some cases (Figure 3.13).

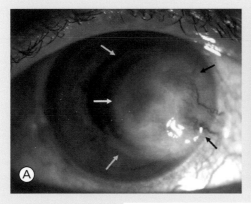
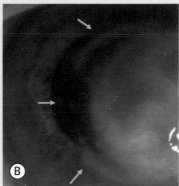
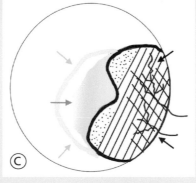

Figure 3.10 Slit lamp photographs (A) showing healing stromal keratitis (white arrow) with neovascularisation (black arrows) and Wessely immune ring (yellow arrows); note the magnified image (B) and corresponding corneal diagram (C).

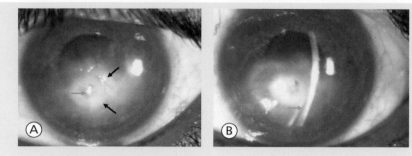

Figure 3.11 Slit lamp photographs showing necrotising stromal keratitis (A) with infiltrates (black arrows) and area of corneal necrosis and melt (green arrow); note the area of shallow anterior chamber (grey arrow) as seen on slit illumination (B).

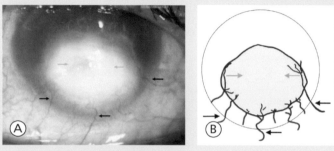

Figure 3.12 Slit lamp photograph (A) and corresponding corneal diagram (B) showing necrotising stromal keratitis with dense infiltrates (yellow arrows) and vascularisation (black arrows).

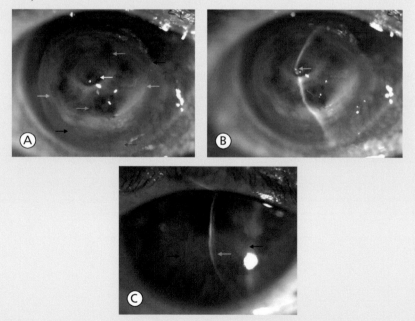

Figure 3.13 Slit lamp photograph showing necrotising stromal keratitis (A) with small central perforation (white arrow). Note the scarring (black arrows), vascularisation (red arrows) and diffuse blood staining (grey arrows) probably resulting from prior vascularisation and the early pseudo-cornea formation (green arrow) as seen on slit illumination (B). The other eye of the same patient revealed healed viral keratouveitis (C) suggested by poor corneal sensations, scarring (black arrows) and differential corneal oedema (grey arrow).

CASE 3.5

CLINICAL FEATURES

A 28-year-old male underwent optical penetrating keratoplasty for visual rehabilitation in the right eye for healed viral keratitis and was kept on oral acyclovir prophylaxis (400 mg twice a day) to prevent recurrence. However, four weeks postoperatively, he presented with pain, redness, watering and diminution of vision. Examination findings and slit lamp appearance are illustrated in Figure 3.14.

KEY POINTS

Diagnosis:
- The above clinical scenario describes a case of recurrence of herpes simplex

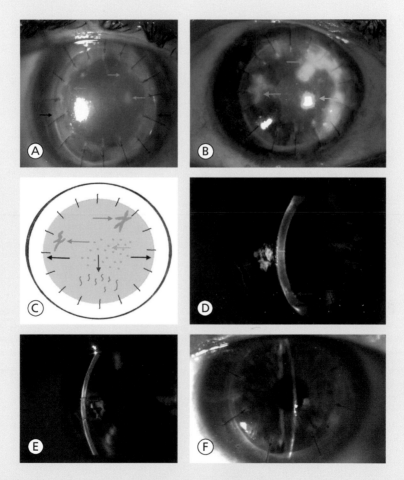

Figure 3.14 Slit lamp photographs (A, B) and corresponding corneal diagram (C) showing recurrence of viral keratitis in a patient post penetrating keratoplasty with diffuse corneal haze and oedema with faintly visible dendrites (grey arrows) near the graft-host junction (black arrows), which are seen distinctly with fluorescein staining under cobalt blue filter. Presence of a distinct area of stromal infiltrates (green arrow), most likely immune-mediated (A) and diffuse punctate staining (yellow arrow) with fluorescein staining (B) is also evident. Slit illumination (D, E) reveals Descemet's folds (red arrows) and stromal oedema (note the increased thickness as depicted by the blue line) involving the host cornea near the graft-host junction as well (E). The patient responded well to treatment; a clear graft was maintained to the last follow-up at one year (F).

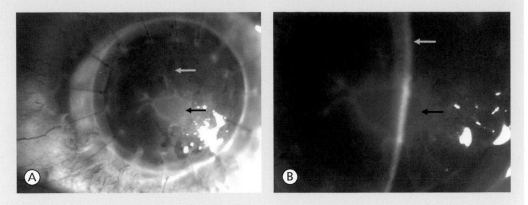

Figure 3.15 Slit lamp photographs (A, B) showing viral keratitis in a patient three months after penetrating keratoplasty with the presence of a central dendritic ulcer (black arrow) with stromal oedema (yellow arrow) involving only the donor tissue.

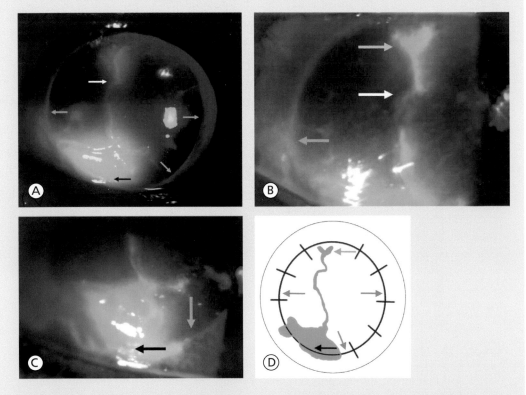

Figure 3.16 Slit lamp photographs (A–C) and corresponding corneal diagram (D) showing viral keratitis in a patient one year after optical keratoplasty (grey arrows pointing towards graft-host junction); note the dendritic ulcer (white arrow) with terminal bulbs (yellow arrow) involving both the graft and host tissue (black arrows).

viral keratitis (presenting primarily as epithelial keratitis) in a corneal graft one month following penetrating keratoplasty.

Treatment:

- The patient was managed with topical acyclovir ointment (3%), topical antibiotic (moxifloxacin 0.5%), cycloplegic (homatropine 2%) and lubricants (preservative-free carboxymethylcellulose 0.5%).
- Topical steroids were withheld till the ulcer healed to prevent the risk of conversion to a geographical ulcer or development of secondary bacterial infection.
- However, a short course of oral steroids (Tab Wysolone 1 mg/kgbw) was given to prevent immune rejection and to control the inflammation.

Outcome:

- The ulcer healed in seven days and thereafter the patient was restarted on topical steroids and kept on close follow-up.
- Oral acyclovir prophylaxis was continued for about 14 months till all sutures were removed and the graft remained clear with no other episodes of recurrence.

Supplementary Information and Additional Tips

- Recurrence is one of the most common complications in a corneal graft following viral keratitis; although mostly seen in the first postoperative year, it can occur at any time.
- It may manifest as small epithelial defect, a classic dendrite or a geographic ulceration (Figures 3.15–3.17).

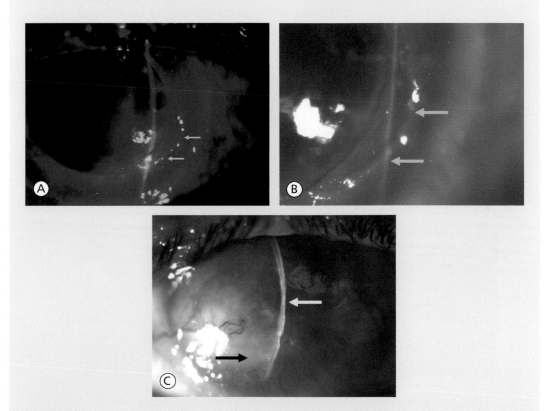

Figure 3.17 Slit lamp photographs (A, B) showing an atypical presentation of recurrence of viral keratitis in a patient one year after optical keratoplasty with sterile stromal melt of the host tissue (yellow arrows); the other eye of the same patient (C) showing healed viral keratitis with differential thinning (white arrow) and a vascularised corneal opacity (black arrow).

CASE 3.6

CLINICAL FEATURES

A 30-year-old male was referred to our outpatient department with diminution of vision, pain and photophobia in both eyes for past one week. He was prescribed topical antibiotics, lubricants and hypertonic saline elsewhere; however, there was no improvement. Examination findings and slit lamp appearance are illustrated in Figure 3.18.

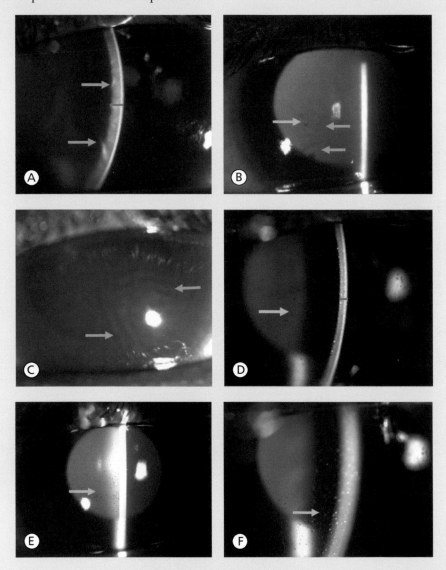

Figure 3.18 Slit lamp photographs showing bilateral diffuse viral endotheliitis with diffuse stromal oedema (A) with increased corneal thickness as visible on slit illumination (orange line) and Descemet's folds (grey arrows) along with keratic precipitates seen well in retro-illumination (yellow arrows) (B). Similar findings were seen in the left eye as well (C). Photographs at follow-up (D–F) showing marked clinical improvement in both eyes one week after treatment, as evidenced by the reduction in corneal oedema and thickness (orange line) and Descemet's folds. Note that the keratic precipitates are more clearly visible (yellow arrows) after the decrease in corneal stromal haze.

KEY POINTS

Diagnosis:

- The above clinical scenario describes a case of bilateral diffuse viral endotheliitis; the tear film PCR tested positive for HSV.

Treatment:

- The patient was managed with topical steroids and cycloplegics along with a course of oral acyclovir (400 mg five times a day) for two weeks.

Outcome:

- The patient responded well to treatment and had significant reduction in corneal oedema with return to normal visual acuity in two weeks.
- A tapering course of topical steroids was continued for about six weeks; a prophylactic dose of oral acyclovir was also recommended.

Supplementary Information and Additional Tips

- Viral endotheliitis may be of disciform (Figure 3.19), linear (Figure 3.20) or diffuse pattern.
- Gradual tapering of topical steroids is warranted and long-term oral antiviral prophylaxis (400 mg twice a day) up to one year is recommended in these cases.

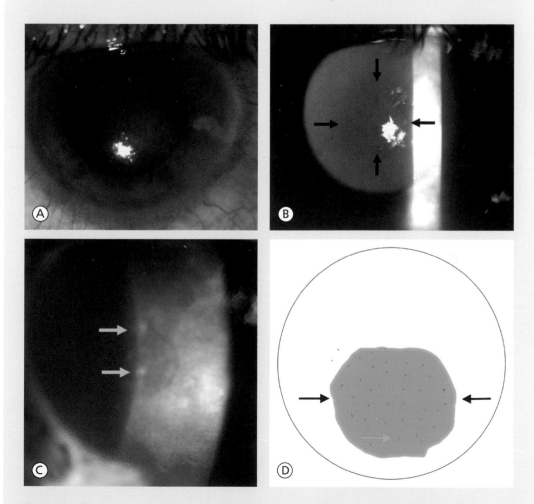

Figure 3.19 Slit lamp photographs (A–C) and corresponding corneal diagram (D) showing disciform viral endotheliitis with localised stromal oedema (black arrows) as seen on diffuse (A) and retro-illumination (B) along with whitish keratic precipitates (yellow arrows) as seen on magnified slit view (C).

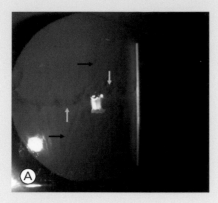
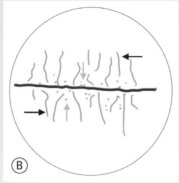

Figure 3.20 Slit lamp photograph (A) and corresponding corneal diagram (B) showing linear viral endotheliitis with Descemet's folds (black arrows) and keratic precipitates (yellow arrows).

CASE 3.7

CLINICAL FEATURES

A 45-year-old male presented to our outpatient department with pain, watering and photophobia in the right eye for the past five days. He gave a history of one similar episode in the past. Examination findings and slit lamp appearance are illustrated in Figure 3.21.

KEY POINTS

Diagnosis:

■ The above clinical scenario describes a case of marginal keratitis, likely owing to viral aetiology. The diagnosis is supported by the presence of a dendrite-like ulcer and a few old keratic precipitates (KPs), possibly

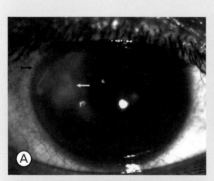
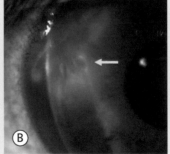

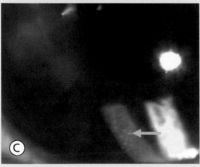

Figure 3.21 Slit lamp photographs (A, B) showing marginal viral keratitis with ciliary congestion, a dendrite-like ulcer (white arrow) in the upper outer periphery along with neovascularisation (black arrow). Also note the few old keratic precipitates inferiorly (yellow arrow) possibly suggestive of a previous episode (C).

suggestive of a previous episode of viral endothelial involvement.

Treatment:
- As this occurs due to active HSV replication, topical antivirals are prescribed; however, topical steroids may be needed to tackle with the intense inflammation and immune response that is often present in these cases.

Outcome:
- The lesion healed with mild nebular scarring in about three weeks.

Supplementary Information and Additional Tips
- HSV marginal keratitis should be differentiated from staphylococcal marginal keratitis; the former usually starts as an ulcer and is followed by the infiltrates (Figure 3.22) and generally progress centrally, while the latter is an immune-mediated keratitis that may be associated with blepharitis and progresses circumferentially (Chapter 6; Figures 6.35 and 6.36).

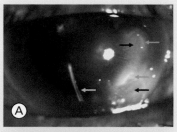
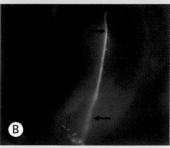

Figure 3.22 Slit lamp photographs (A, B) showing marginal viral keratitis with epithelial defect with underlying stromal thinning (black arrows), stromal infiltrates (green arrows) along with few keratic precipitates (yellow arrow).

CASE 3.8

CLINICAL FEATURES

A 60-year-old male presented to our outpatient department with pain, watering and photophobia in the right eye for the previous two days. He gave a history of painful skin lesions on the right forehead and nose ten days prior to this episode. Examination findings and slit lamp appearance are illustrated in Figure 3.23.

KEY POINTS

Diagnosis:
- The above clinical scenario describes a case of varicella zoster keratitis with pseudo-dendrites.

Investigations:
- As the diagnosis can be mostly established based on history and examination findings, investigations are not usually needed; Tzanck smear or Wright stain, PCR, IF and viral culture can be done.

Treatment:
- The patient was treated with oral acyclovir 800 mg TDS for ten days that was already initiated by a dermatologist for skin lesions. In addition, a topical antibiotic, cycloplegics and lubricants were given.

Outcome:
- The lesion healed with no scarring in about one week.

Supplementary Information and Additional Tips
- Herpes zoster keratitis can also present as punctate epithelial keratitis, pseudo-dendrites, stromal keratitis, disciform keratitis (Figure 3.24), endotheliitis/keratouveitis (Figure 3.25), peripheral ulcerative keratitis (Figure 3.26) or sclerokeratitis (Figure 3.24).

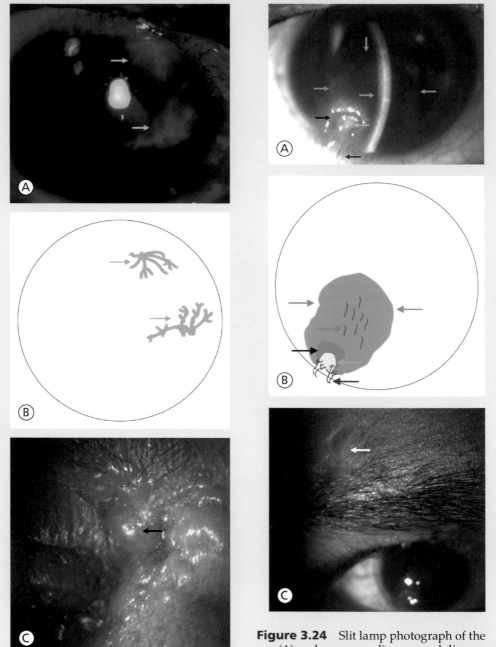

Figure 3.23 Slit lamp photograph of the eye (A) and corresponding corneal diagram (B) showing herpes zoster viral keratitis with dendrite-like ulcers (yellow arrows) stained with fluorescein stain; note that there are no terminal bulbs or dichotomous branching (as in HSV dendrites). External photograph of the face (C) showing healing vesicular skin lesion on lateral aspect of nose (black arrow).

Figure 3.24 Slit lamp photograph of the eye (A) and corresponding corneal diagram (B) showing herpes zoster sclerokeratitis along with disciform keratitis; note marginal epithelial defect and stromal lysis (black arrow), stromal infiltrates (yellow arrow) and neovascularisation (red arrow) along with mild stromal oedema (demarcated with green arrows) and Descemet's folds (grey arrow). The external photograph (C) reveals the healed scar (white arrow) from previous herpes zoster lesion on the face.

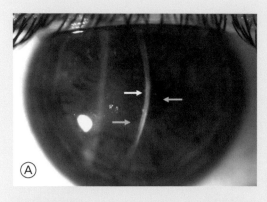
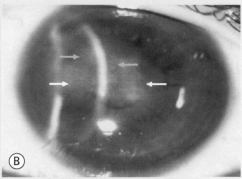

Figure 3.25 Slit lamp photographs showing two different cases (A, B) with herpes zoster keratouveitis with presence of localised stromal oedema (white arrows) and keratic precipitates (yellow arrows).

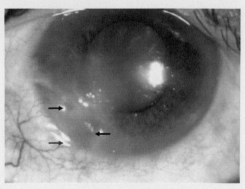

Figure 3.26 Slit lamp photograph showing herpes zoster peripheral ulcerative keratitis with presence of peripheral thinning (black arrows) and vascularisation (red arrow).

CASE 3.9

CLINICAL FEATURES

A 25-year-old female presented to our outpatient department with recurrent episode of pain, watering, photophobia and diminution of vision in the right eye. She had a history of painful skin lesions on the right forehead and nose two months prior which resolved following treatment. Examination findings and slit lamp appearance are illustrated in Figure 3.27.

KEY POINTS

Diagnosis:
- The above clinical scenario describes a case of neurotrophic keratopathy post-varicella zoster keratitis.

Treatment:
- The patient was initially treated with preservative-free lubricants and intermittent patching; however, after no response was seen for about two weeks, she was prescribed autologous serum eye drops following which an initial healing response was seen (Figure 3.27B).
- A mild reduction in size of the ulcer was noted after two weeks of the above therapy; the patient was eventually taken for amniotic membrane transplantation (AMT).

Outcome:
- The lesion completely healed in about 10 weeks with two sittings of AMT

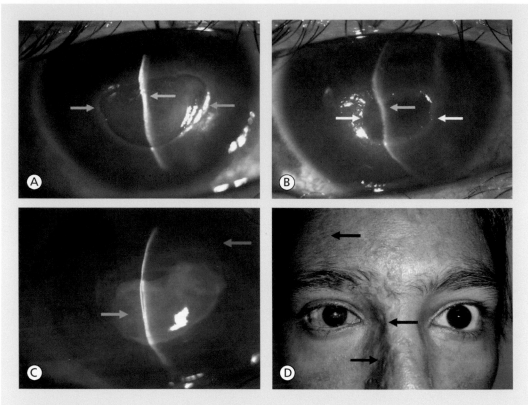

Figure 3.27 Slit lamp photographs showing herpes zoster neurotrophic keratitis at presentation (A) with a central ulcer with sharp demarcated edges (grey arrows) and stromal thinning (yellow arrow), which showed some resolution with treatment with decrease in size of the ulcer (B). Note the unhealthy appearance of the healing epithelium at the margins of ulcer (white arrows). After unsatisfactory response to medical management, multilayered amniotic membrane transplantation (AMT) was performed (C); note the amniotic membrane fashioned to fill in the area of defect (green arrow) and also to cover the entire cornea as a patch (blue arrow). The external face photograph (D) of the same patient showing healed scars (black arrows) post herpes zoster infection.

and aggressive lubricating therapy, leaving behind a central macular corneal scar.

Supplementary Information and Additional Tips

- Neurotrophic keratopathy is one of the most frequent long-term complications of herpes zoster ophthalmicus; therefore, adequate ocular surface support should be given.
- Other sequelae of herpes zoster keratitis are persistent corneal oedema, corneal scar, secondary bacterial infection (Figure 3.28), lipid keratopathy (Figure 3.29) and corneal melt and perforation (Figure 3.30).

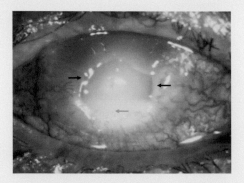

Figure 3.28 Slit lamp photograph showing secondary bacterial infection post herpes zoster keratitis with a large central ulcer (black arrows) with well-defined margins with secondary infiltrates (green arrow).

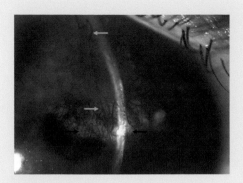

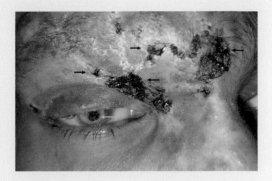

Figure 3.29 Slit lamp photograph showing a case of lipid keratopathy with the arborising vessels (grey arrows) along with lipid deposition along their course (black arrows).

Figure 3.30 External photograph of the face showing a severe case of herpes zoster ophthalmicus in a male with central perforation and iris tissue prolapse (yellow arrow) along with active skin lesions (black arrows).

CASE 3.10

CLINICAL FEATURES

A 32-year-old male presented to our outpatient department with a history of diminution of vision and photophobia in both his eyes for the past three days. He also gave history of pain, watering and redness in the left eye for ten days, and two days following that in the right eye. Patient was prescribed cold compresses, topical antibiotics, lubricants and oral non-steroidal anti-inflammatory drugs (NSAIDs) by a local ophthalmologist. Examination findings and slit lamp appearance are illustrated in Figure 3.31.

KEY POINTS

Diagnosis:
- The above clinical scenario describes a case of bilateral adenoviral keratoconjunctivitis.
- Diagnosis is most often based on clinical features vis-à-vis presence of acute conjunctivitis and one of the following features: follicles on the inferior tarsal conjunctiva, preauricular lymphadenopathy, associated upper respiratory infection or recent contact with a person with a red eye.

Investigations:
- While cell culture with confirmatory immunofluorescence staining (CC-IFA)

is the historical gold standard, there is a trend towards the newer and more rapid PCR techniques.
- Rapid diagnostic tests that can be applied directly to conjunctival swabs of infected eyes are also available.

Treatment:
- The treatment of adenoviral conjunctivitis mainly includes providing symptomatic relief (cold compresses, lubricants, NSAIDs) and prevention of transmission and complications.
- The patient was additionally treated with topical steroids (fluorometholone 0.1%) as the subepithelial immune infiltrates (SEI) involved the visual axis, in addition to topical antibiotic and preservative-free lubricants.

Outcome:
- The lesions resolved in about two weeks of treatment; steroids were gradually tapered, while lubricants were continued for about two months.

Supplementary Information and Additional Tips

- Corneal involvement in adenoviral conjunctivitis may be in the form of early epithelial vesicle-like elevations,

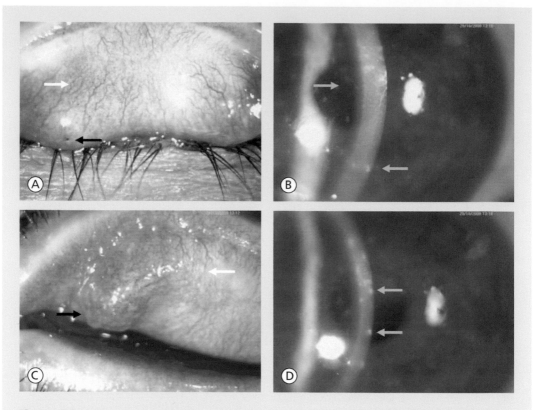

Figure 3.31 Slit lamp photographs showing bilateral adenoviral keratoconjunctivitis in a 32-year-old male showing conjunctival hyperemia (white arrows) and chemosis with few follicles (black arrows) with sub-epithelial infiltrates (yellow arrows) in the right (A, B) and left eye (C, D).

superficial or deep epithelial punctate keratitis (Figure 3.32), nummular keratopathy, SEI (Figure 3.33) or nebular corneal opacities.

- The usage of topical corticosteroids is controversial; however, their use is justified in membranous or pseudomembranous conjunctivitis, iridocyclitis, severe keratitis and persistent SEIs involving the visual axis.
- Uveitis has also been reported in a few cases; however, it is uncommon and usually self-limiting.
- An extremely rare presentation is adenoviral endotheliitis (Figure 3.34), reported only in handful number of cases. A young woman who presented to us with primary complaints of unilateral photophobia and mild diminution of vision in her right eye was found to have localised corneal oedema and epithelial bullae in the concerned eye and a few endothelial guttae-like lesions and

fine pigment dusting in both eyes. A provisional diagnosis of bilateral corneal endothelial dystrophy with right herpetic endotheliitis was made; however, there was no improvement

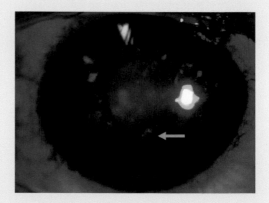

Figure 3.32 Slit lamp photograph showing a case with adenoviral conjunctivitis with superficial punctate epithelial keratitis (green arrow).

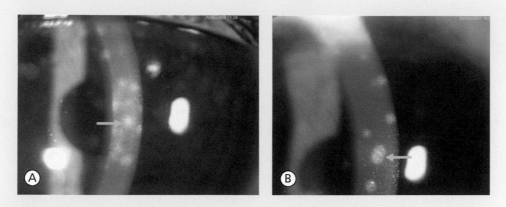

Figure 3.33 Slit lamp photographs showing a case of bilateral adenoviral keratoconjunctivitis (A, B) with large sub-epithelial infiltrates (yellow arrows).

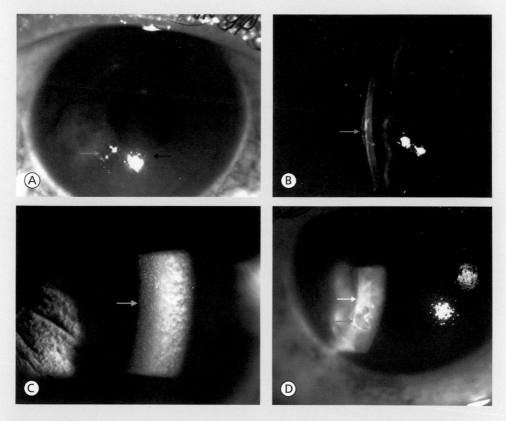

Figure 3.34 Slit lamp photographs of a 29-year-old female with localised corneal oedema (black arrow) and epithelial bullae (grey arrow) in the right eye (A); the latter can be seen clearly on slit illumination (B). The left eye of the same patient (C) showed few endothelial guttae-like lesions and fine pigment dusting (yellow arrow). A provisional diagnosis of bilateral corneal endothelial dystrophy with right herpetic endotheliitis was made (D) with an increase in scarring (white arrow) noted along with ruptured bulla (grey arrow) after two weeks of acyclovir treatment.

even after two weeks of acyclovir treatment with an increase in scarring (white arrow) along with ruptured bulla (grey arrow). Tear film and

aqueous humour PCR were then sent, which turned out to be positive for adenoviral DNA and negative for HSV DNA.

CASE 3.11

CLINICAL FEATURES

A 43-year-old female presented to our outpatient department with a history of painful diminution of vision and photophobia in her right eye for the past two weeks. The patient was already taking topical antibiotics (moxifloxacin),

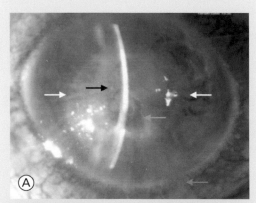
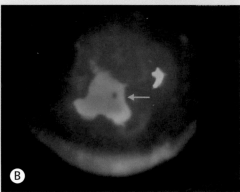

Figure 3.35 Slit lamp photograph showing a case with CMV viral endotheliitis (A) with disciform-like stromal oedema (white arrows), ciliary congestion (grey arrow), epithelial keratitis (yellow arrow) and a few small, disc-shaped keratic precipitates (black arrow); the epithelial defect is better visualised with fluorescein staining under cobalt blue filter (B).

cycloplegic and lubricants prescribed by a local ophthalmologist; however, there was no significant improvement. Examination findings and slit lamp appearance are illustrated in Figure 3.35.

KEY POINTS

Diagnosis:
- The patient was provisionally diagnosed as a case of a mixed variety of herpetic keratitis with epithelial keratitis and underlying stromal, endothelial involvement and iritis.

Investigations:
- As the diagnosis was primarily clinical, a tear film PCR to test for HSV and cytomegalovirus (CMV) was sent only after the patient did not show any improvement despite the addition of topical and oral acyclovir for five days; the sample tested positive for CMV DNA and negative for HSV DNA.
- PCR from the aqueous humour from an anterior chamber tap is considered a reliable method for the diagnosis of CMV endotheliitis and iritis.

Treatment:
- Topical and oral acyclovir were stopped, and the patient was instead prescribed topical ganciclovir 0.15% gel (starting five times a day and tapered as per response thereafter) and oral valacyclovir (900 mg twice daily).
- Acyclovir, both topical and oral, has also shown clinical benefit in cases of CMV keratitis and uveitis; however, as there was no initial improvement in this case with the same, the patient was shifted to other antiviral drugs.

Outcome:
- The epithelial keratitis resolved in about seven days of treatment, after which topical steroids were added

and gradually tapered as per clinical response.

■ The stromal keratitis, endotheliitis and iritis resolved in about four weeks, leaving behind macular corneal opacity with Descemet's scarring.

Supplementary Information and Additional Tips

■ Anterior segment manifestations of CMV are rare; they include acute catarrhal conjunctivitis, epithelial keratitis, nonulcerative dendrites, stromal keratitis, endotheliitis and iritis.

■ Although the disease is rare, making a clinical diagnosis is often difficult; corneal endotheliitis with the presence of fine- to medium-sized, coin-shaped KPs, sometimes arranged in a ring or linear pattern (Figure 3.36), and association with high IOP and corticosteroid-recalcitrant inflammation could be used as indicators for CMV-related anterior segment infection.

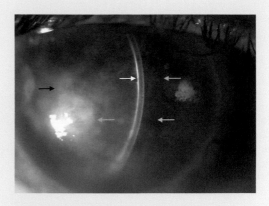

Figure 3.36 Slit lamp photograph of a 40-year-old male with recurrent CMV viral keratouveitis and secondary fungal keratitis showing cornea stromal oedema with scarring (black arrow) along with feathery infiltrates (yellow arrow). Note the diffuse Descemet's scarring (white arrow) as a result of repeated attacks of viral endotheliitis and multiple pigmented coin-like keratic precipitates (green arrows). The mixed aetiology in this case was proven by tear film PCR (positive for CMV) and confocal microscopy that showed the presence of fungal hyphae.

REFERENCES

1. Holland EJ, Schwartz GS, Shah KJ. CHAPTER 77. Herpes Simplex Keratitis. In: Cornea; Volume 1 – Fundamentals, Diagnosis and Management. 4th ed. USA: Elsevier; 2017; 909–41.
2. Lee WB. CHAPTER 78. Herpes Zoster Keratitis. In: Cornea; Volume 1 – Fundamentals, Diagnosis and Management. 4th ed. USA: Elsevier; 2017; 942–55.
3. Golen JR, Chern KC. CHAPTER 79. Less Common Viral Corneal Infections. In: Cornea; Volume 1 – Fundamentals, Diagnosis and Management. 4th ed. USA: Elsevier; 2017; 956–63.
4. Wilhelmus KR, Gee L, Hauck WW, Herpetic Eye Disease Study. A controlled trial of topical corticosteroids for herpes simplex stromal keratitis. Ophthalmology. 1994; 101: 1883–96.
5. Barron BA, Gee L, Hauck WW, Herpetic Eye Disease Study. A controlled trial of oral acyclovir for herpes simplex stromal keratitis. Ophthalmology. 1994; 101: 1871–82.

4 Bacterial Keratitis

Yogita Gupta, Ritika Mukhija, Aishwarya Rathod, Noopur Gupta

INTRODUCTION

Any alteration in corneal anatomy, immunity or defence mechanisms may be a risk factor for the development of keratitis. Causative bacterial organisms can be Gram-positive or Gram negative. Gram-positive organisms (e.g. *Staphylococcus aureus, Staphylococcus, Streptococcus* species) usually cause well-localised lesions. Gram-negative organisms (e.g. *Pseudomonas, Neisseria* species, *Enterobacter*) may cause fulminating suppurative lesions. A few virulent bacteria (e.g. *Neisseria* species, *Haemophilus* species) may penetrate through an intact cornea. The severity and progression of bacterial keratitis is thus dependent upon the virulence of the pathogenic organism and host factors such as pre-existing contact lens wear, ocular surface disease, eye injury, immunocompromised status and systemic disease.[1–3]

CASE 4.1

CLINICAL FEATURES

A 29-year-old male presented with pain, redness, photophobia and foreign body sensation in the right eye of two weeks duration. He did not give any prior history of such episodes, contact lens wear, ocular injury or any other ocular or systemic disease. Visual acuity at presentation was 6/18 with accurate projection of rays. Examination findings and slit lamp appearance are illustrated in Figure 4.1.

KEY POINTS

Diagnosis:
- The clinical scenario describes a case of microbial corneal ulcer, diagnosed after careful history taking and examination.

Investigations:
- Microbiological investigations were performed from corneal scrapings: Gram stain, Giemsa stain, calcofluor white stain, KOH mount, bacterial culture on blood agar, fungal culture on Sabouraud dextrose agar and thioglycollate broth, and drug sensitivity testing. A bacterial corneal ulcer was established as the laboratory diagnosis for this patient, due to

Staphylococcus epidermidis growth in culture media.

Treatment:
- As the ulcer was small and superficial and the patient ensured compliance to treatment and follow-up, he was started on topical moxifloxacin hydrochloride 0.5% and cycloplegics. The antibiotic was prescribed hourly for the first 24 hours, then every two hours for 48 hours (round the clock), then given every four hours for one week, then every six hours for a week and then tapered.

Outcome:
- The infiltrates were noted to resolve with treatment on follow-up. The signs of resolution in a bacterial corneal ulcer are usually healing epithelial defects, decreasing size and density of infiltrates, decreasing conjunctival injection and reduced surrounding corneal oedema. The final visual acuity was 6/9 which improved with refractive correction, leaving behind a faint residual corneal opacity. The organism can cause a more severe keratitis as shown in Figures 4.2 and 4.3 that usually resolves with a residual corneal opacity (Figure 4.4).

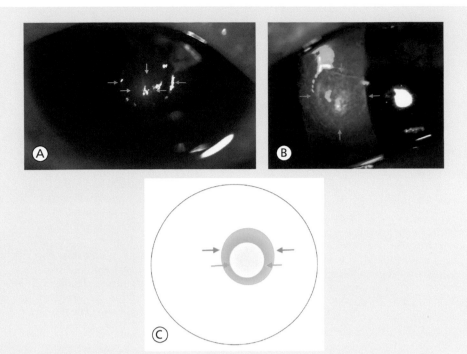

Figure 4.1   Slit lamp photograph of a case of infective keratitis caused by *Staphylococcus epidermidis*. Note that the ulcer (A) is small and central with confluent infiltrates (yellow arrows) and distinct margins (grey arrows). Anterior chamber inflammation is conspicuously absent. Fluorescein staining demonstrates (B) the well-demarcated margins of the small and central epithelial defect (grey arrows) when examined under cobalt blue filter. The corresponding corneal diagram (C) demonstrates the small, central and superficial corneal ulcer with few infiltrates.

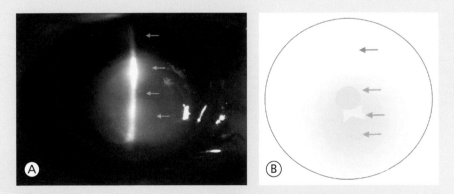

Figure 4.2   Slit lamp photograph demonstrating (A) extensive ulceration of the central cornea with involvement of the deeper corneal layers with obscuration of anterior chamber details beneath the area of the ulcer. Dense, creamy white exudates (yellow arrows) with thinning of corneal layers (green arrow) is evident (*Staphylococcus epidermidis* colonies grown on culture). Note that the surrounding peripheral cornea has maintained its transparency with a clear view of iris tissue (grey arrow) despite the severe ulceration. Marked ciliary and conjunctival congestion demonstrate the severity of the bacterial infection. Corresponding corneal diagram (B) of the clinical picture illustrating the extent of corneal ulcer, size of epithelial defect, corneal thinning and presence of exudates.

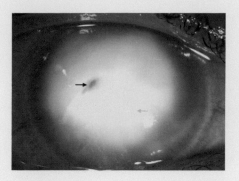

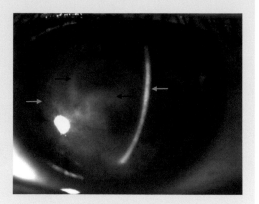

Figure 4.3 Slit lamp photograph of a case of corneal ulcer caused by *Staphylococcus* species presenting as deep corneal stromal abscess (yellow arrows) with central corneal thinning. The progressive thinning has contributed to the impending corneal perforation (black arrow). The peripheral corneal rim beyond the boundaries of the corneal abscess appear hazy and the infiltrates have reached the limbus in the inferior quadrants. Ciliary congestion is also evident.

Figure 4.4 Slit lamp photograph demonstrating the final outcome in a case of healed keratitis with full-thickness diffuse corneal scarring (grey arrows) associated with vascularisation. Anterior chamber details can be seen through the maculo-leucomatous corneal opacity (black arrows).

CASE 4.2

CLINICAL FEATURES

A 67-year-old diabetic male presented with pain and redness in the left eye of three weeks' duration. He gave a history of cataract surgery performed 12 years before with good gain of vision following surgery. He gave a history of use of some traditional eye medications of unknown composition, following which the pain and redness worsened. Examination findings and slit lamp appearance are illustrated in Figure 4.5.

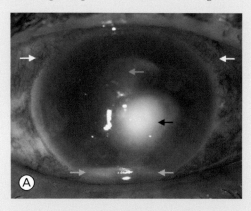

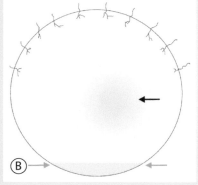

Figure 4.5 Slit lamp photograph of microbial keratitis (A) and corresponding corneal diagram (B) caused by *Streptococcus pneumoniae* showing well-defined, central corneal ulcer (black arrow) involving the visual axis, dense yellowish infiltrates, surrounding corneal haze, inferior mobile hypopyon of 1.5-mm height (yellow arrows), moderate anterior chamber inflammation along with profuse conjunctival injection (white arrows) in a pseudophakic patient (grey arrow).

KEY POINTS

Diagnosis:

- The clinical picture describes a case of microbial corneal ulcer in the left eye. After investigating further, the diagnosis of bacterial corneal ulcer was established for this patient, caused by *Streptococcus pneumoniae*.

Investigations:

- Corneal scrapings were sent for microbiological investigations: Gram stain, Giemsa stain, calcofluor white stain, KOH mount, bacterial culture on blood agar, fungal culture on Sabouraud dextrose agar and thioglycollate broth, and drug sensitivity testing.

Treatment:

- This case was managed with topical fortified antibiotics (cefazolin 5% and tobramycin 1.3%), started hourly and tapered slowly as per response. Oral antibiotics (ciprofloxacin 500 mg twice a day) were added due to the presence of hypopyon and the diabetic status of the patient.

Outcome:

- The hypopyon resolved within 48 hours of starting antibiotics. The infiltrate reduced in size and density over two weeks and vascularisation

appeared in three weeks after initiation of therapy, leaving a vascularised residual corneal opacity (Figure 4.6).

Supplementary Information and Additional Tips

- *Streptococcus pneumoniae* causes a suppurative reaction in the corneal stroma. Severe hypopyon and anterior uveitis are commonly associated.

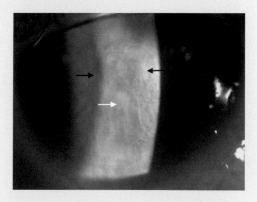

Figure 4.6 Slit lamp photograph of a case of vascularised corneal opacity formed after complete resolution of bacterial keratitis. Diffuse superficial corneal scarring (white arrow) along with formation of early ghost vessels (black arrows) can be seen.

CASE 4.3

CLINICAL FEATURES

A 39-year-old female presented with pain and redness in the right eye of two weeks' duration. The patient complained of a burning sensation, mucopurulent discharge and matting of eyelashes for two weeks. She did not give any prior history of such episodes or any other ocular or systemic disease. Examination findings and slit lamp appearance are illustrated in Figure 4.7.

KEY POINTS

Diagnosis:

- The clinical scenario describes a case of microbial corneal ulcer, diagnosed after careful history taking and examination.

Investigations:

- Microbiological investigations were performed from corneal scrapings: Gram stain, Giemsa stain, calcofluor white stain, KOH mount, bacterial culture on blood agar, fungal culture on Sabouraud dextrose agar and thioglycollate broth, and drug sensitivity testing. A bacterial corneal ulcer was established as the laboratory diagnosis for this patient, due to *S. aureus* growth in culture media.

Treatment:

- Fortified topical antibiotics (cefazolin 5% and tobramycin 1.3%) were started due to involvement of visual axis and presence of hypopyon. They were

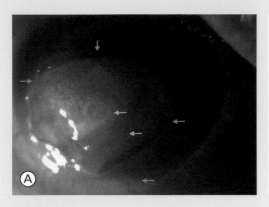
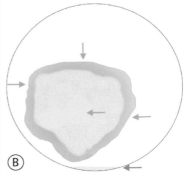

Figure 4.7 Slit lamp photograph (A) and corresponding corneal diagram (B) demonstrating a well-demarcated bacterial corneal ulcer (culture growth suggestive of *Staphylococcus aureus*) with a large epithelial defect (green arrows), diffuse infiltrates (yellow arrows), corneal oedema and minimal inflammatory hypopyon (grey arrow). Note the clarity of the uninvolved surrounding cornea.

given hourly for the first 24 hours, then every two hours for 48 hours (round the clock), then every four hours for one week, then every six hours for another week and then tapered as per the response.

Outcome:

■ The infiltrates were noted to resolve with treatment on follow-up. The epithelial defect decreased in size with reduced conjunctival injection and the surrounding corneal oedema resolved with timely institution of appropriate therapy.

Supplementary Information and Additional Tips

■ Gross clinical features in a case of bacterial keratitis include matting of eyelashes, eyelid oedema, mucoid discharge, diffuse conjunctival injection, chemotic and inflamed conjunctiva with occasionally erythematous changes on the lid margins and skin of the upper and lower eyelid (Figures 4.8 and 4.9).

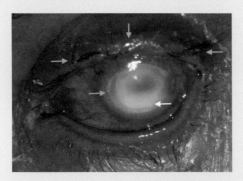

Figure 4.8 External photograph of a case of bacterial keratitis with matting of eyelashes (yellow arrows), eyelid oedema, mucoid discharge (black arrow), diffuse conjunctival injection, diffuse circumferential corneal infiltrates (green arrow) and hypopyon (white arrow). There is some evidence of central corneal thinning.

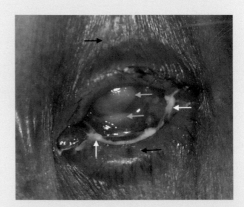

Figure 4.9 External photograph of a case of central corneal ulcer (yellow arrow) with hypopyon (green arrow) in a 70-year-old female. Note the string of mucoid discharge (white arrows), chemotic and inflamed conjunctiva with erythematous changes on the lid margins and skin of the upper and lower eyelids (black arrows).

CASE 4.4

CLINICAL FEATURES

A 25-year-old male presented with pain and redness in the right eye of four weeks' duration. He gave a history of some foreign particle entering the eye, following which he rubbed the eye vigorously. He did not give any history of prior similar episodes. Previous treatment history revealed use of topical steroids prescribed by a local medical practitioner for redness following the fall of foreign body in the eye. Examination findings and slit lamp appearance are illustrated in Figure 4.10.

KEY POINTS

Diagnosis:
- The clinical scenario describes a case of microbial corneal ulcer presenting as dense stromal abscess with hypopyon.

Investigations:
- Corneal scrapings were collected on the first day of presentation before starting empirical antibiotics.
- Microbiological investigations were performed: Gram stain, Giemsa stain, calcofluor white stain, KOH mount, bacterial culture on blood agar, fungal culture on Sabouraud dextrose agar and thioglycollate broth, and drug sensitivity testing.
- The diagnosis of **bacterial corneal ulcer** was established for this patient, due to *S. epidermidis* growth on blood agar.

Treatment:
- Fortified topical antibiotics (cefazolin 5% and tobramycin 1.3%) were started and maintained and tapered as per clinical response. Oral ciprofloxacin (500 mg BID) was added due to the presence of hypopyon and dense abscess.
- Partial response was noted with a decrease in size of the epithelial defect, reduction in infiltrates with mild improvement in corneal clarity and decrease in the size of the hypopyon (black arrows). Corneal thinning, however, worsened with treatment.
- Considering the clinical presentation and presumed polymicrobial aetiology, confocal imaging was performed that revealed the presence of septate fungal hyphae. Oral and topical antifungal therapy was added. Response to therapy was noted and resulted in a marked decrease in the size and density of infiltrates, clearing of the surrounding cornea, disappearance of hypopyon and appearance of corneal scarring.

Outcome:
- Best corrected visual acuity (BCVA) of 6/60 was achieved at the end of three months and a residual opacity involving the visual axis.

Supplementary Information and Additional Tips
- Gram-positive organisms, e.g. *S. aureus, S. epidermidis, Streptococcus* species, often cause well-localised lesions. *Staphylococcus epidermidis* causes ulcers with white-grey to creamy white stromal infiltrates that may later form a stromal abscess.

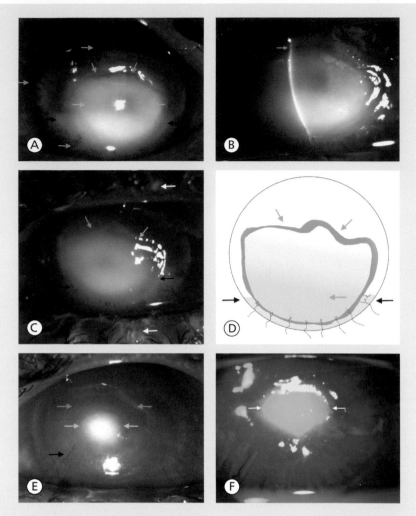

Figure 4.10 Slit lamp photograph of a large microbial ulcer (A) with diffuse stromal infiltrates (yellow arrows), large epithelial defect, stromal lysis as demonstrated by severe corneal thinning (green arrows), surrounding corneal oedema, large hypopyon (black arrows) and diffuse limbal injection with superficial vessels invading the corneal tissue beyond the limbus inferiorly (grey arrows) (*Staphylococcus epidermidis* grown on culture). The circumferential corneal thinning (green arrows) was more evident on slit illumination (B) with total obscuration of the view of anterior chamber and iris details. Treatment with fortified antibiotics as per the microbiological sensitivity report resulted in a marginal response with decrease in size of the epithelial defect (C), reduction in infiltrates (yellow arrow) with mild improvement in corneal clarity and decrease in size of the hypopyon (black arrows). Corneal thinning, however, worsened (green arrows) with treatment. Note the mucoid discharge and matted eye lashes (white arrows). Corresponding corneal diagram of the clinical presentation in (C) is shown in (D). Considering the clinical presentation and presumed polymicrobial aetiology (later confirmed hyphal elements seen on confocal imaging), antifungal therapy was started. Response to therapy was noted and the clinical picture after three weeks of therapy (E) reveals marked decrease in size and density of infiltrates (yellow arrows), clear surrounding cornea, disappearance of hypopyon, presence of early scarring (grey arrows) in areas of previous corneal thinning and appearance of superficial corneal vascularisation as a sign of healing (black arrow). Note that the limbal and conjunctival injection has reduced markedly with the clinical response. Decrease in the size of the epithelial defect (white arrows) was noted with fluorescein staining under cobalt blue filter (F).

CASE 4.5

CLINICAL FEATURES

A 27-year-old male presented with a sudden onset of pain and profuse watering in his left eye for the previous three days. He gave a history of extended-wear soft contact lens use for the past year. Examination findings and slit lamp appearance are illustrated in Figure 4.11.

KEY POINTS

Diagnosis:
- The clinical scenario describes a case of infective keratitis caused by *Pseudomonas aeruginosa* in a contact lens user.

Investigations:
- The case was investigated. Corneal scrapings, contact lens with its case and solution were sent for microbiological investigations. Ultrasonography B-scan was done for posterior segment examination. Haemogram and fasting blood sugar were also checked.

Treatment:
- The case responded well to topical antibiotics: polymyxin-B sulphate (7500 IU/ml) and fortified tobramycin (1.3%) started hourly for 24 hours, then every two hours for 48 hours and then tapered according to response. Oral vitamin C, oral doxycycline

and topical cycloplegics were also administered. The hypopyon resolved within the first 48 hours of therapy. Corneal vascularisation and scarring (signs suggestive healing of corneal ulcer) was observed after three weeks of therapy.

Outcome:
- An optical keratoplasty was performed six months after formation of the corneal opacity, with improvement of BCVA to 6/12 after surgery.

Supplementary Information and Additional Tips

- In such cases, the contact lens case solution, contact lenses and corneal scrapings specimen should be sent for microbiological investigations to improve the yield of bacterial culture.
- *Pseudomonas* keratitis, as well as keratitis caused by other Gram-negative bacilli like *Proteus* species, *Klebsiella* and *Escherichia*, often progresses very rapidly, as was evident in this case.
- Suppurative lesions often with hypopyon and mucopurulent discharge are noted. These cases present with fulminant bacterial keratitis and progressive stromal thinning (Figure 4.12) which may

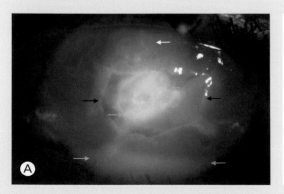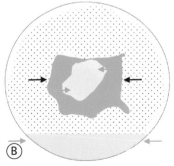

Figure 4.11 Slit lamp photograph (A) and corresponding corneal diagram (B) of a large bacterial corneal ulcer that grew *Pseudomonas aeruginosa* on culture presenting with a large central epithelial defect (black arrows), dense creamy white infiltrates (yellow arrows) and mobile hypopyon (green arrows). Note the diffuse haze in the surrounding cornea extending up to the limbus (white arrow).

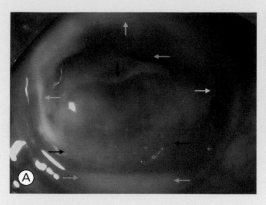
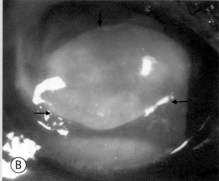

Figure 4.12 Slit lamp photograph of a patient presenting with fulminant bacterial keratitis (culture grew *Escherichia coli*) and a large necrotising corneal ulcer (A) with immune infiltrates arranged in a ring (yellow arrows), epithelial defect (black arrows), better demarcated on cobalt blue filter (B), and hypopyon (green arrows). Progressive stromal thinning, corneal vascularisation (grey arrow) and conjunctival congestion are also evident.

progress to sloughing and melting of the corneal layers, perforation with uveal tissue prolapse (Figure 4.13) along with displacement or extrusion of the crystalline lens (Figure 4.14) and scleral necrosis and eventually panophthalmitis (Figure 4.15) in some cases, despite treatment.

- Tectonic keratoplasty is required for cases presenting with corneal perforation and iris tissue prolapse in these severe necrotising ulcers.

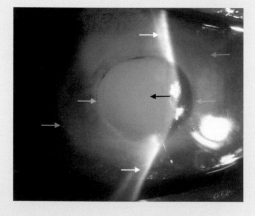

Figure 4.14 Slit lamp photograph of a long-standing bacterial ulcer with central corneal melt (yellow arrows) with prolapse of the anterior hyaloid phase of the vitreous humour (black arrow) in a patient with healing keratitis, evident by the surrounding scarring (grey arrows). Note that the anterior chamber is flat as seen on slit illumination (white arrows). Iris chafing with thin, atrophied iris tissue is evident due to the chronic infection and inflammation. The patient was referred for tectonic penetrating keratoplasty from a private clinic with a soft bandage contact lens in situ that is preventing the vitreous from completely prolapsing.

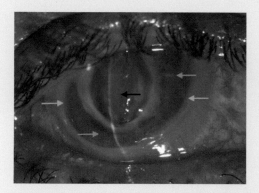

Figure 4.13 Slit lamp photograph of a case of severe infective keratitis with large corneal melt (green arrows) and sloughed off corneal tissue, iris prolapse (grey arrows) and crystalline lens prolapsing through the central pupillary area (black arrow). Circumcorneal congestion with matting of eyelashes is also evident.

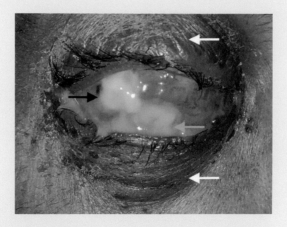

Figure 4.15 External photograph of a case with severe infective keratitis that progressed to panophthalmitis as a result of fulminant multi-drug resistant Gram-negative bacteria. Note the diffuse corneal abscess with sloughing (yellow arrow) along with areas of scleral involvement (black arrow), boggy and inflamed conjunctiva, copious mucopurulent discharge and diffuse skin oedema, erythema and excoriation on upper and lower lids (white arrows) likely due to prolonged inflammation and topical drug use.

CASE 4.6

CLINICAL FEATURES

A 34-year-old male presented with gradual development of pain and diminution of vision in his left eye for the previous six weeks. He gave a history of watering from the left eye for the previous four months and a history of trivial trauma to the left eye sustained during a fall on the ground two months prior. Examination findings and slit lamp appearance are illustrated in Figure 4.16.

KEY POINTS

Diagnosis:
- The clinical scenario describes a case of chronic, slowly progressive microbial ulcer caused by keratitis, most likely caused by an organism with an indolent course.

Investigations:
- Corneal scrapings did not reveal any organism on Gram stain or KOH mount and no growth was noted on culture media. This is quite common in cases where the patient has already been taking anti-microbial treatment.
- The patient was also diagnosed with acquired nasolacrimal duct obstruction in the left eye on performing syringing and probing under aseptic precautions.
- Ultrasonography B-scan performed for posterior segment examination was within normal limits.

Treatment:
- After poor clinical response to conservative management in the first week of treatment with topical fortified antibiotics, vis-à-vis vancomycin 5% and tobramycin 1.3%, surgical debridement of the plaque and debulking of infiltrates was performed under topical anaesthesia.
- The scraped material revealed growth of *Streptococcus viridans* on bacterial culture.
- Thereafter, topical fortified antibiotics, topical cycloplegics, oral antibiotics

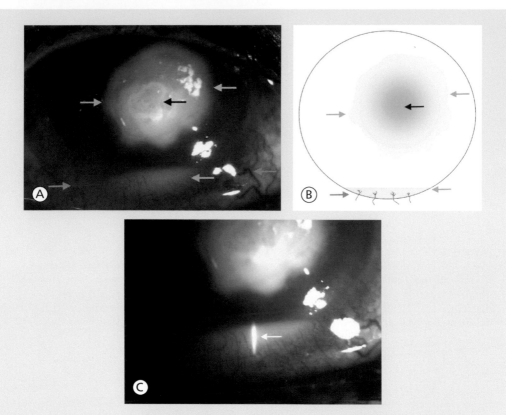

Figure 4.16 Slit lamp photograph (A) and corresponding corneal diagram (B) of a patient with a bacterial ulcer presenting as a deep stromal abscess, surrounding dense infiltrates (yellow arrows), early plaque formation (black arrow), hypopyon (green arrow) and limbal injection (grey arrows). The height of the hypopyon can be measured with a small vertical slit (C) using the measuring graticule of the slit lamp (white arrow) and this can be monitored on follow-up to assess response to therapy.

(ciprofloxacin 500 mg twice a day) and anti-glaucoma (Tab acetazolamide 250 mg three times a day) were prescribed.

Outcome:
■ The hypopyon resolved within a week of therapy and the ulcer healed with leucomatous corneal scarring after around ten weeks of therapy.

Supplementary Information and Additional Tips
■ Withdrawal of all anti-microbial drugs for 24–48 hours followed by corneal scraping may be helpful in identifying the causative organism in such cases.
■ Suture or punch biopsy in case of deep infiltrates and debridement in cases with thick plaques are also useful.

CASE 4.7

CLINICAL FEATURES

A 48-year-old diabetic woman presented with painful, progressive diminution of vision in the left eye associated with redness, watering and photophobia of five days' duration. A past history of recurrent redness and watering was reported by the patient over 15 years. Visual acuity in the right eye was 6/24 and 3/60 in the left eye. Slit lamp biomicroscopy of the right eye revealed multiple, irregular grey-white opacities with indistinct borders extending to the corneal periphery and intervening haze consistent with the diagnosis of macular corneal dystrophy (Figure 4.17). This was confirmed with confocal microscopy. The left eye demonstrated an irregular surface along with a central corneal epithelial defect of 10×6 mm with a 2.5-mm mobile hypopyon and raised intraocular pressure.

KEY POINTS

Diagnosis:

- The clinical picture describes a case of microbial corneal ulcer in a case of corneal dystrophy with poor ocular surface. After investigating further, the diagnosis of bacterial corneal ulcer was established for this patient, caused by *S. pneumoniae*.

Investigations:

- Corneal scrapings were sent for microbiological investigations: Gram stain, Giemsa stain, calcofluor

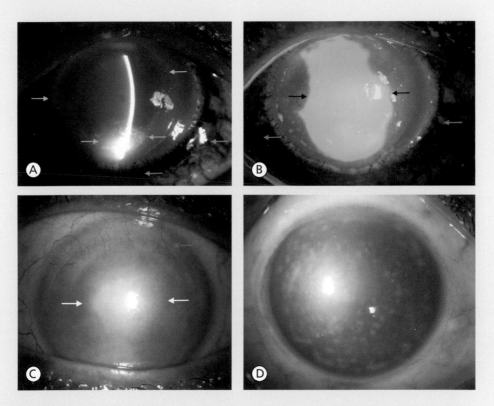

Figure 4.17 Slit lamp photograph of the left eye of a patient with macular dystrophy and diabetes mellitus showing (A) multiple peripheral infiltrates (yellow arrows), mucoid discharge, sloughing (green arrow), corneal thinning and severe limbal injection with angry red vessels (grey arrows). Diffuse corneal oedema, anterior chamber inflammation and pigments can also be seen. Note the large epithelial defect (black arrows) as seen on fluorescein staining under cobalt blue filter (B) and noticeable, tortuous conjunctival vessels highlighting the intense inflammatory response due to keratitis. The patient responded to antibiotic therapy and completely healed (C) around ten weeks later with resultant central corneal scarring (white arrows) and vascularisation (red arrows). Clinical examination of the right eye of the same patient (D) revealed multiple, irregular grey-white opacities in the corneal stroma extending out into the peripheral cornea up to the limbus suggestive of macular corneal dystrophy.

white stain, KOH mount, bacterial culture on blood agar, fungal culture on Sabouraud dextrose agar and thioglycollate broth, and drug sensitivity testing.

Treatment:

- A growth of *S. pneumoniae* was verified. This case was managed with topical fortified antibiotics (cefazolin 5% and tobramycin 1.3%), started hourly and tapered slowly as per response. Homatropine 2% and anti-glaucoma medication were also administered. Oral antibiotics (ciprofloxacin 500 mg BID) were added due to the presence of hypopyon and the diabetic status of the patient.

Outcome:

- The hypopyon resolved within 48 hours of starting antibiotics. The infiltrate reduced in size and density over two weeks and vascularisation appeared in three weeks after initiation of therapy, leaving a vascularised residual corneal opacity (Figure 4.17).

REFERENCES

1. Lin A, Rhee MK, Akpek EK, Amescua G, Farid M, Garcia-Ferrer FJ, Varu DM, Musch DC, Dunn SP, Mah FS; American Academy of Ophthalmology Preferred Practice Pattern Cornea and External Disease Panel. Bacterial Keratitis Preferred Practice Pattern®. Ophthalmology. 2019 Jan;126(1): P1–P55.

2. Tam ALC, Côté E, Saldanha M, Lichtinger A, Slomovic AR. Bacterial Keratitis in Toronto: A 16-Year Review of the Microorganisms Isolated and the Resistance Patterns Observed. Cornea. 2017 Dec;36(12): 1528–1534.

3. Hong AR, Shute TS, Huang AJW. CHAPTER 75. Bacterial Keratitis. In: Cornea; Volume 1 – Fundamentals, Diagnosis and Management. 4th ed. USA, Elsevier; 2017; 875–901.

5 Fungal Keratitis

Pooja Kumari, T Monikha, Rashmi Singh, Ritika Mukhija

INTRODUCTION

Keratomycosis or fungal keratitis is an important corneal cause of ocular morbidity. It is more commonly seen in tropical regions of the world. Fungal organisms can penetrate through the corneal stroma without perforation of the cornea resulting in an infectious hypopyon or the formation of an endothelial plaque.[1] The management becomes challenging as the majority of antifungal drugs exhibit poor corneal penetration properties. Unlike bacterial keratitis, the corneal epithelium overlying a stromal fungal infection can heal despite the presence of active infection once treatment is initiated and should not, by itself, be used as a guide to successful therapy.[2]

CASE 5.1

CLINICAL FEATURES

A 23-year-old male presented with sudden onset of redness and diminution of vision of the right eye. A history of injury with a wooden stick was elicited. He did not give any prior history of such episodes, contact lens wear or any other ocular or systemic disease. Visual acuity at presentation was 6/18 with accurate projection of rays. Examination findings and slit lamp appearance are illustrated in Figure 5.1.

KEY POINTS

Diagnosis:
- The above clinical scenario describes a case of fungal corneal ulcer with the classic dry-looking appearance and feathery margins. Satellite lesions surrounding the central lesion were also noted.

Investigations:
- Microbiological investigations were performed from corneal scrapings. In these cases, the diagnosis is confirmed by KOH mount of the specimen obtained through corneal scraping followed by fungal culture on Sabouraud dextrose agar and thioglycollate broth and drug sensitivity testing. Culture grew colonies of *Cladosporium* species.

Treatment:
- The patient was treated with natamycin ophthalmic suspension (5%) one hourly

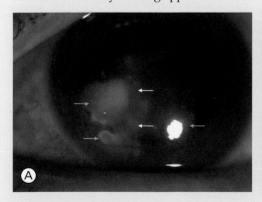
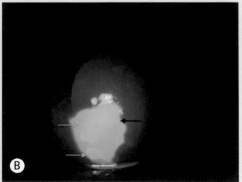

Figure 5.1 Slit lamp photograph of the right eye demonstrating fungal corneal ulcer (A) with greyish white, fluffy, dry-looking infiltrates (yellow arrows) and feathery margins (white arrows). Note the characteristic satellite lesion (green arrow) with similar morphology as the main lesion. The epithelial defect (B) overlying the infiltrates (yellow arrows) is clearly visible on staining with fluorescein dye when examined with cobalt blue filter on slit lamp examination (black arrow).

for 48 hours followed by tapering the frequency based on the clinical response, prophylactic topical antibiotic (moxifloxacin hydrochloride 0.5% four times a day), cycloplegic (homatropine hydrobromide 2% three times a day) and lubricants (preservative-free carboxymethylcellulose 0.5% six times a day).

Outcome:
- The infiltrates were noted to resolve with treatment on follow-up. The lesion responded to treatment and healed within a month of starting therapy without any residual corneal opacity and final visual acuity of 6/6.

CASE 5.2

CLINICAL FEATURES

A 67-year-old male, a farmer by occupation, underwent right penetrating keratoplasty eight months ago for trachomatous keratopathy with preoperative poor ocular surface. He was prescribed topical steroids following corneal grafting and was using prednisolone phosphate 1% twice a day. He presented with redness, foreign body sensation and diminution of vision in the operated eye. On examination, there was a small, superficial, paracentral corneal ulcer with well-defined margins and few central infiltrates on the donor cornea (Figure 5.2). The surrounding cornea was relatively clear with surface irregularity and corneal xerosis. Examination of the other eye revealed a small, paracentral leucomatous opacity with poor ocular surface. Visual acuity in the right and left eye was 6/24 and 6/18, respectively.

KEY POINTS

Diagnosis:
- The above clinical scenario describes a case of fungal corneal ulcer following prolonged topical steroid use following penetrating keratoplasty in the setting of corneal xerosis and compromised ocular surface.

Investigations:
- Microbiological investigations were performed from corneal scrapings. In this case, the diagnosis was confirmed by KOH mount of the specimen. Fungal culture demonstrated growth of *Alternaria* species.

Treatment:
- The patient was treated with natamycin ophthalmic suspension (5%) one hourly for 48 hours followed by tapering the frequency based on the clinical response, prophylactic topical antibiotic (moxifloxacin hydrochloride 0.5% four times a day), cycloplegic (homatropine hydrobromide 2% three times a day) and copious lubricants (preservative-free carboxymethylcellulose 1% every two hours with ointment hydroxypropylmethyl cellulose 0.3% at night).

Outcome:
- The lesion responded to treatment and healed with a nebulo-macular corneal scar in around four weeks. The ocular surface also improved with medication. Best corrected visual acuity was recorded to be 6/9.

Supplementary Information and Additional Tips

- *Alternaria* is a filamentous fungus from the Dematiaceae family, a group of darkly pigmented moulds that are ubiquitous in soil, plants, food and indoor air environments. It is a relatively uncommon fungus causing keratitis and may have varied clinical presentations and may present without macroscopic pigmentation. It occurs with increased propensity in patients with compromised ocular surface, previous surgery and trauma.

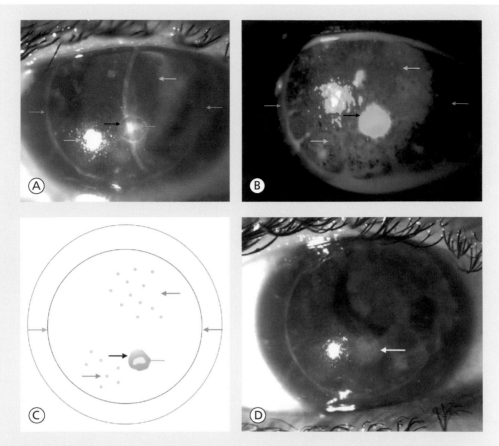

Figure 5.2 Slit lamp photograph of a patient who underwent penetrating keratoplasty (green arrows pointing towards graft-host junction) 18 months ago for trachomatous keratopathy with preoperative poor ocular surface. He presented with a small, paracentral corneal ulcer (A) with well-defined margins (black arrow) with few central infiltrates (yellow arrow). Note the poor ocular surface (grey arrows) evident as punctate staining (B) under cobalt blue filter. Schematic representation (C) of the clinical picture reveals the same findings. The ulcer healed (D) with timely treatment with antifungals, leaving behind a residual nebulo-macular corneal scar (white arrow).

CASE 5.3

CLINICAL FEATURES

A 47-year-old male farmer presented with a history of trauma with a cow's tail to the right eye while working on a milk farm. He sought treatment at a local hospital for sudden onset pain, redness and discharge. He was prescribed topical medications for symptomatic relief. His symptoms worsened over a period of one week. He presented to our tertiary-care hospital with the clinical picture and slit lamp appearance as illustrated in Figure 5.3.

KEY POINTS

Diagnosis:
- The above clinical scenario describes a case of a non-healing fungal corneal ulcer. The ulcer involved all the corneal layers with evidence of feathery morphology, fluffy

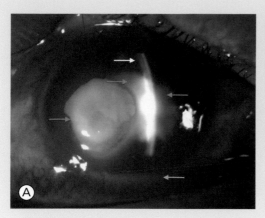
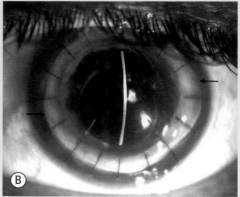

Figure 5.3 Slit lamp photograph of a patient (A) presenting with a localised fungal corneal abscess (green arrow) with evidence of an endothelial plaque (grey arrows) along with surrounding corneal oedema (white arrow). Note the feathery morphology, fluffy exudates and a small, fixed hypopyon (yellow arrow), characteristic of fungal keratitis. The patient underwent therapeutic keratoplasty (B) for a non-healing corneal ulcer and non-response to maximal medical therapy due to poor penetration of antifungals in a case with deeper corneal involvement with the fungal organism. A clear graft cornea with well-apposed graft-host junction (black arrows) and intact sutures (blue arrows) is seen after successful surgery.

exudates, endothelial plaque and fixed hypopyon characteristic of fungal keratitis.

Investigations:
- Microbiological investigations were performed from corneal scrapings. In this case, the diagnosis was confirmed by fungal culture that demonstrated growth of *Aspergillus flavus*.

Treatment:
- This patient was managed with topical and systemic antifungals. He did not demonstrate any improvement with medical management. Topical antiglaucoma medication in the form of timolol maleate 0.5% and brimonidine tartrate 0.1% along with oral acetazolamide 250 mg three times a day was prescribed for control of intraocular pressure consequent to inflammatory glaucoma.
- He underwent therapeutic penetrating keratoplasty for the same with successful functional and morphological outcome.
- The postoperative care comprised frequent topical instillation of antifungal agents and oral ketoconazole for two weeks. Assessment was made for any recurrence during the first two postoperative weeks and initiation of topical corticosteroids (prednisolone acetate 1%) every six hours was done after a period of 14 days only when the eye was noted to have no evidence of residual or recurrent infection on clinical slit lamp examination.

Outcome:
- The therapeutic keratoplasty was successful in controlling the fungal infection with a final visual acuity of 6/36 at a six-month follow-up visit. The patient was kept on topical antifungals for three months post keratoplasty.

CASE 5.4

CLINICAL FEATURES

A 30-year-old diabetic female presented with sudden onset pain, redness and diminution of vision. She gave a history of the fall of a foreign body into the eye. After removal of the foreign body at a local hospital, her symptoms persisted and worsened over time. Visual acuity at presentation was 6/24 with accurate projection of rays. Examination findings and slit lamp appearance are illustrated in Figure 5.4.

KEY POINTS

Diagnosis:
- The above clinical scenario describes a case of fungal corneal ulcer with an indolent course.

Investigations:
- Microbiological investigations were performed from corneal scrapings. In this case, the diagnosis was confirmed by a KOH mount that revealed budding yeasts and fungal culture that demonstrated growth of *Candida albicans*.

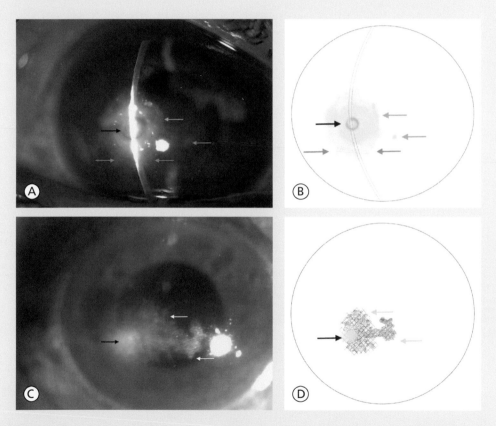

Figure 5.4 Slit lamp photograph of a patient presenting with (A) a paracentral, discrete fungal corneal ulcer (*Candida albicans*) with pearly-white infiltrates (yellow arrow) and indistinct feathery borders (grey arrows). A small satellite lesion (green arrow) is also seen. The overlying slit shows corneal thinning at the base of the ulcer (black arrow) that is also depicted in the corresponding schematic diagram (B). Patient responded well after treatment with topical antifungals and the healing of the epithelial defect (C) with a reduction in the size of infiltrates (black arrow) and the appearance of scarring was noted (white arrows); similar findings illustrated in the schematic diagram (D).

Treatment:

- The patient was managed with topical amphotericin 0.15% eye drops and oral ketoconazole 400 mg twice a day, cycloplegic (homatropine hydrobromide 2% three times a day) and antiglaucoma therapy.

Outcome:

- The lesion responded well to treatment and healed with a nebulo-macular corneal scar with a final visual acuity of 6/12 with rigid gas-permeable contact lens.

CASE 5.5

CLINICAL FEATURES

A 50-year-old female with uncontrolled diabetes mellitus presented with sudden onset pain, redness and diminution of vision after instillation of over-the-counter drops for irritation of eyes. Her vision dropped suddenly with severe pain and discharge although she had been symptomatic for a month. The clinical picture and slit lamp appearance are shown in Figure 5.5.

KEY POINTS

Diagnosis:

- The above clinical scenario describes a case of severe hypopyon fungal corneal ulcer with impending perforation occurring in a diabetic patient.

Investigations:

- A corneal scraping specimen from the ulcer base and margins revealed septate hyphae with V-shaped branching on the KOH mount. The diagnosis was confirmed by a culture that demonstrated growth of *A. flavus*.
- Glycosylated Haemoglobin (HbA1c) level at the time of presentation was 6.5.

Treatment:

- The patient was managed with topical and systemic antifungals but the clinical picture worsened with progressive corneal thinning in spite of maximal medical therapy.
- Endocrinologist opinion was sought and the patient was shifted to injectable insulin therapy for better

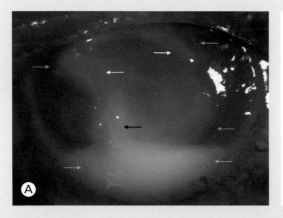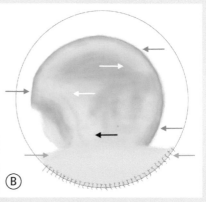

Figure 5.5 Slit lamp photograph demonstrating (A) a fulminant, large fungal corneal ulcer with diffuse infiltrates (white arrows) that are denser in certain areas (black arrow) along with circumferential thinning (green arrows), diffuse ciliary congestion and a large hypopyon (yellow arrow). (B) Corresponding schematic diagram illustrates the same findings.

glycaemic control and need for surgical intervention.
- Owing to the impending perforation and limbus to limbus involvement, the patient underwent therapeutic penetrating keratoplasty and was maintained on topical antifungals for around three months.

Outcome:
- The corneal graft tissue remained clear for three months and she was kept on close follow-up. No recurrence of infection was noted on follow-up and strict diabetic control was ensured.

CASE 5.6

CLINICAL FEATURES

A 25-year-old male presented with pain, redness and diminution of vision after a trauma to the right eye while playing with a wooden stick (local game of Gulli-Danda). He went to a local practitioner and started topical medications. After a month, he noticed brownish discoloration of the lesion present over his eyes. The examination findings and slit lamp appearance are shown in Figure 5.6.

KEY POINTS

Diagnosis:
- The above clinical scenario describes a case of slowly progressing dematiaceous fungal corneal ulcer.

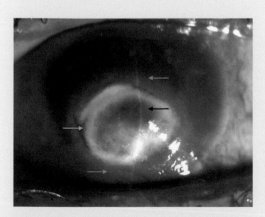

Figure 5.6 Slit lamp photograph of a patient presenting with an indolent, dematiaceous fungal corneal ulcer with infiltrates (yellow arrow), feathery margins and overlying brown pigmentation (black arrow) with surrounding corneal haze (grey arrows). Note the conjunctival and ciliary congestion is mild in nature.

Investigations:
- A corneal scraping specimen from the ulcer base and margins revealed septate branching fungal filaments on a KOH mount. Smears of corneal scrapings on culture media showed dematiaceous fungal growth within one week.

Treatment:
- The patient was managed with therapeutic corneal scraping to promote penetration of topical antifungals and removal of pigmented top layer. An oral antifungal, Tab ketoconazole 200 mg twice a day, was also prescribed.
- Along with antifungal therapy, antiglaucoma medication and cycloplegics were also prescribed.

Outcome:
- The patient responded well to treatment and gradually healed with scarring.

Supplementary Information and Additional Tips
- Melanin in the cell walls of dematiaceous hyphae and conidia resist killing and could be involved in pathogenicity. Macroscopic and microscopic pigmentation of corneal infiltrates in the form of raised plaques is a characteristic of dematiaceous fungal keratitis.
- Characteristic clinical features include dry, thick and raised corneal surface, stromal infiltrates with feathery margins, typical satellite lesions, dense hypopyon (Figure 5.7), deep

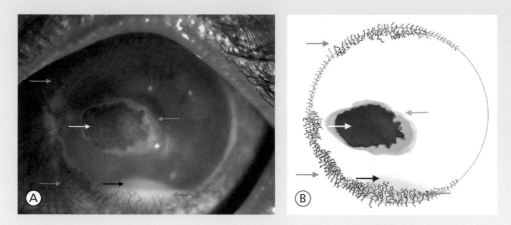

Figure 5.7 Slit lamp photograph demonstrating (A) diffuse conjunctival and ciliary congestion in a case of dematiaceous fungal corneal ulcer (yellow arrow) with overlying brown pigmentation (white arrow), a fixed hypopyon (green arrow) having a convex upper meniscus (black arrow) and diffuse limbal injection (grey arrows). Note that the surrounding cornea is clear and not affected by the infective process. The findings are also depicted in (B) a schematic diagram.

stromal infiltration and corneal perforation (Figure 5.8). Because of the pigmented nature of the lesions, it may mimic a foreign body or uveal tissue, in which case it may give the false impression of corneal perforation and uveal tissue prolapse (Figure 5.9). Hence, accurate diagnosis and careful, timely management are critical in these cases.

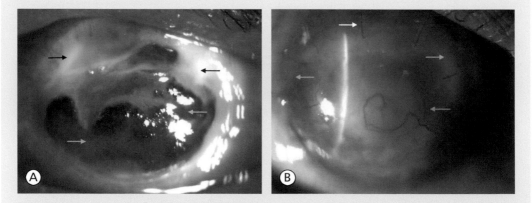

Figure 5.8 Slit lamp photograph demonstrating (A) a case of severe corneal involvement by dematiaceous fungi occurring post trauma with vegetative matter. Involvement of the entire cornea from limbus to limbus with infiltrates (black arrows) and pigmented fungal growth (yellow arrows) with corneal thinning and corneal vascularisation is noted. The patient was a farmer by occupation with multiple episodes of agricultural trauma which was evident by the other eye (B) showing an optically failed graft with diffuse vascularised corneal opacity (grey arrow) and a few corneal sutures (white arrow) at the graft-host junction (green arrows) that was performed for non-responding infective keratitis.

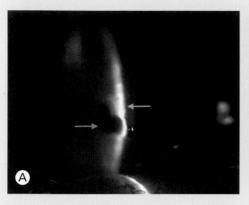
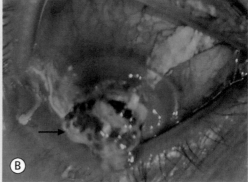

Figure 5.9 Slit lamp photograph demonstrating (A) a small localised epicorneal and corneal fungal ball (yellow arrow) mimicking a foreign body (grey arrow) occurring due to infection with a dematiaceous fungus and (B) showing an external photograph of large pigmented mycetoma caused due to *Acremonium* species, a pigmented fungus, masquerading as a perforated corneal ulcer with massive uveal prolapse (black arrow) and overlying exudative material.

CASE 5.7

CLINICAL FEATURES

A 50-year-old female presented with sudden onset redness and diminution of vision after trauma to right eye with vegetative matter while working in the field. She took treatment from a local ophthalmologist for infective keratitis, who had prescribed her topical antifungals, as per the corneal scraping report. After two weeks of therapy, she noted marginal improvement with increase in the whiteness of the corneal opacity, hence she presented to our tertiary care centre. Examination findings and slit lamp appearance are illustrated in Figure 5.10.

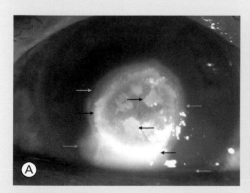
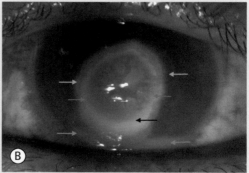

Figure 5.10 Slit lamp photograph of a patient (A) with a moderately sized fungal corneal ulcer (yellow arrows) with extensive drug deposits (black arrows) of topical natamycin 5%. It also features a hypopyon (green arrow), diffuse infiltrates and an endothelial plaque (grey arrow). Therapeutic corneal scraping was done following which the ulcer showed a healing response (B). The ulcer decreased in size (yellow arrows) with decrease in infiltrates (blue arrows) and reduction in drug deposits (black arrow) and size of endothelial plaque (grey arrow) due to better drug penetration following therapeutic scraping and removal of drug deposits.

KEY POINTS

Diagnosis:
- The above clinical scenario describes a case of fungal corneal ulcer with drug deposits.

Investigations:
- Corneal scraping culture report demonstrated *Aspergillus fumigatus* after removal of drug deposits. The KOH mount gave negative results.

Treatment:
- Therapeutic corneal scraping was done following which the ulcer showed a healing response.
- The ulcer decreased in size with a decrease in infiltrates and a reduction in drug deposits and size of endothelial plaque due to better drug penetration following therapeutic scraping and removal of drug deposits.
- Patient was started on topical and oral antifungals and on follow-up drug deposits were present over the ulcer.
- Alternate day scraping of the lesion was done to allow better penetration of the drug.

Outcome:
- The lesion healed with scarring over a period of three months. Best corrected visual acuity was 6/12.

Supplementary Information and Additional Tips

- Other topical medications like fluoroquinolones (ciprofloxacin, ofloxacin) used to treat corneal infections may also cause drug deposits.

CASE 5.8

CLINICAL FEATURES

A 65-year-old female presented with sudden onset redness and pain of right eye. She was a diagnosed case of neovascular glaucoma (NVG) with uncontrolled diabetes. The clinical picture revealed features of long-standing corneal oedema due to raised intraocular pressure. Examination findings and slit lamp appearance are illustrated in Figure 5.11.

KEY POINTS

Diagnosis:
- The above clinical scenario describes a case of a small, discrete corneal ulcer occurring in a patient of NVG with chronic corneal oedema, poor ocular surface and poor ocular defence mechanisms.

Investigations:
- Corneal scraping culture report demonstrated *C. albicans*.

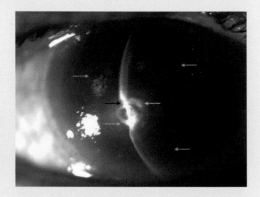

Figure 5.11 Slit lamp photograph of a 65-year-old female with uncontrolled diabetes and neovascular glaucoma (NVG) demonstrating a small fungal corneal ulcer (*Candida albicans*) with minimal conjunctival congestion. Note the few whitish infiltrates (yellow arrows) with marked corneal thinning on slit illumination (black arrow). Diffuse corneal oedema (grey arrows) and inferior hyphaema with endothelial staining (green arrow) can be attributed to the bleed from neovascularisation of the iris and angle in NVG.

Treatment:
- The patient was initially treated with topical amphotericin 0.15% eye drops.
- A mild reduction in size of the ulcer was noted after two weeks of the above therapy.

- Antiglaucoma drugs were also added to reduce the intraocular pressure.

Outcome:
- The lesion completely healed in about six weeks leaving behind a central macular corneal scar.

CASE 5.9

CLINICAL FEATURES

A 70-year-old diabetic male presented with sudden onset redness and pain of the left eye following trauma with vegetative matter. He presented with a large fungal corneal ulcer with dense infiltrates (black arrows) and necrotic slough (Figure 5.12).

KEY POINTS

Diagnosis:
- The above clinical scenario describes a case of a severe fungal corneal ulcer with extensive necrosis of the corneal tissue. B-Scan ultrasonography revealed vitreous exudates suggestive of endophthalmitis.

Investigations:
- The excised corneal specimen was subjected to microbiological evaluation and demonstrated growth of *Fusarium solani* in the culture media.

Treatment:
- Diabetic control was achieved.
- The patient was initially treated with topical and systemic antifungals after the diagnosis but the patient was non-responsive to medical therapy.
- He underwent therapeutic penetrating keratoplasty but due to ongoing infection and inflammation with co-existing endophthalmitis, the graft failed.

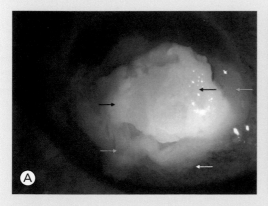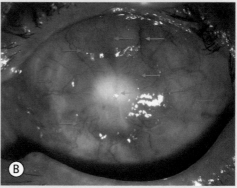

Figure 5.12 Slit lamp photograph of a diabetic patient (A) presenting with a large, fulminant fungal corneal ulcer with dense infiltrates (black arrows) and necrotic slough (yellow arrows) extending up to the lower limbus (white arrow). Note the extensive sloughing and chemosed conjunctiva with intense injection. The patient underwent therapeutic keratoplasty to control the infection and salvage the globe and eventually presented with (B) failed graft and atrophic bulbi three months after surgery. Note the diffuse corneal scarring (grey arrow), residual exudates in the anterior chamber (yellow arrow), multiple loose sutures (blue arrows), and 360° corneal vascularisation (green arrows) with the red arrows pointing towards graft-host junction.

Outcome:

- Graft failure and the recurrence of infection led to the development of atrophic bulbi. Structural integrity could be restored in this case, but the patient did not gain any useful vision.

Supplementary Information and Additional Tips

- *Fusarium* species characteristically are known to cause severe involvement

with corneal thinning. Clinically, the presentation is similar to fulminant bacterial keratitis and a high level of suspicion for polymicrobial aetiology or a mixed fungal and bacterial aetiology should always be kept in mind.

- Poor response to medical therapy is usually encountered in these cases, wherein the role of early surgical intervention becomes important.

CASE 5.10

CLINICAL FEATURES

A 40-year-old male presented with sudden onset pain, redness and diminution of vision. He gave a history of the fall of a foreign body into the eye. After removal of the foreign body at a local hospital, his symptoms persisted and worsened over time. Visual acuity at presentation was 4/60 with accurate projection of rays. Examination findings and slit lamp appearance are illustrated in Figure 5.13.

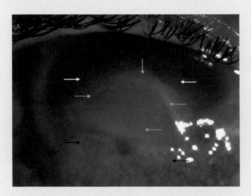

Figure 5.13 Slit lamp photograph demonstrating features of a resolving fungal corneal ulcer with neurotrophic keratopathy likely as a result of prolonged epitheliotoxic drugs. Note the well-defined epithelial defect (green arrows) with punched out margins and few diffuse infiltrates (yellow arrows). Also note the surrounding area of early scarring (white arrows) with inferior vascularisation (black arrows), both indicating the healing phase of the ulcer.

On close examination, there was a mild lagophthalmos with inferior corneal exposure due to a lower lid injury in childhood.

KEY POINTS

Diagnosis:

- The above clinical scenario describes a case of fungal corneal ulcer with neurotrophic component due to defective lid closure. Corneal sensations were reduced.

Investigations:

- Microbiological investigations were performed from corneal scrapings. In this case, the diagnosis was confirmed by a KOH mount that revealed fungal elements and fungal culture that demonstrated growth of *A. flavus*.

Treatment:

- The patient was managed with topical natamycin 5% eye drops and preservative-free carboxymethylcellulose 1% every two hours, cycloplegic (homatropine hydrobromide 2% three times a day) and antiglaucoma therapy. Ointment vitamin A at night was prescribed. Surgical tarsorrhaphy was performed to promote healing.

Outcome:

- The lesion responded to treatment after withdrawal of epitheliotoxic drugs and performing surgical tarsorrhaphy. Healing was noted with formation of a leucomatous corneal

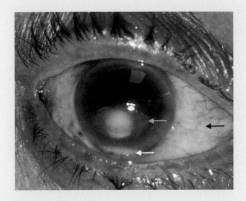

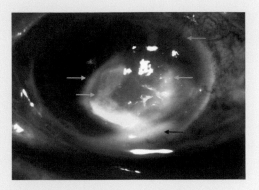

Figure 5.14 External photograph of a patient with fungal keratitis showing a large epithelial defect (yellow arrow), infiltrates with feathery margin and a small hypopyon (white arrow). Note that there is no significant discharge or conjunctival congestion (black arrow) which favours a fungal aetiology.

Figure 5.15 Slit lamp photograph of a moderate-sized fungal corneal ulcer revealing an irregular epithelial defect (green arrow) with surrounding infiltrates (yellow arrows), fixed hypopyon (black arrow) and superficial corneal vascularisation (grey arrow).

scar with a best corrected visual acuity of 6/60 achieved with a rigid gas-permeable contact lens.

Supplementary Information and Additional Tips

- The classic presentation of a fungal corneal ulcer is characterised by more signs than symptoms (Figure 5.14).

- Classical signs in a moderate-sized fungal keratitis include an irregular epithelial defect with surrounding infiltrates with feathery margins and fixed hypopyon (Figure 5.15).
- It may present in a more severe form with a large epithelial defect with limbus-to-limbus involvement and dense localised corneal infiltrates with progressive corneal thinning (Figure 5.16).

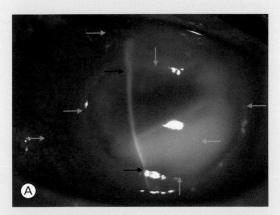

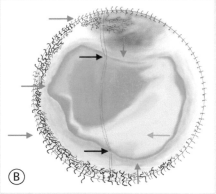

Figure 5.16 Slit lamp photograph demonstrating severe fungal keratitis (A) with a large epithelial defect (green arrows) with discrete margins, dense localised corneal infiltrates (yellow arrow) along with progressive thinning as seen on slit illumination (black arrows). Note the superior area of dense corneal vascularisation (grey arrow) and intense perilimbal injection. (B) Schematic diagram representing the clinical picture of severe fungal keratitis.

CASE 5.11

CLINICAL FEATURES

A 30-year-old male with retroviral disease and chronic viral keratouveitis presented with sudden onset pain, redness and diminution of vision after instillation. He was on chronic, low dose topical steroid therapy for the same. The clinical picture and slit lamp appearance are shown in Figure 5.17.

KEY POINTS

Diagnosis:
- The above clinical scenario describes an unusual presentation of chronic viral keratouveitis with secondary fungal stromal keratitis.

Investigations:
- A corneal scraping specimen could not be obtained as there was no epithelial defect and the infection was confined to the stromal layers.

- Confocal microscopy revealed the presence of branching fungal hyphae.

Treatment:
- The patient was managed with topical and systemic antifungals for two weeks, but partial response was observed. Topical steroids were discontinued.
- Intrastromal voriconazole 50 µg/0.1 ml was injected in five divided doses around the infiltrate to form a depot of the drug around the circumference of the fungal lesion.

Outcome:
- The cornea cleared with a reduction in stromal infiltrates and corneal oedema, as exhibited on anterior segment optical coherence tomography.

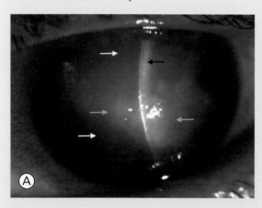 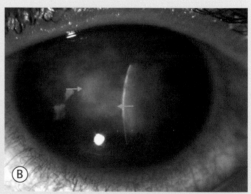

Figure 5.17 Slit lamp photograph of (A) a patient with recurrent viral keratouveitis on chronic topical steroid therapy. Secondary fungal infection was noted in this case with the appearance of flocculent, diffuse infiltrates (yellow arrows), corneal oedema (white arrows), better visualised on the illuminated slit (black arrow). Response to topical antifungal therapy along with cessation of topical steroids was noted after three weeks as seen on slit lamp examination (B) demonstrating reduction in stromal infiltrates (yellow arrows) and corneal oedema.

CASE 5.12

CLINICAL FEATURES

A 55-year-old male patient with uncontrolled diabetes mellitus and concomitant hypertension and chronic renal failure presented with pain, redness and diminution of vision after instillation of over-the-counter drops for irritation of eyes. His vision dropped suddenly with severe pain, following a fall of sand particles in his eyes during driving. The clinical picture revealed a stromal abscess, fluffy exudates on the corneal endothelium and cotton ball exudates in the anterior chamber (Figure 5.18).

KEY POINTS

Diagnosis:
- The above clinical scenario describes a case of fungal ball with a hypopyon occurring in a diabetic patient.

Investigations:
- Corneal scraping specimen could not be obtained.
- Anterior chamber aspirate revealed growth of *A. flavus* on culture.
- The HbA1c level at the time of presentation was 6.5.

Treatment:
- The patient was managed with topical and systemic antifungals along with intracameral voriconazole (50 μg/0.1 ml).
- Endocrinologist opinion was sought and the patient was shifted to injectable insulin therapy for better glycaemic control.

Outcome:
- After the intracameral injection, corneal and anterior chamber lesions were reduced in size and density that completely resolved within four weeks.

Supplementary Information and Additional Tips

- Fungal keratitis may also present as a localised stromal abscess with Descemet's folds (Figure 5.19), hypopyon, endothelial plaque (Figure 5.20) and extensive corneal thinning, that can progress to formation of a descemetocele (Figure 5.21).

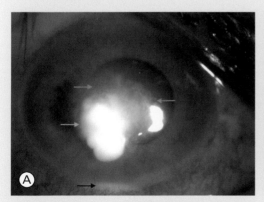
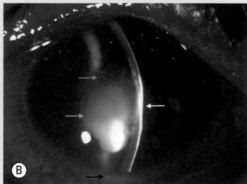

Figure 5.18 Slit lamp photograph of a patient with (A) fungal keratitis and exudates in the anterior chamber (fungal ball) (yellow arrow), endothelial plaque (grey arrows) and a small hypopyon (black arrow). Corneal thinning (white arrow) can be clearly visualised on (B) slit illumination. Note that the surrounding cornea is relatively clear and uninvolved.

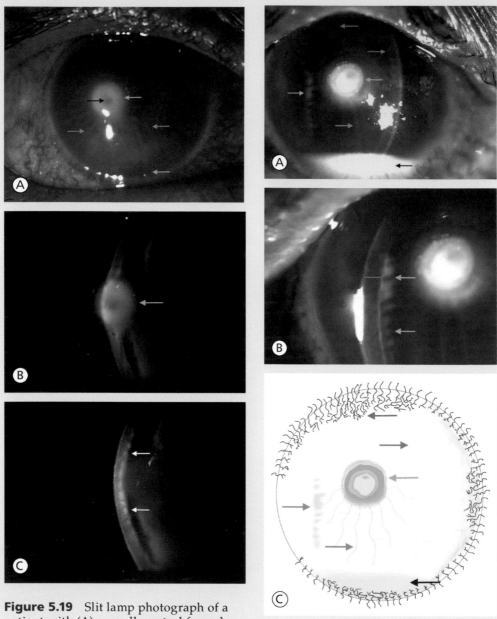

Figure 5.19 Slit lamp photograph of a patient with (A) a small, central fungal corneal ulcer post trauma with vegetative matter wherein a localised stromal abscess (yellow arrow) has formed. An area of central thinning (black arrow) with radial Descemet's folds (grey arrows) and minimal hypopyon (green arrow) can be seen. The magnified view reveals (B) a slit view of the dense stromal infiltrates (yellow arrow) and (C) endothelial involvement (white arrows).

Figure 5.20 Slit lamp photograph of (A) a central fungal corneal ulcer (yellow arrow) with a large fixed hypopyon (black arrow), radial Descemet's folds (grey arrow), endothelial plaque (green arrow), surrounding stromal oedema (blue arrow) and peripheral corneal vascularisation (red arrow). Magnified slit view (B) clearly shows the surrounding stromal oedema (blue line) and endothelial plaque (green arrows). The corresponding schematic diagram (C) reveals the salient findings in this case of fungal keratitis.

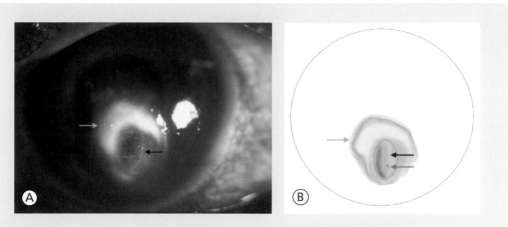

Figure 5.21   Slit lamp photograph (A) showing a long-standing fungal corneal ulcer (yellow arrow) with severe thinning and descemetocele formation (black arrow); the same findings are shown in (B) the corresponding schematic diagram. Note a foreign body (blue arrow) lying over the corneal ulcer bed.

REFERENCES

1. Miller D, Galor A, Alfonso EC. CHAPTER 80. Fungal Keratitis. In: Cornea; Volume 1 – Fundamentals, Diagnosis and Management. 4th ed. USA: Elsevier; 2017; 964–75.

2. FlorCruz NV, Evans JR. Medical interventions for fungal keratitis. Cochrane Database Syst Rev. 2015; (4):CD004241.

6 Protozoal Keratitis and Other Atypical Infections

Ritika Mukhija, Rashmi Singh, Vipul Singh, Shubhi Jain, Radhika Tandon

INTRODUCTION

Infective keratitis is a major cause of ocular morbidity and it is extremely important to manage these cases appropriately and in a timely manner.[1] A majority of cases are caused by a handful of pathogens; however, there are a few atypical organisms that the ophthalmologist should be aware of. Apart from viral, bacterial and fungal causes, keratitis can occur due to a variety of micro-organisms such as protozoa (*Acanthameoba, Microsporidia, Entamoeba*), filamentous bacteria (*Actinomyces, Nocardia, Mycobacterium*), Spirochaetes (*Borrelia,*

Treponema) and other rare organisms like *Pythium insidiosum*.[2–4] While it is not entirely possible to reach a conclusive diagnosis based on clinical findings alone, it is important to suspect unusual organisms and unusual presentations so that appropriate investigations can be ordered to enable early institution of appropriate therapy for achieving improved outcomes in such cases. It is also important to differentiate noninfective causes from infective ones.[5,6] This chapter includes a few clinical scenarios detailing the presentation and practical aspects of their diagnosis and treatment.

CASE 6.1

CLINICAL FEATURES

A 34-year-old male presented with a history of redness, pain, photophobia and diminution of vision in his left eye for the past two weeks. He gave a history of bathing in sea water a few days before the onset of pain. Examination findings and slit lamp appearance are illustrated in Figure 6.1.

KEY POINTS

Diagnosis:

- The above clinical scenario describes a case of early *Acanthamoeba* keratitis (AK) with a partial ring ulcer.

Investigations:

- A fresh wet mount of corneal scraping specimens, which revealed *Acanthamoeba* trophozoites on

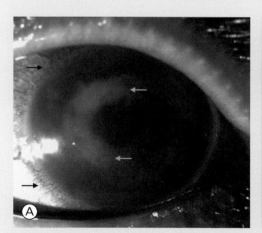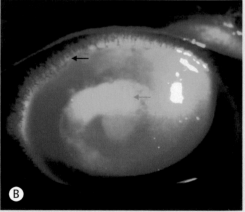

Figure 6.1 Slit lamp photograph of a patient with early *Acanthamoeba* keratitis (A) showing severe ciliary congestion (black arrows) and corneal ring infiltrates arranged in a semi-circular pattern (yellow arrows); (B) shows the epithelial defect (grey arrow) as visualised with fluorescein staining under cobalt blue filter.

Giemsa-Wright staining in this case and/or a positive culture of organisms on *Escherichia coli*-enriched non-nutrient agar are helpful for diagnosis.

■ In vivo confocal microscopy (IVCM), a non-invasive test, is particularly useful in cases where microbiological investigations yield inconclusive results.

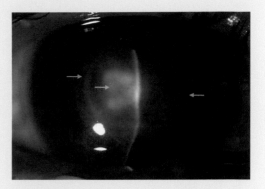

Figure 6.2 Slit lamp photograph of a patient with *Acanthamoeba* keratitis which was previously misdiagnosed as viral stromal keratitis; note the localised area of stromal infiltrates (yellow arrow) with excavation (black arrow) and early ring infiltrates (grey arrows).

Treatment:

■ The patient was managed with topical propamidine (0.1%) and topical polyhexamethylene biguanide (PHMB, 0.02%), initially started at an hourly frequency round the clock, along with a topical broad-spectrum antibiotic (chloramphenicol 0.5% four times a day) and cycloplegic (homatropine hydrobromide 2%) TDS. The fortified drops were tapered as per clinical response.

Outcome:

■ The patient showed marked symptomatic improvement within the first 48 hours followed by a gradual decrease in corneal infiltrates.

■ A complete resolution with macular corneal scarring was noted at two months; however, topical PHMB was continued for six months to prevent any recurrence.

Supplementary Information and Additional Tips

■ Early cases of AK may present as include epithelial erosions, microcysts or ridges, pseudo-dendrites and localised stromal keratitis and/or shallow excavation. Due to non-specific initial presentation, misdiagnosis as herpes simplex keratitis or even bacterial or fungal keratitis is not uncommon (Figures 6.2 and 6.3).

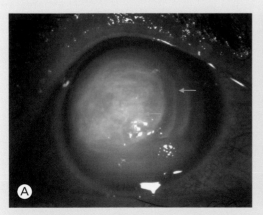

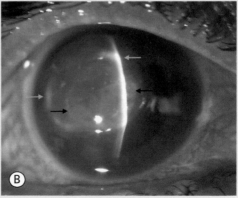

Figure 6.3 Slit lamp photograph of a patient with *Acanthamoeba* keratitis with super-added bacterial infection (*Staphylococcus epidermidis*) who was previously misdiagnosed with fungal keratitis (A) showing dry-looking infiltrates (yellow arrow) and a large epithelial defect (green arrow). A good response was noted with anti-amoebic and antibacterial drugs; a clinical picture two weeks after starting medications (B) shows regression in size and density of infiltrates (yellow arrows) and a healing epithelial defect (black arrows).

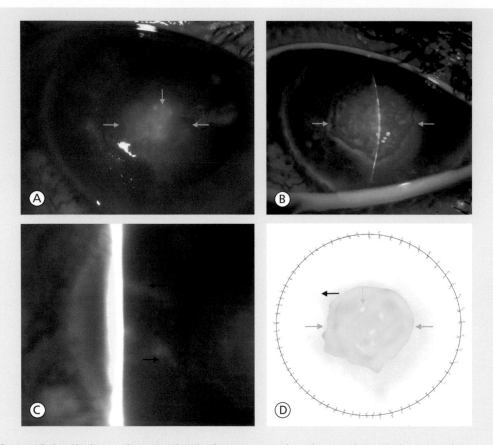

Figure 6.4 Slit lamp photograph (A) of a patient with early *Acanthamoeba* keratitis showing an ill-defined ring ulcer with epithelial defect (green arrows) and localised dry-looking stromal infiltrates (yellow arrow); the epithelial defect (green arrows) can be well-demarcated as visualised with fluorescein staining under cobalt blue filter (B). A magnified image (C) shows radial keratoneuritis (black arrows), which helped in clinching the diagnosis in this case; the corresponding schematic corneal diagram (D) illustrates the various findings.

■ Radial keratoneuritis, i.e. linear radial, branching infiltration by the parasites along corneal nerves in the anterior stroma, is a characteristic sign and may be helpful in picking up cases early (Figure 6.4); it is also responsible for the excruciating pain present in some patients (Figure 6.5).

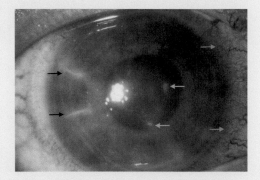

Figure 6.5 Slit lamp photograph of a patient with early *Acanthamoeba* keratitis showing ciliary congestion (grey arrows), few localised stromal infiltrates (yellow arrows) and the characteristic radial keratoneuritis (black arrows).

CASE 6.2

CLINICAL FEATURES

A 40-year-old female, a farmer by occupation, presented with a six-week history of severe pain, photophobia and diminution of vision in her right eye. The symptoms first started six months ago when she was diagnosed elsewhere as viral keratitis and treated with topical antivirals and antibiotics and an intermittent course of topical steroids. The symptoms resolved for some time; however, they recurred after a few weeks and were worse than before. Examination findings and slit lamp appearance are illustrated in Figure 6.6.

KEY POINTS

Diagnosis:
- The above clinical scenario highlights the classical protracted waxing and waning course of AK with a well-defined corneal ring ulcer.

Investigations:
- All microbiological investigations, including Gram stain, Giemsa-Wright stain and KOH fresh wet mount, were inconclusive.
- IVCM was performed, which demonstrated classical *Acanthamoeba* cysts; IVCM is a non-invasive test and particularly useful in such cases where microbiological investigations yield inadequate results (Figure 6.7).

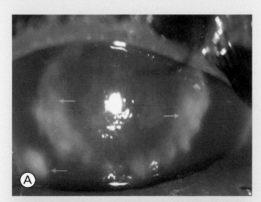

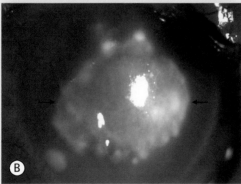

Figure 6.6 Slit lamp photograph of a patient with *Acanthamoeba* keratitis (A) showing a large classical ring ulcer (yellow arrows) and a satellite lesion (grey arrow); photograph (B) shows the clinical picture one week after starting medications with regression of infiltrates and appearance of defined margins (black arrows).

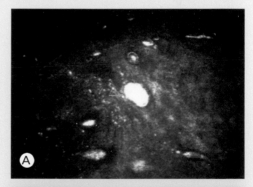

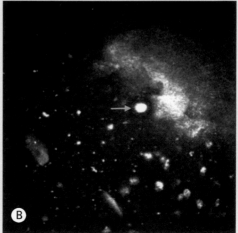

Figure 6.7 In vivo confocal microscopy pictures (A, B) showing hyperreflective round to oval *Acanthamoeba* cysts (yellow arrows).

Treatment:

- The patient was treated with topical propamidine (0.1%) and topical polyhexamethylene biguanide (PHMB, 0.02%), topical broad-spectrum antibiotic (chloramphenicol 0.5% QID) and cycloplegic (homatropine hydrobromide 2%) TDS.
- Although a good response was seen initially, a therapeutic penetrating keratoplasty had to be performed to control the infection (Figure 6.8).

Outcome:

- Patient was prescribed anti-amoebic drugs (PHMB) for six months after surgery, and no recurrence was noted.
- She also developed visually significant cataract around six months after the keratoplasty and underwent a successful phacoemulsification with posterior chamber intraocular lens implantation; the graft remained clear till the last follow-up at one year.

Supplementary Information and Additional Tips

- Misdiagnosis in early cases is extremely common, and a high rate of clinical suspicion is warranted, especially in cases with known risk factors, such as poor contact lens hygiene, significant water exposure or contaminated trauma, or with features in history that are suggestive of AK, vis-à-vis chronicity, multiple referrals, microbiologically inconclusive scrapings, poor response to standard therapy and previous corticosteroid use.
- Even though the disease has an indolent course, long-standing or severe cases may present with corneal melting (Figures 6.9 and 6.10).
- Response to medical management is often unsatisfactory and recurrences are common even after keratoplasty.

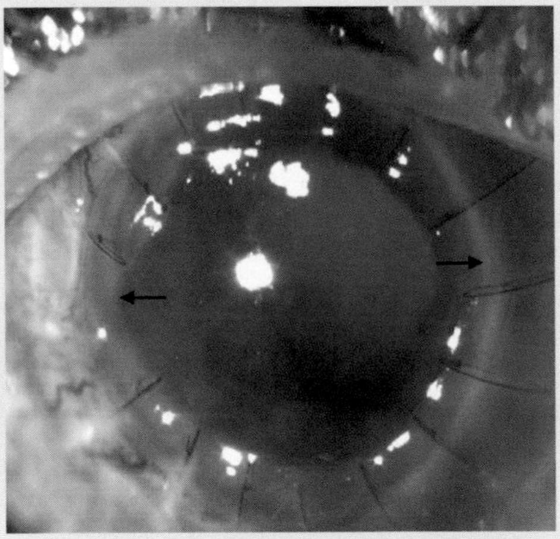

Figure 6.8 Slit lamp photograph of the above patient two months after therapeutic keratoplasty showing a clear eccentric graft and a well-apposed graft-host junction (black arrows) with cataractous lens.

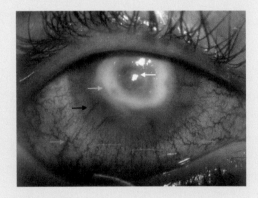

Figure 6.9 Slit lamp photograph of a patient with long-standing *Acanthamoeba* keratitis showing a well-defined ring ulcer (yellow arrow) with an area of central stromal melt (white arrow) and intense surrounding corneal neovascularisation (black arrow).

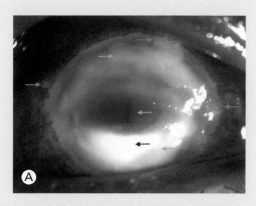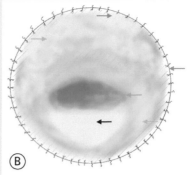

Figure 6.10 Slit lamp photograph (A) and corresponding corneal diagram (B) of a patient with severe *Acanthamoeba* keratitis showing a diffuse ciliary congestion and a large ring ulcer (yellow arrows) along with areas of dense stromal infiltration (black arrow), limbal involvement (grey arrows) and stromal melting (green arrow).

CASE 6.3

CLINICAL FEATURES

An 18-year-old healthy male presented with symptoms of redness, photophobia, watering and mild diminution of vision for the past four days. There was no history of trauma or prior such episodes; however, there was history of tap water splashing in the eye. Examination findings and slit lamp appearance are illustrated in Figure 6.11.

KEY POINTS

Diagnosis:
- The above clinical scenario describes a case of microsporidial keratoconjunctivitis, which is caused by Microsporidia, a group of obligate intracellular parasites.

Investigations:
- Diagnosis was made clinically by noting the superficial, multifocal, raised punctuate keratopathy and confirmed by identifying characteristic small oval spores on modified acid-fast stain.

Treatment:
- The patient was treated with topical ciprofloxacin (0.3%) and gatifloxacin (0.3%) eye ointment at bedtime along with cycloplegics and lubricants.
- A variety of other anti-microbials such as albendazole, fumagillin, itraconazole have also been used with success.
- Topical corticosteroids should not be used as they may worsen the disease.

Outcome:
- The patient showed good response to treatment and most of the infiltrates disappeared with a return to normal visual acuity after two weeks of treatment.

Supplementary Information and Additional Tips

- Microsporidial keratoconjunctivitis occurs more often in immunocompromised patients; however, it can occur in healthy

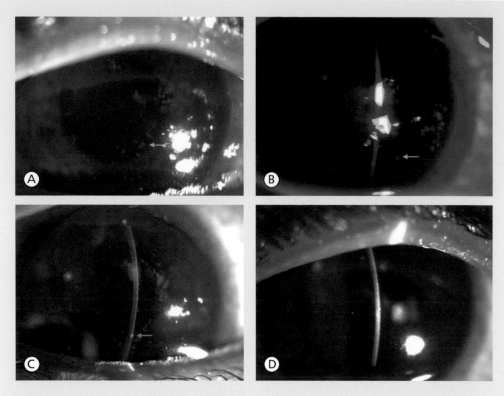

Figure 6.11 Slit lamp photograph of a case of microsporidial keratitis (A) showing multiple superficial coarse raised lesions (yellow arrow), better appreciated on cobalt blue filter with fluorescein staining (B); note that the lesions are intraepithelial (grey arrow) as seen on the parallelepiped view (C). Photograph after two weeks of treatment (D) shows marked improvement with significant clearing of the cornea.

individuals. They need to be differentiated from epidemic keratoconjunctivitis or other causes of superficial punctuate keratitis.
- A history of trauma or exposure to contaminated water is most commonly noted.

- Another form of the infection is stromal microsporidiosis, which is found more commonly in immunocompetent patients as a chronic, progressive keratitis resembling a herpetic disciform disease with pain and decreased vision.

CASE 6.4

CLINICAL FEATURES

A 38-year-old male presented with complaints of pain, redness and watering along with gradually progressive diminution of vision for the past six weeks. He was a field-construction worker by occupation and recalled some trivial trauma while working two months back. There was no other relevant ocular or systemic history. Examination findings and slit lamp appearance are illustrated in Figure 6.12.

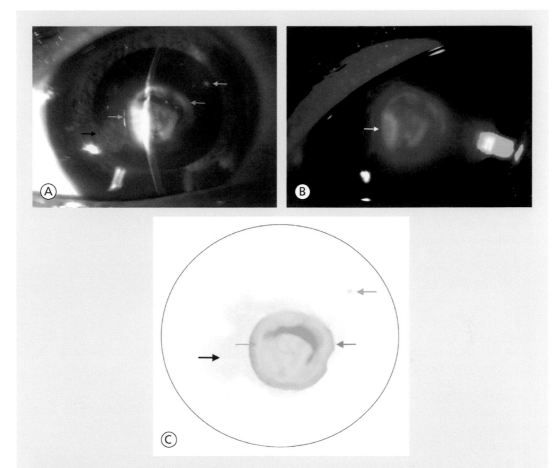

Figure 6.12 Slit lamp photograph of a patient of *Nocardia* keratitis showing (A) a localised central corneal ulcer (grey arrow) with raised infiltrates (yellow arrow) arranged in a wreath-like pattern along with feathery stromal involvement (black arrow) and a small satellite lesion (green arrow); fluorescein staining under cobalt blue filter (B) helps delineate the epithelial defect (white arrow). The corresponding schematic corneal diagram (C) illustrates the same findings.

KEY POINTS

Diagnosis:
- The above clinical scenario highlights a case of *Nocardia* keratitis, occurring most likely in the setting of minor trauma.

Investigations:
- Corneal scraping from the ulcer revealed Gram-positive bacillus in branching filaments and growth of *Nocardia* was found on routine bacterial culture.
- *Nocardia* species can also be identified in smears with Giemsa stain, 10% KOH wet mount and acid-fast stain using 1% sulfuric acid (modified Kinyoun method) and grow in a variety of culture media, including blood agar, chocolate agar and Sabouraud dextrose agar (without antibiotics).

Treatment:
- Patient was treated with topical amikacin 2.5%, along with cycloplegics and night-time gatifloxacin eye ointment.

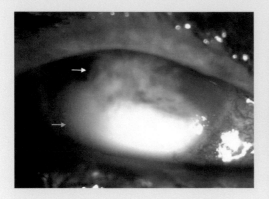

Figure 6.13 Slit lamp photograph of a patient with *Nocardia* keratitis showing central feathery stromal infiltrates (white arrow) with a disproportionately large and dense hypopyon (yellow arrow).

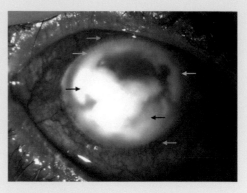

Figure 6.14 Slit lamp photograph of a patient with *Nocardia* sclerokeratitis showing diffuse conjunctival and ciliary congestion (grey arrows), diffuse deep stromal infiltrates (black arrows) with scleral involvement (yellow arrows) in around three quadrants.

Outcome:

- Patient responded well to treatment and the ulcer healed in four weeks leaving behind a central nebular corneal opacity.

Supplementary Information and Additional Tips

- *Nocardia* are usually indolent organisms and often run a prolonged or a waxing and waning course; history of minor trauma or exposure to contaminated soil may be present.
- They can cause both keratitis and/ or scleritis; the former may be in the form of small, raised pin-head infiltrates arranged in a wreath-like configuration, patchy infiltrates predominantly in the anterior stroma, satellite lesions, anterior chamber reaction or hypopyon (Figure 6.13).
- Scleritis is often associated with keratitis (Figure 6.14), although isolated scleral involvement (Figure 6.15) has also been reported.

- Treatment with fluoroquinolones (moxifloxacin, gatifloxacin) and PHMB has also proven to be effective. The role of systemic antibiotics is unclear; they may be helpful in cases with scleral involvement.

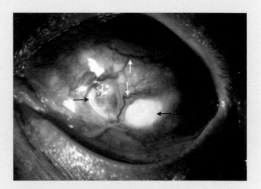

Figure 6.15 Slit lamp photograph of a patient with *Nocardia* scleritis showing an area of scleral abscess with necrosis (black arrows) along with thinning and uveal show (yellow arrow) and engorged episcleral vessels (white arrows).

CASE 6.5

CLINICAL FEATURES

A 58-year-old male was referred as a case of non-healing corneal ulcer after poor response to treatment with antibiotic (gatifloxacin, tobramycin, fortified cefazolin) and antifungal eye drops (natamycin) for around three weeks. Patient gave a history of an episode of trauma with a stone prior to the development of symptoms. Examination findings and slit lamp appearance are illustrated in Figure 6.16.

KEY POINTS

Diagnosis:
- The above clinical scenario describes a case of *Pythium* keratitis, which is caused by *P. insidiosum*, a fungus-like, aquatic oomycete.

Investigations:
- A diagnosis was reached with the help of polymerase chain reaction (PCR), which is one of the main methods used for the identification of this pathogen.
- Microbiology results of direct microscopy with various stains (10% potassium hydroxide, Gram stain, acridine orange) and culture on potato dextrose agar, Sabouraud dextrose agar and chocolate agar are also useful.

Treatment:
- The patient was treated with a combination of topical antibiotics (topical linezolid 0.2%) and antifungals (topical voriconazole 1% and itraconazole 1%) along with oral azithromycin (500 mg OD for 14 days).

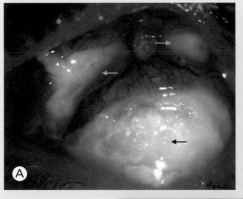
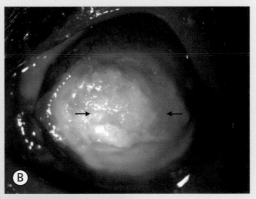
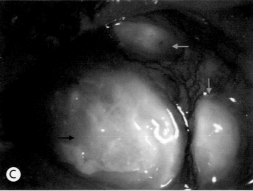

Figure 6.16 Slit lamp photographs of a case of *Pythium* keratitis (A–C) showing total corneal abscess with dense infiltrates (black arrows) as seen with the eye in primary gaze (B); note the multiple pockets of scleral infiltration and melt (yellow arrows) in the superotemporal quadrant (A) and superotemporal quadrant (C) visualised well with the eye in respective down-gaze.

Outcome:

- There was poor response to treatment and rapid worsening with development of total corneal melt (Figure 6.17), following which evisceration had to be performed for control of infection.

Supplementary Information and Additional Tips

- A variety of treatment options, including topical antibacterial drugs (linezolid, azithromycin) and antifungal drugs (natamycin, voriconazole, itraconazole) have been tried, with some success; however, there is no specific drug of choice for *Pythium* keratitis.
- Although rare, it has an extremely high morbidity rate due to poor response to medical therapy, even with a prompt diagnosis.

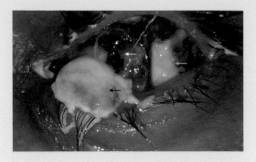

Figure 6.17 Slit lamp photograph of the above case of *Pythium* keratitis showing total corneal melt (black arrow) with uveal prolapse (white arrow) and scleral infiltration and melt (yellow arrow); note the diffuse matting of eyelashes with mucopurulent discharge.

CASE 6.6

CLINICAL FEATURES

A 42-year-old male presented with complaints of painful diminution of vision associated with gradually progressing whitening of his left eye for the past six weeks. He recalled a history of trivial trauma with a soiled object while working around three months back, following which he had mild redness for a day. Since the onset of symptoms, he was seeking medical care with a local ophthalmologist and was receiving empirical treatment in the form of fortified antibiotics and antifungal eye drops. Despite that, there was progressive worsening of symptoms. Examination findings and slit lamp appearance are illustrated in Figure 6.18.

KEY POINTS

Diagnosis:

- The above clinical scenario highlights a case of nontuberculous mycobacterial keratitis.

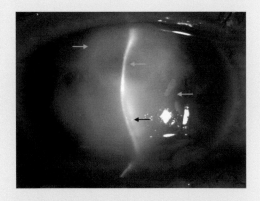

Figure 6.18 Slit lamp photograph of a case of nontuberculous mycobacterial keratitis showing diffuse stromal infiltrates (yellow arrows) in mid-to-deep stroma; on the parallelepiped view, it can be seen that the overlying epithelium appears intact with relatively clear sub-epithelial area (black arrow) in certain areas along with a localised area of stromal necrosis and thinning (green arrow) superiorly.

Investigations:

- As the previous corneal scrapings performed by the local ophthalmologist, prior to starting treatment, did not reveal any micro-organism and as the patient was already on multiple antimicrobial drugs, all topical medications were stopped for 24 hours, and repeat corneal scarping was performed.
- While Gram stain and KOH mount did not reveal anything, bright red, thin rods were noted on Ziehl-Neelson (ZN) acid-fast stain; further, culture on Löwenstein-Jensen medium also revealed growth of nontuberculous mycobacteria (NTM) in a week.
- Anterior segment optical coherence tomography was also performed in this case to document the depth of infiltrates and thinning of the cornea.

Treatment:

- The previous treatment, consisting of topical fortified cefazolin, tobramycin and natamycin, was stopped prior to scarping; based on identification of NTM on ZN staining, the patient was prescribed topical amikacin (2.5%) and ciprofloxacin (0.3%) alternating round the clock.

- Additionally, oral antibiotics (clarithromycin), topical cycloplegic and antiglaucoma therapy were prescribed.

Outcome:

- The patient started responding to the modified treatment with regression of the margins of infiltrates; however, he eventually underwent therapeutic keratoplasty after three weeks in view of sub-optimal outcomes with medical management alone.

Supplementary Information and Additional Tips

- NTM keratitis, although uncommon, continues to pose as a diagnostic and therapeutic enigma for ophthalmologist; a combination of treatment modalities is often needed.
- Common risk factors that should be kept in mind include a history of minor trauma and prior ocular surgery, particularly following laser in situ keratomileusis (LASIK); NTM are considered as the most frequently isolated organisms in late-onset post LASIK keratitis.

CASE 6.7

CLINICAL FEATURES

A 62-year-old male presented with complaints of rapidly progressive and painful diminution of vision in his right eye for the past ten days; associated redness and discharge were also present. Patient was a known case of diabetes mellitus which was controlled on oral hypoglycaemic agents and insulin. There was no history of any preceding trauma or contact lens use. Examination findings and slit lamp appearance are illustrated in Figure 6.19.

KEY POINTS

Diagnosis:

- The above clinical scenario highlights a case of fulminant infective keratitis caused by *Proteus* species.

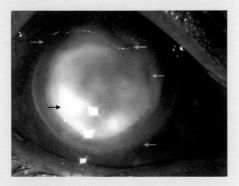

Figure 6.19 Slit lamp photograph of a case of bacterial keratitis showing a large ulcer with infiltrates arranged in a diffuse, ring-shaped pattern (black arrow) along with diffuse ciliary congestion (grey arrow) and areas of stromal thinning (green arrows).

Investigations:

- Corneal scraping revealed Gram-negative rods and bacterial culture was found to be positive for growth of *Proteus* species.

Treatment:

- The patient was initially treated with fluoroquinolones (gatifloxacin) and fortified tobramycin eye drops round the clock, along with topical cycloplegic drops.
- On availability of antibiotic sensitivity reports after 72 hours, the patient was shifted to fortified amikacin in place of gatifloxacin drops, and additionally, oral ciprofloxacin was added.

Outcome:

- Regression in the margins of the infiltrates was achieved with medical management; thereafter, a penetrating keratoplasty was performed in view of the large ulcer and infective load and impending perforation.

Supplementary Information and Additional Tips

- While *Pseudomonas* is the most common Gram-negative bacteria isolated from corneal ulcers, it is important to identify other Gram-negative organisms, such as *Proteus*, *Serratia*, *Moraxella* and *Haemophilus*, as many of these may not respond well to the conventional empirical therapy for infective keratitis.
- Many of these organisms are known to cause fulminant keratitis with development of rapid stromal thinning, necrosis and consequent corneal perforations (Figure 6.20); however, some may have an indolent course or present with localised stromal infiltrates, ring ulcer or hypopyon (Figures 6.21 and 6.22).

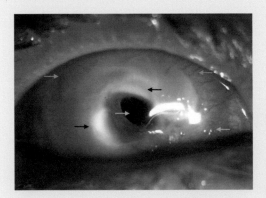

Figure 6.20 Slit lamp photograph of a case of recurrent viral keratitis with secondary bacterial infection (*Klebsiella* species) showing central corneal abscess (black arrows) with a large perforation (yellow arrow), diffuse superficial vascularisation (grey arrows) and conjunctival congestion (green arrow).

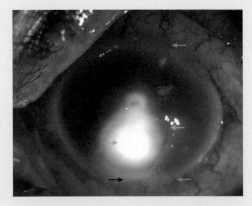

Figure 6.21 Slit lamp photograph of a case of *Moraxella* keratitis in a patient with pre-existing dry eye showing a localised corneal ulcer (green arrow) with dense stromal infiltrates (yellow arrow), a small hypopyon (black arrow) and early superficial corneal vascularisation (grey arrows).

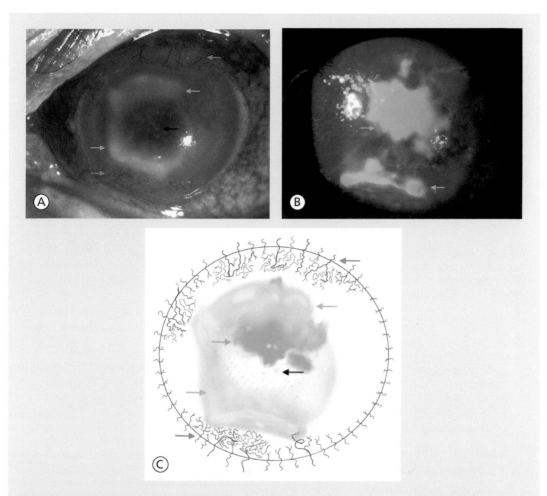

Figure 6.22 Slit lamp photograph of a case of *Serratia* keratitis showing (A) infiltrates arranged in a ring-shaped fashion (yellow arrows) along with keratic precipitates (black arrow) and corneal neovascularisation (grey arrows); photograph under cobalt blue filter with fluorescein staining (B) shows the extent of epithelial breakdown (green arrows). The corresponding schematic corneal diagram (C) illustrates the same findings.

CASE 6.8

CLINICAL FEATURES

A 45-year-old male presented with complaints of pain, redness, discharge and diminution of vision in his left eye following trauma with a soiled stick while farming around 10 weeks previously. There was no other relevant ocular or systemic history. Examination findings and slit lamp appearance are illustrated in Figure 6.23.

KEY POINTS

Diagnosis:
- The above clinical scenario highlights a case of rapidly progressing infective keratitis caused by *Bacillus cereus*.

Investigations:
- Corneal scraping did not reveal any organism on Gram stain or KOH mount; however, *B. cereus* was identified morphologically in the bacterial cultures.

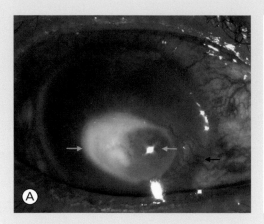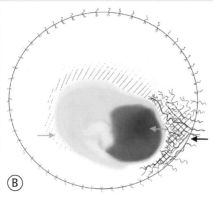

Figure 6.23 Slit lamp photograph (A) and corresponding corneal diagram (B) of a case of *Bacillus cereus* keratitis showing a localised corneal abscess (yellow arrow) along with areas of severe stromal necrosis and descemetocele formation (green arrow) and early corneal neovascularisation (black arrow).

Treatment:

- The patient was treated with topical fortified tobramycin (1.5%) and ciprofloxacin (0.3%) along with twice daily atropine (1%) ointment.
- In addition, a course of oral doxycycline and vitamin C were prescribed.

Outcome:

- The ulcer showed good response to medical management and healed with development of an adherent leucoma in about two months.

Supplementary Information and Additional Tips

- *Bacillus cereus* is a Gram-positive bacillus and can cause fulminant and devastating keratitis following trauma or wound contamination.
- It can present as a distinct stromal ring, stromal abscess, perforation or hypopyon.

CASE 6.9

CLINICAL FEATURES

A 43-year-old male presented with complaints of redness, pain, watering and diminution of vision for the past two weeks. Patient had a history of undergoing penetrating keratoplasty two years prior for healed keratitis; however, he had poor compliance to follow-up and treatment. Examination findings and slit lamp appearance are illustrated in Figure 6.24.

KEY POINTS

Diagnosis:

- The above clinical scenario describes a case of severe late-onset graft infection resulting from a polymicrobial infection.

Investigations:

- Corneal scraping was not performed in view of the presence of corneal melt and the patient was taken for an emergency tectonic re-graft. Corneal

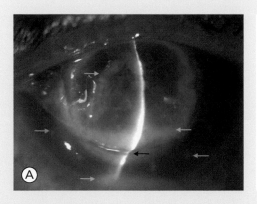
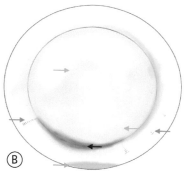

Figure 6.24 Slit lamp photograph (A) and corresponding corneal diagram (B) of a case of polymicrobial keratitis (coagulase-negative *Staphylococcus* and *Cladosporium* species) in a patient with operated penetrating keratoplasty showing infiltrates involving the entire graft-host junction (yellow arrows) with areas of early stromal melt leading to inferior graft dehiscence (black arrow); also note the small hypopyon (green arrow) and suture marks from the prior surgery (grey arrows).

specimens sent for microbiological investigations revealed growth of coagulase-negative *Staphylococcus* and *Cladosporium* species.

Treatment:
- After the surgery, the patient was prescribed topical moxifloxacin 0.5% and voriconazole 1% in addition to cycloplegics and lubricants.

Outcome:
- There was no recurrence of infection and the graft remained clear up until the last follow-up of the patient at six months following surgery.

Supplementary Information and Additional Tips
- Polymicrobial infections, particularly a combination of bacteria and fungi, are not uncommon; suspicion may be warranted in cases with mixed clinical features, inadequate response to therapy and prior topical steroid use (Figure 6.25).

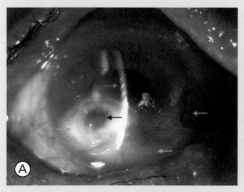
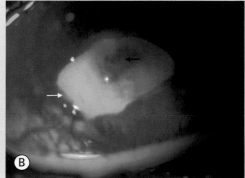

Figure 6.25 Slit lamp photograph of a case of polymicrobial keratitis (*Staphylococcus aureus* plus *Alternaria* species) showing (A) peripheral corneal infiltrates (green arrow) with an area of thinning and pigmentation (black arrow) and a dense hypopyon (yellow arrow); also note the Descemet's folds (blue arrow) and the pseudo-pterygium (grey arrow). Photograph under cobalt blue filter with fluorescein staining (B) delineates the epithelial defect (white arrow).

- They may present with relatively more aggressive features and are often more difficult to treat.
- *Cladosporium* is a filamentous, septate fungus and reported to be a rare causative organism for fungal keratitis; some other uncommon causes of fungal keratitis in humans are *Scedosporium*, *Curvularia* and *Helminthosporium* (Figure 6.26).

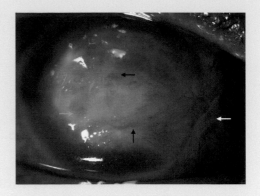

Figure 6.26 Slit lamp photograph of a case of resolving keratitis caused by *Helminthosporium* species showing infiltrates (yellow arrow) with areas of surrounding scarring, dense vascularisation (black arrows) and peripheral conjunctivalisation (white arrow).

CASE 6.10

CLINICAL FEATURES

A 65-year-old male presented with a long-standing history of a localised, non-healing, deep stromal abscess as per his previous clinical records. No organisms were cultured on corneal scarping and confocal microscopy was inconclusive. The patient underwent a lamellar patch graft to remove the infective foci; however, the infection recurred and the patient had to be taken for a full-thickness keratoplasty within three weeks of the first surgery. Two weeks after the second surgery, the patient presented with pain, watering and photophobia in the same eye. Patient was a known case of type II diabetes mellitus that was well controlled on oral hypoglycaemic agents. Examination findings and slit lamp appearance are illustrated in Figure 6.27.

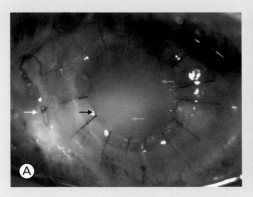
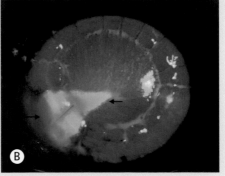

Figure 6.27 Slit lamp photograph of a case of refractory fungal keratitis caused by *Rhodotularia* species presenting as a recurrent graft infection showing (A) corneal ulcer involving both the graft and host cornea (black arrow) and surrounding stromal infiltrates (green arrows) along with diffuse graft oedema and haze (grey arrow). Examination under cobalt blue filter after fluorescein staining (B) delineates the epithelial defect clearly (black arrows).

KEY POINTS

Diagnosis:

- The patient was diagnosed as a case of refractory fungal keratitis with *Rhodotularia* as the causative organism.

Investigations:

- Lamellar host corneal button, which was sent for microbiological analysis, revealed growth of *Rhodotularia* in fungal culture; *Staphylococcus epidermidis* was also isolated, which was most likely a secondary bacterial infection from the patient's own flora.

Treatment:

- Patient was treated with combination of topical antifungals (voriconazole 1% and amphotericin 0.15%) in addition to oral voriconazole.
- Apart from these, topical antibiotics (moxifloxacin 0.5%), cycloplegics, lubricating drops and oral vitamin C were also prescribed.

Outcome:

- The ulcer gradually healed with formation of macular leucomatous opacity in the involved area in about four months; however, consequently, the patient developed an optically failed graft.

Supplementary Information and Additional Tips

- Long-standing or recurrent corneal ulcers, as in this case, may require prolonged therapy and repeated surgical interventions.
- Occasionally, corneal ulceration develops in the setting of an old adherent leucoma, due to degenerative changes; this is sometimes referred to as an atheromatous corneal ulcer (Figure 6.28).

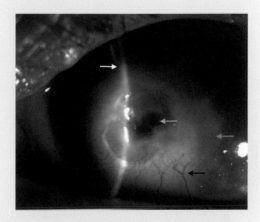

Figure 6.28 Slit lamp photograph of a patient with old adherent leucoma with atheromatous corneal ulcer showing corneal melt (yellow arrow) with surrounding corneal scarring (grey arrow) and vascularisation (black arrow); note the calcific degenerative changes and the nearly flat anterior chamber (white arrow) on parallelepiped view.

CASE 6.11

CLINICAL FEATURES

A 40-year-old female was referred from the Dermatology department for ocular complaints of redness, discharge and diminution of vision in her right eye for two weeks. She was being investigated for multiple poorly healing cutaneous ulcers over the face, legs and trunk and was diagnosed initially as a case of pyoderma gangrenosum. However, following poor response to steroids and immunosuppressants, a palatal biopsy was performed which was suggestive of

histoplasmosis. Examination findings and clinical appearance at presentation to the ophthalmology department are illustrated in Figure 6.29.

KEY POINTS

Diagnosis:

- The above scenario highlights a case of severe infective keratitis and scleritis in the setting of systemic histoplasmosis, caused by the fungus *Histoplasma capsulatum*.

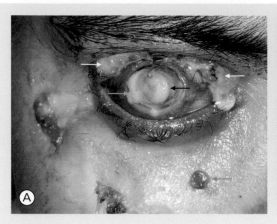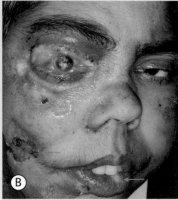

Figure 6.29 Clinical photograph of a patient with histoplasmosis showing (A) severe infective keratitis (black arrow) and scleritis (yellow arrow); note the multiple cutaneous lesions (grey arrows) and areas of upper lid and tarsal conjunctival necrosis (white arrows). Photograph (B) shows the presentation on follow-up; worsening of the ocular features with total corneal melt and uveal tissue prolapse (blue arrow) along with multiple cutaneous lesions (grey arrows) can be noted.

Investigations:

- Ocular discharge and necrotic debris were sent for microbiological investigations; however, no organism could be identified.
- A careful B-scan ultrasonography was performed, which revealed posterior segment involvement in the form of vitreous exudates.
- The left eye was screened for any features of presumed ocular histoplasmosis syndrome (POHS) such as atrophic chorioretinal scars (Histo spots) and peripapillary atrophy.

Treatment:

- Patient was already receiving systemic amphotericin and itraconazole as prescribed by the dermatology team. Topical treatment in the form of amphotericin drops, broad-spectrum antibiotics, itraconazole eye ointment and cycloplegics was added.

Outcome:

- There was poor response to therapy, and total corneal melt along with restriction of extra-ocular movements was noted at subsequent follow-up. An evisceration had to be eventually performed for control of infection.

CASE 6.12

CLINICAL FEATURES

A 50-year-old female presented with complaints of painful diminution of vision, redness and discharge in her left eye for the last two months. She was diagnosed elsewhere as a case of bacterial keratitis and was being treated for the same. There was significant improvement in her symptoms in the first month; however, she started developing progressive white opacity with further diminution of vision for the past four weeks. Examination findings and slit lamp appearance are illustrated in Figure 6.30.

KEY POINTS

Diagnosis:

- The above clinical scenario highlights a case of drug deposits in a case of healing keratitis.

Investigations:

- Anterior segment optical coherence tomography was performed and the

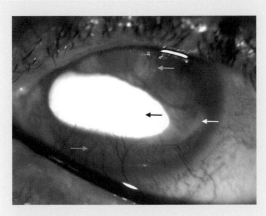

Figure 6.30 Slit lamp photograph of a patient with resolving keratitis showing dense fluoroquinolone drug deposits (black arrow); note the various signs of healing: surrounding corneal scarring (white arrow) with vascularisation (grey arrow) and intrastromal lipid deposits (yellow arrow).

deposits were found to be mostly in the anterior stroma.

Treatment:
- Patient was advised to stop all topical antibiotics (ciprofloxacin and tobramycin); she was instead prescribed preservative-free lubricating eye drops and prophylactic topical chloramphenicol (0.5% TDS).

Outcome:
- There were no signs of improvement in the first week, following which a gentle debridement was performed under topical anaesthesia; specimens were sent for histopathological and microbiological investigations to rule out infection, and they did not reveal any micro-organism.
- After the debridement, the same treatment was continued and there was a significant resolution in the symptoms and signs.

Supplementary Information and Additional Tips
- Drug deposits, although rare, are an important cause of ocular morbidity in patients on prolonged topical therapy. Fluoroquinolones (ciprofloxacin and ofloxacin) are the most frequently encountered drugs and they result in the deposition of a chalky white precipitates; other drugs such as natamycin may also be implicated (Figure 6.31).
- Withdrawal of the drug is sufficient in most cases; however, surgical intervention in the form of debridement or even lamellar or penetrating keratoplasty may be required in few cases (Figure 6.32).
- It is important to differentiate such cases from plaque-like corneal ulcers; the latter usually occur in long-standing keratitis, where low virulence micro-organisms are often entrapped in the plaque (Figure 6.33).

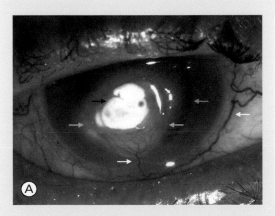
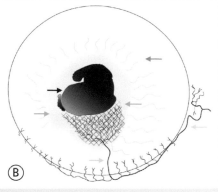

Figure 6.31 Slit lamp photograph (A) and corresponding corneal diagram (B) of a patient with resolving fungal keratitis showing central drug deposits (black arrow) likely due to natamycin drops; note the resolving infiltrates (green arrows), radiating Descemet's folds (grey arrow) and corneal and limbal vascularisation (white arrows).

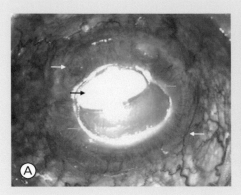
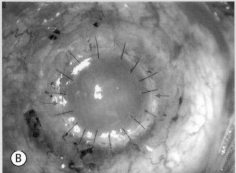

Figure 6.32 Clinical intra-operative photographs showing (A) refractory keratitis with dense drug deposits (black arrow); note the large epithelial defect with distinct margins and stromal tissue loss (yellow arrows) along with diffuse corneal neovascularisation (white arrows). Photograph at the end of therapeutic lamellar keratoplasty (B) showing the well-apposed graft (blue arrows) with all sutures in place.

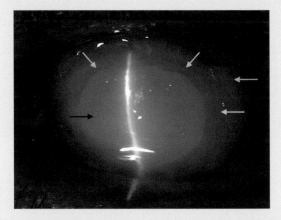

Figure 6.33 Slit lamp photograph of a case of *Acremonium* keratitis with probable secondary bacterial infection showing a large ulcer with thick plaque (black arrow) overlying the area of ulceration (yellow arrow); note the deep stromal infiltrates (grey arrow) with areas of thinning (green arrows).

CASE 6.13

CLINICAL FEATURES

A 10-year-old girl presented with complaints of redness, photophobia and watering in her right eye for the past one week. Parents also gave a history of a slowly growing mass in her right lower lid and that there was a history of a similar mass in her friend at school. There was no history of ocular trauma or any similar mass lesions elsewhere in the body.

Examination findings and clinical appearance are illustrated in Figure 6.34.

KEY POINTS

Diagnosis:
- The above clinical scenario highlights a case of a peripheral corneal ulcer in a patient with a pustular lid mass at the same site.

Investigations:
- Shave excision of lid mass was done by the oculoplastic team; histopathological and microbiological examination was suggestive of ocular rhinosporidiosis.
- An ENT referral was also sought to rule out nasal polyps.

Treatment:
- Patient was empirically treated with topical moxifloxacin and tobramycin along with cycloplegics and lubricants.

Outcome:
- She responded well to treatment and the ulcer started healing within one week of initiation of therapy. At one-month follow-up, a small peripheral nebular corneal opacity was noted.

Supplementary Information and Additional Tips
- Ocular rhinosporidiosis is a rare entity caused by *Rhinosporidium seeberi*. It can present as a polypoidal mass arising from palpebral conjunctiva or peri-orbital skin, recurrent chalazion, conjunctival cyst, peripheral keratitis and scleritis.

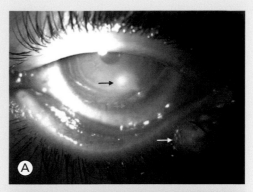

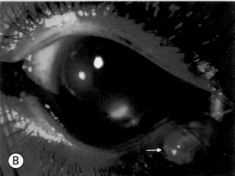

Figure 6.34 Clinical photograph of a young girl with rhinosporidiosis (A) showing the lid mass (white arrow) along with a peripheral corneal ulcer (black arrow) with adjoining inflamed conjunctiva (grey arrow). Photograph under cobalt blue filter with fluorescein staining (B) shows the corneal ulcer and epithelial defect (black arrow).

CASE 6.14

CLINICAL FEATURES

A 32-year-old male presented with bilateral redness, watering and photophobia for the previous four days. Patient gave a history of recurrent foreign body sensation and itching in both his eyes for the past six months for which he was using lubricating eye drops as prescribed. Examination findings and slit lamp appearance are illustrated in Figure 6.35.

KEY POINTS

Diagnosis:
- The above clinical scenario highlights a case of bilateral staphylococcal blepharokeratoconjunctivitis; the diagnosis was quite straightforward based on typical features of staphylococcal blepharitis along with the presence of corneal infiltrates at 2-, 4-, 8- and 10-o'clock positions suggestive of immune-mediated marginal keratitis.

Investigations:
- Investigations may be required to rule out other differential diagnoses, such as infective keratitis, including herpetic marginal keratitis or peripheral ulcerative keratitis.

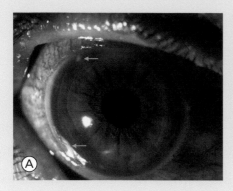
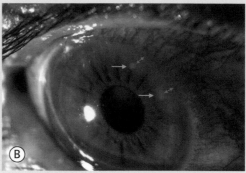

Figure 6.35 Slit lamp photograph of a case of bilateral staphylococcal marginal keratitis in a patient with blepharitis (right eye: A; left eye: B) showing ciliary congestion, peripheral corneal infiltrates (yellow arrows) at characteristic location (2-, 4-, 8-, 10 o'clock) with a clear area (lucid interval) between the infiltrates and limbus (blue arrows).

Treatment:

- The patient was advised of lid hygiene measures and hot fomentation along with a course of oral doxycycline for management of blepharitis.
- In addition, a short course of low-potency topical corticosteroids (loteprednol) along with night-time antibiotic ointment was prescribed.

Outcome:

- Complete resolution of infiltrates was noted within two weeks of starting the treatment; however, treatment of blepharitis was continued.

Supplementary Information and Additional Tips

- Staphylococcal marginal keratitis occurs as an immune response to the staphylococcal antigen, which leads to peripheral stromal infiltrates; these tend to occur at the points of contact between eyelids and cornea, as in the above case.
- The infiltrates spread circumferentially (Figure 6.36) and there is presence of a lucid interval between infiltrates and limbus; these features are helpful when differentiating from herpetic marginal keratitis (Chapter 3, Figures 3.21 and 3.22).

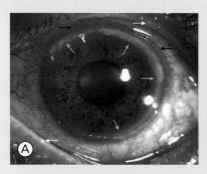
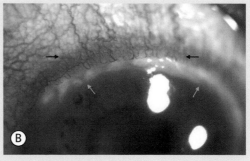

Figure 6.36 Slit lamp photograph of a case of advanced staphylococcal marginal keratitis (A) showing the circumferential spread of the infiltrates (yellow arrows) with associated ciliary congestion (black arrows); the magnified image (B) depicts the same findings clearly.

CASE 6.15

CLINICAL FEATURES

A 25-year-old female presented with complaints of recurrent episodes of redness, pain, watering and photophobia for the past two years. There was no history of any systemic disease. Examination findings and slit lamp appearance are illustrated in Figure 6.37.

KEY POINTS

Diagnosis:
- The above clinical scenario highlights a case of Thygeson's superficial punctate keratitis.

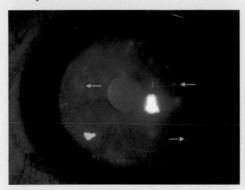

Figure 6.37 Slit lamp photograph of a case of Thygeson's superficial punctate keratitis showing multiple, small, intraepithelial, whitish-grey corneal lesions (yellow arrows).

Investigations:
- Diagnosis was based primarily on clinical presentation; no specific investigation was performed.

Treatment:
- Patient was prescribed preservative-free lubricating eye drops (carboxymethyl cellulose 0.5% 4–6 times a day).

Outcome:
- Patient reported some improvement in symptoms with regular use of artificial tears and was asked to continue the same.

Supplementary Information and Additional Tips

- Thygeson's superficial punctate keratitis usually presents as bilateral, asymmetric involvement with multiple, small, intraepithelial, whitish-grey lesions involving mostly central or pupillary area which stain minimally with fluorescein.
- A short course of low-potency topical steroids may be prescribed; topical ciclosporin is reserved for cases requiring long-term treatment.

REFERENCES

1. Ung L, Bispo PJM, Shanbhag SS, Gilmore MS, Chodosh J. The persistent dilemma of microbial keratitis: global burden, diagnosis, and antimicrobial resistance. Surv Ophthalmol. 2019; 64(3):255–71.
2. Tu EY. CHAPTER 81. Acanthamoeba and Other Parasitic Corneal Infections. In: Cornea; Volume 1 – Fundamentals, Diagnosis and Management. 4th ed. USA: Elsevier; 2017; 976–85.
3. Biber JM. CHAPTER 76. Nontuberculous Mycobacteria Keratitis. In: Cornea; Volume 1 – Fundamentals, Diagnosis and Management. 4th ed. USA: Elsevier; 2017; 902–8.
4. Hasika R, Lalitha P, Radhakrishnan N, Rameshkumar G, Prajna NV, Srinivasan M. Pythium keratitis in South India: incidence, clinical profile, management, and treatment recommendation. Indian J Ophthalmol. 2019; 67(1):42–7.
5. Srinivasan M, Mascarenhas J, Prashanth CN. Distinguishing infective versus noninfective keratitis. Indian J Ophthalmol. 2008; 56(3):203–7. doi:10.4103/0301-4738.40358.
6. Chung G, Iuorno JD. CHAPTER 91. Phlyctenular Keratoconjunctivitis and Marginal Staphylococcal Keratitis. In: Cornea; Volume 1 – Fundamentals, Diagnosis and Management. 4th ed. USA: Elsevier; 2017; 1076–81.

SECTION C

CORNEAL INFLAMMATORY DISORDERS

7 Peripheral Ulcerative Keratitis

Noopur Gupta, Yogita Gupta, M Vanathi, Radhika Tandon

INTRODUCTION

Peripheral ulcerative keratitis (PUK) occurs as a result of immune-mediated or inflammatory melting of the peripheral corneal stroma (keratolysis) due to an interplay between the anatomical and physiological characteristics of the peripheral cornea, extrinsic environmental factors and intrinsic host factors.[1] PUK may occur in association with underlying ocular conditions such as bacterial, viral and fungal infections, ocular trauma, keratoconjunctivitis sicca, neurotrophic keratitis, Mooren's ulcer and other ectatic disorders. Systemic associations include infections, autoimmune diseases like Wegener's granulomatosis, rheumatoid arthritis, systemic lupus erythematosus, rosacea, inflammatory bowel disease and malignancy.[2,3] PUK may sometimes be the first sign of an underlying systemic condition and may herald exacerbation of the systemic disease. Various presentations and management outcomes of PUK are being discussed in this chapter.

CASE 7.1

CLINICAL FEATURES

A 56-year-old male presented with pain and redness in the left eye for four weeks. The best corrected visual acuity (BCVA) was 6/60 and 6/9 in the right and left eye, respectively. He did not give any history of prior similar episodes. There was history of pain and tenderness in the small joints of the hand for two years (recurrent episodes of pain in the wrist, interphalangeal joints and tarsometatarsal joints). He was diagnosed to have rheumatoid arthritis after consultation with the rheumatologist. The examination findings and slit lamp appearance are shown in Figure 7.1.

KEY POINTS

Diagnosis:
- The above clinical scenario describes a case of PUK in a patient with rheumatoid arthritis disease.

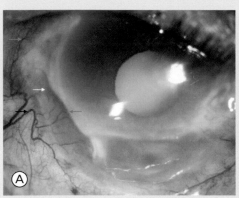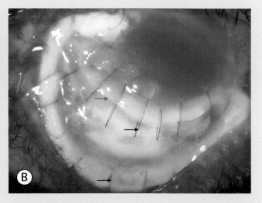

Figure 7.1 Slit lamp photograph of peripheral ulcerative keratitis (PUK) in a case of rheumatoid arthritis, showing (A) an extensive peripheral corneal ulcer (white arrow), extending for almost six clock hours of limbus, caused by significant 'keratolysis' due to inflammatory mediators reaching the limbus, seen with overhanging edges (yellow arrow) and surrounding conjunctival congestion (grey arrow) and dilated scleral vessels (black arrow). The patient underwent (B) a crescentic corneal patch graft transplantation wherein the donor cornea with a rim of sclera was sutured using 10-0 monofilament nylon sutures (black arrows). The graft-host junction (green arrow) was well apposed.

Investigations:

- Meticulous systemic workup was performed, including the following laboratory investigations tailored as per clinical presentation: complete haemogram with erythrocyte sedimentation rate (ESR), Mantoux test, chest X-ray, baseline kidney and liver function tests, peripheral blood smear, urine routine and microscopic evaluation and rheumatoid factor (RF).
- RF was elevated in this case.

Treatment:

- The patient was managed with crescentic corneal patch graft surgery along with oral (1 mg/kg prednisolone) and topical steroids (1% prednisolone acetate drops six times a day and tapered over Six to eight weeks) for the autoimmune condition and to halt the immune-mediated keratolysis. The patient was treated by the rheumatologist for management and control of the systemic disease.

Outcome:

- Adequate healing (anatomical outcome) and BCVA of 6/9 (functional outcome) was achieved at six weeks postoperative period.

Supplementary Information and Additional Tips

- PUK due to autoimmune systemic diseases may or may not be associated with scleritis.
- Peripheral corneal ulceration, stromal thinning and peripheral corneal vascularisation with stromal haze are usual signs of inflammation in PUK (Figure 7.2).

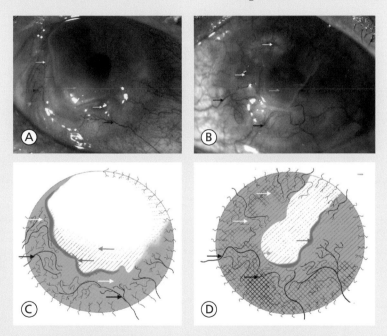

Figure 7.2 Slit lamp photograph in a case of PUK showing (A) peripheral corneal thinning extending from 3 to 11 o'clock (white arrows), peripheral corneal vascularisation (black arrows), overhanging edges created due to active stromal destruction (green arrow) and corneal stromal haze (yellow arrow) progressing from periphery to the centre of the cornea in the right eye. Examination of the left eye revealed (B) extensive corneal thinning (white arrows) extending 360 degrees of the limbus, stromal haze (yellow arrow) approaching the centre of the cornea with extensive 360 degrees of peripheral corneal vascularisation (black arrows) and raised edges of the uninvolved central cornea (green arrow) marking the edge of the destroyed peripheral corneal stroma. Corresponding schematic images of the right eye (C) and the left eye (D) depict the same findings of peripheral corneal thinning (white arrows), peripheral corneal vascularisation (black arrows), areas with stromal destruction (green arrows) and corneal stromal haze (yellow arrows).

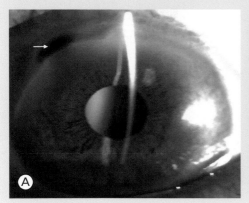
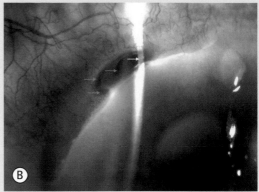

Figure 7.3 Slit lamp photograph of a patient with senile furrow degeneration showing (A) peripheral corneal thinning (white arrow) noted at 11 o'clock position of the limbus. The magnified view reveals (B) peripheral corneal thinning (white arrow) well appreciated in slit examination, with localised furrowing (yellow arrow) with raised edges (grey arrows) in the peripheral cornea. Inflammation and stromal haze are characteristically absent unlike PUK.

- Important differential diagnoses for PUK include marginal keratitis, senile furrow degeneration (Figure 7.3) and Terrien's marginal degeneration, which may also present with peripheral corneal thinning and perforation (Figure 7.4).

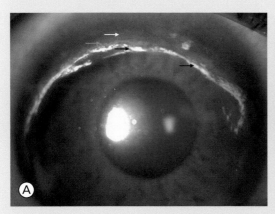
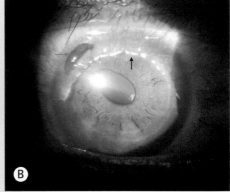

Figure 7.4 Slit lamp photograph of Terrien's marginal degeneration (TMD) demonstrating (A) peripheral corneal thinning (yellow arrow) mostly located in superior limbus with vascularisation (white arrow) and occasional secondary lipid deposition (black arrows) at the site of thinning. There is absence of any stromal haze or inflammation. The peripheral corneal thinning in TMD may sometimes progress to corneal perforation (B) with uveal tissue prolapse (grey arrow). Note the areas of superior vascularisation (white arrow), lipid deposition (black arrow) and superior ectasia (yellow arrow). The pupillary margins are distorted due to plugging of the iris tissue superotemporally at the perforation site.

CASE 7.2

CLINICAL FEATURES

A 39-year-old male presented with a history of pain and watering in his right eye for the past three weeks. He did not give any history of prior similar episodes. There was a history of mouth ulcers and skin rashes three months back. The BCVA was hand movements close to face with accurate projection of rays in the right eye and 6/9 in the left eye. The examination findings and slit lamp appearance at presentation and after management have been shown in Figure 7.5.

KEY POINTS

Diagnosis:

- The above clinical scenario describes a case of PUK with secondary bacterial infection in a case of syphilis.

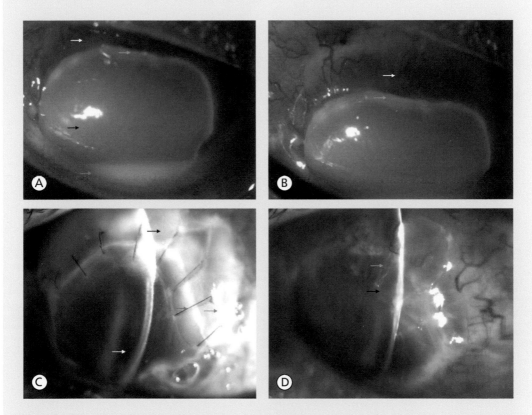

Figure 7.5 Slit lamp photograph of infective PUK in a patient with syphilis demonstrating (A) peripheral ulcer (white arrow) with overhanging edges (green arrow), surrounding corneal oedema (black arrow) and hypopyon (yellow arrow). A magnified slit lamp view of the superior peripheral cornea (B) shows the peripheral ulceration with corneal thinning and vascularisation (white arrow) along with overhanging edges (green arrow). After systemic infection control, corneal patch graft (C) secured with sutures was performed along with amniotic membrane graft (AMG) placement. The banana-shaped donor cornea (black arrow) was seen sutured with 10-0 nylon monofilament sutures (yellow arrow), with a well-formed anterior chamber (white arrow) seen in thin slit illumination and well-positioned AMG (grey arrow). The postoperative clinical photograph revealed (D) peripheral healing of the ulceration with well-apposed graft-host junction (black arrow) and vascularisation of the peripheral cornea (yellow arrow).

Investigations:

- Systemic investigations were done: complete haemogram with ESR, viral serology (tests for human immunodeficiency virus, hepatitis B and C), VDRL (Venereal Disease Research Laboratory test for screening of syphilis), Mantoux test, chest X-ray, baseline kidney and liver function tests, peripheral blood smear, blood culture and urine routine and microscopic evaluation. Additional tests included RF, serum antinuclear antibodies (ANA), antineutrophil cytoplasmic antibodies (cANCA and pANCA), anti-SSA and anti-SSB antibodies, serum calcium and serum angiotensin converting enzyme (ACE). All other underlying causes of PUK were ruled out.
- A positive VDRL test was obtained. An internist referral was taken and a TPHA test (treponemal palladium haemagglutination test with higher specificity for syphilis pathogen) was then performed, which was reported to be positive.

Treatment:

- The patient was managed with systemic penicillin in consultation with the internist.

- After systemic infection control, a crescentic corneal patch graft transplantation surgery with amniotic membrane graft was performed for the patient.

Outcome:

- There was gain of visual acuity postoperatively with aBCVA of 6/12 attained two months after the surgery.

Supplementary Information and Additional Tips

- Patients with PUK cases may be managed surgically with tectonic keratoplasty with full-thickness or partial-thickness annular grafts (Figure 7.6), corneoscleral patch grafts (Figure 7.7) or crescentic and banana-shaped patch grafts (Figure 7.8). The 'match and patch' surgical technique for PUK involves matching the cornea patch graft to the size of defect in PUK, followed by placement of the customised corneal graft fashioned from the donor cornea (Figure 7.8).

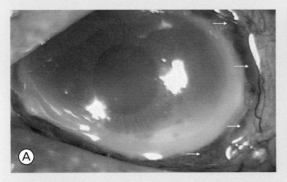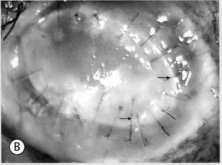

Figure 7.6 Slit lamp photograph of a case of peripheral ulcerative keratitis presenting (A) with circumferential thinning (white arrows) of the peripheral cornea spreading all around 360 degrees of the limbus with adjoining stromal haze and conjunctival congestion. The patient was managed by transplanting (B) an annular corneal graft so as to provide tectonic support for extensive corneal thinning with a doughnut shaped corneal graft (grey arrow) fashioned as per the pattern of corneal thinning seen intraoperatively and sutured with 10-0 monofilament sutures (black arrows).

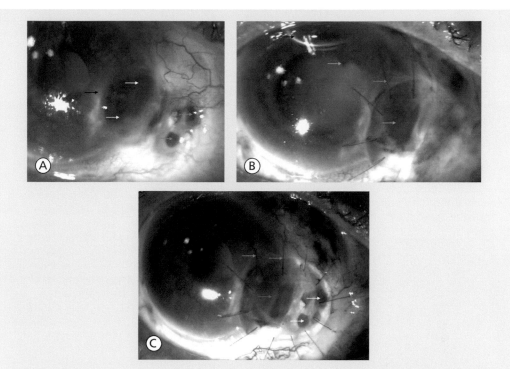

Figure 7.7 Slit lamp photograph of a case of PUK with (A) sectoral thinning of peripheral corneal stroma (white arrows) along with sclera (yellow arrows). Note the surrounding stromal haze (black arrow) at the junction of normal and affected cornea with prominent scleral vessels. The patient underwent tectonic keratoplasty with (B) a circular corneoscleral patch graft (green arrow) sutured with 10-0 monofilament nylon sutures (yellow arrow). An air bubble (black arrow) is seen superiorly in anterior chamber with a pharmacologically dilated pupil with a focal posterior synechiae (grey arrow). The late postoperative image (C) reveals the same case after six months with areas of recurrence of scleral thinning (white arrows), intact sutures (yellow arrows), well-apposed graft-host junction with the corneal graft in place (green arrow).

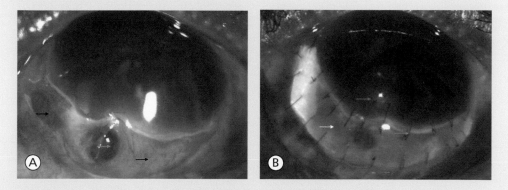

Figure 7.8 Slit lamp photograph of a patient with inferior peripheral ulcerative keratitis showing (A) peripheral corneal thinning (black arrows) extending up to six clock hours of limbus, stromal haze approaching the corneal centre (green arrow) and an area of descemetocele (grey arrow) formation. The patient underwent customised tectonic lamellar keratoplasty and the postoperative photograph reveals (B) a crescentic corneal graft with mild haze (white arrow) and intact sutures (yellow arrow). The adjoining stromal haze in the host cornea has resolved (green arrow) after the surgery.

CASE 7.3

CLINICAL FEATURES

A 44-year-old female, a known case of systemic lupus erythematosus, presented with a history of pain, watering, photophobia and foreign body sensation in her right eye for the past three weeks. There was history of malar rash and progressive nephropathy in the past. She was on intermittent treatment for dry eye disease. The examination findings and slit lamp appearance are shown in Figure 7.9.

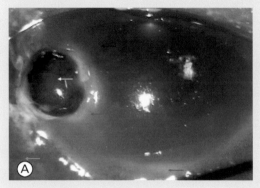

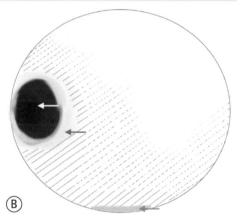

Figure 7.9 Slit lamp photograph of a case of peripheral ulcerative keratitis showing (A) small corneal perforation of nearly 3 mm in diameter (white arrow), pupillary peaking (black arrow) towards the site of perforation, surrounding stromal haze and infiltrates (green arrow), mild inferior hypopyon (grey arrow) and adjacent scleritis (yellow arrow). The corresponding schematic image (B) shows the same findings.

KEY POINTS

Diagnosis:
- The above clinical scenario describes a case of peripheral corneal perforation in a patient with systemic lupus erythematosus.

Investigations:
- Systemic investigations in consultation with a rheumatologist including a complete haemogram with ESR, viral serology (tests for HIV, hepatitis B and C), VDRL (test for screening for syphilis), Mantoux test, chest X-ray, baseline kidney and liver function tests, peripheral blood smear, blood culture and urine routine and microscopic evaluation were sent. Additional tests included RF, serum ANA, antineutrophil cytoplasmic antibodies (cANCA and pANCA), anti-SSA and anti-SSB antibodies, serum calcium and serum ACE.

Treatment:
- The patient was managed with systemic immunosuppressive treatment including oral prednisolone 60 mg once daily as advised by the rheumatologist.
- The patient was managed with topical fortified antibiotics (cefazolin 5% and tobramycin 1.3%) one hourly, homatropine 2% thrice a day and timolol 0.5% twice a day.
- A corneal patch graft transplantation secured with sutures was performed to seal the defect after systemic treatment was initiated.

Outcome:
- There was gain of BCVA which was recorded as 6/9 four months after the corneal surgery.

Supplementary Information and Additional Tips

- Progressive corneal thinning and impending corneal perforation are an important indication for emergency keratoplasty in patients with PUK.

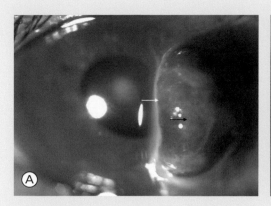
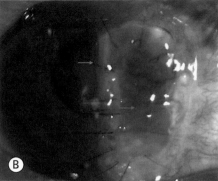

Figure 7.10 Slit lamp photograph of a case of PUK showing (A) corneal perforation of nearly 5 mm in length in the vertical dimension (white arrow) plugged by iris tissue (black arrow). The perforation was sealed with (B) an oval-shaped oblong graft (green arrow) of customised shape that was sutured with 10-0 monofilament nylon sutures (yellow arrow). The exposed iris tissue was abscissed.

- Perforations in PUK may be small, as seen in Case 3 or large (Figure 7.10) depending on the underlying aetiology, timing of presentation and severity of disease.
- Large corneal perforations may be associated with scleritis and vascularisation of the host bed

that may need to be repaired with a corneal patch graft along with a scleral rim. Peripheral lamellar 'C'-shaped grafts can effectively restore tectonic integrity, while maintaining a reasonable corneal contour to enhance visual acuity (Figure 7.11).

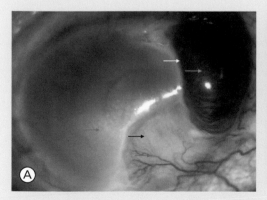
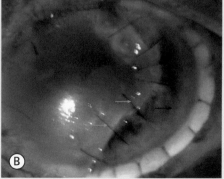

Figure 7.11 Slit lamp photograph of a patient with sclerokeratitis presenting as (A) peripheral ulceration, thinning and perforation (white arrow) plugged by iris tissue (yellow arrow). The site of peripheral corneal thinning (black arrow) demonstrated a vascularised, corneal bed (green arrow) with surrounding stromal haze (grey arrow). The postoperative clinical picture demonstrated (B) a crescentic corneoscleral patch graft (black arrow) well secured by sutures (yellow arrows) with well-apposed graft-host junction.

CASE 7.4

CLINICAL FEATURES

A 75-year-old male presented with a history of pain, redness and watering in his right eye for the past three weeks, for which he was on treatment from a local ophthalmologist. He reported that he developed the symptoms following an insect falling in the eye for which he had splashed tap water into the eye. The examination findings and slit lamp appearance at presentation are shown in Figure 7.12.

KEY POINTS

Diagnosis:
- The above clinical scenario describes an acute presentation of post-traumatic PUK with corneal perforation along with co-existing central infective keratitis.

Investigations:
- A comprehensive systemic evaluation was performed and none of the investigations were positive for any autoimmune disease.
- Ultrasound B-scan was anechoic.
- Microbiological investigations were performed from corneal scrapings: Gram stain, Giemsa stain, calcofluor white stain, KOH mount, bacterial culture on blood agar, fungal culture on Sabouraud dextrose agar and thioglycolate broth, and drug sensitivity testing. A bacterial corneal ulcer was established as the laboratory diagnosis for this patient, due to *Staphylococcus epidermidis* growth in culture media.
- An anterior segment optical coherence tomography (AS-OCT) was performed to look for any full-thickness defect in the central cornea. AS-OCT showed oedema in the central cornea (with thickness ~795 μm).

Treatment:
- The patient was managed with topical fortified antibiotics (cefazolin 5% and tobramycin 1.3%) due to involvement of the visual axis and the presence of hypopyon. They were given hourly for the first 24 hours, then every two hours for 48 hours (round the clock), then given every four hours for one week, then every six hours for a week and then tapered as per the response. Antibiotic ointment and anti-glaucoma medication were also prescribed.

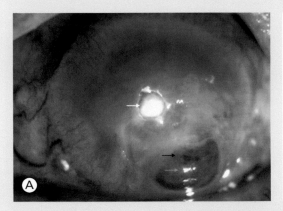
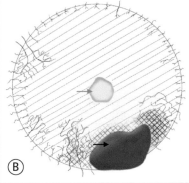

Figure 7.12 Slit lamp photograph of a case of peripheral ulceration showing (A) central infective keratitis with ulceration (white arrow) along with peripheral inferonasal corneal perforation (black arrow) and iris tissue prolapse (yellow arrow) at the site of PUK due to severe thinning and weak peripheral cornea. Peripheral corneal vascularisation and conjunctival congestion can also be appreciated. The schematic corneal diagram (B) highlights the same findings.

- A circular corneal patch graft was transplanted to close the peripheral perforation.

Outcome:
- Final postoperative visual acuity was 6/24 with a central residual corneal opacity.

Supplementary Information and Additional Tips
- AS-OCT is an important tool to investigate and manage PUK. It helps document corneal thickness and images stromal infiltrates, if any.
- Certain cases of fungal keratitis may be associated with peripheral corneal thinning and scleritis, thus may present as PUK (Figure 7.13).

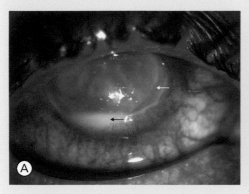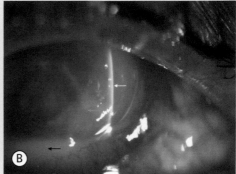

Figure 7.13   Slit lamp photograph of a case of PUK with fungal keratitis revealing (A) peripheral ulceration and thinning (white arrow), inferior hypopyon (black arrow), diffuse corneal oedema (yellow arrow) and surrounding conjunctival congestion (green arrow). The slit view (B) highlights the same findings of peripheral corneal thinning (white arrow), hypopyon (black arrow) and surrounding infiltrates (yellow arrow).

CASE 7.5

CLINICAL FEATURES

A 65-year-old male presented with pain and redness in the right eye of two weeks' duration. He did not give any history of prior similar episodes. There was no history of fever, rash or joint pain. The examination findings and slit lamp appearance at presentation and follow-up are illustrated in Figure 7.14.

KEY POINTS

Diagnosis:
- The above clinical scenario describes a case of peripheral corneal ulcer and all causes of PUK were ruled out on the basis of history and laboratory investigations. The diagnosis of Mooren's ulcer was made after

exclusion of all systemic and ocular conditions that may possibly cause PUK.

Investigations:
- A meticulous systemic workup was performed, including laboratory investigations like a complete haemogram with ESR, viral serology (tests for HIV, hepatitis B and C), VDRL test for syphilis, Mantoux test, chest X-ray, baseline kidney and liver function tests, peripheral blood smear, blood culture and urine routine and microscopic evaluation. Additional tests included RF, serum ANA, antineutrophil cytoplasmic antibodies (cANCA and pANCA), anti-SSA and anti-SSB antibodies, serum

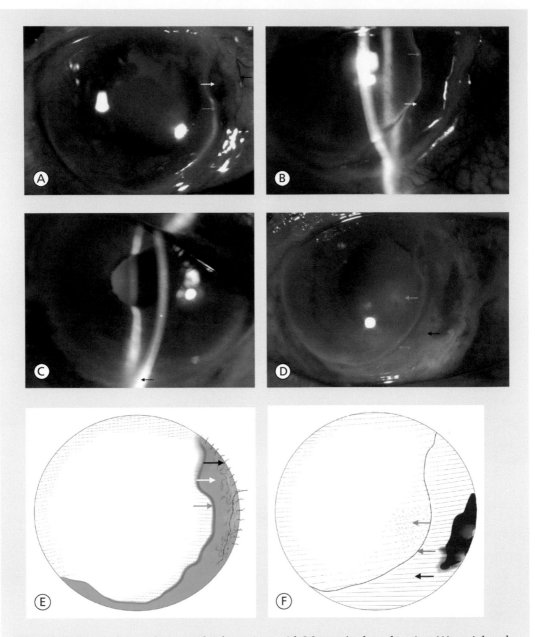

Figure 7.14 Slit lamp photograph of a patient with Mooren's ulcer showing (A) peripheral corneal ulcer (white arrow) appearing like a localised furrow with overhanging edges (yellow arrow), five clock hour extent of stromal and epithelial thinning with surrounding congestion (black arrow). The slit view (B) highlights peripheral corneal thinning (white arrow), with bending of the slit beam, overhanging edges and surrounding congestion (black arrow). Overhanging edges, absence of scleritis and excruciating pain (out of proportion to signs) favour the diagnosis of Mooren's ulcer. Examination of the other eye (C) was within normal limits with normal peripheral corneal thickness (black arrow). The patient underwent tectonic keratoplasty (D) using a crescentic donor corneal graft (black arrow) secured with fibrin glue and a healthy and a well-apposed graft-host junction (yellow arrow) with few endothelial pigments in the adjacent cornea (grey arrow). The preoperative (E) and postoperative (F) clinical picture highlighted through the schematic corneal diagrams showing the same findings.

calcium and serum ACE. All possible etiological conditions associated with PUK were ruled out.

Treatment:

- The patient was managed on topical steroids: prednisolone acetate (1%) drops (started at every four hours for first week then every six hours for two weeks then tapered slowly according to clinical response), cycloplegic thrice a day, topical antibiotics (moxifloxacin 0.5% QID for two weeks) and topical lubricants (carboxymethylcellulose 0.5% every two hours). A crescentic lamellar corneal patch graft secured with fibrin-aprotinin glue along with amniotic membrane transplantation was performed.

Outcome:

- There was adequate healing noted in the postoperative period with a final BCVA of 6/9 attained six weeks after surgery.

Supplementary Information and Additional Tips

- Clinical presentations of Mooren's ulcer have been divided into three types depending on presentation and outcome, namely, unilateral Mooren's ulcer that usually presents in old age, bilateral aggressive Mooren's ulcer that usually presents in young males and the bilateral indolent Mooren's ulcer that is seen in middle aged and elderly individuals and shows good response to treatment.
- Bilateral Mooren's ulcer in the elderly usually has an indolent course and heals with appropriate management to leave a residual peripheral corneal opacity with a clear visual axis. Recurrence is uncommon in these cases.

CASE 7.6

CLINICAL FEATURES

A 22-year-old male presented with sudden onset of severe pain, redness and diminution of vision in the right eye for one week. The other eye had a history of no symptoms. He did not give any history of prior similar episodes. There was no history of fever or rash or joint pain; no history suggestive of any rheumatological disease. The examination findings and slit lamp appearance are shown in Figure 7.15.

KEY POINTS

Diagnosis:

- The above clinical scenario describes a case of fast progressing, unilateral severe PUK. The diagnosis of aggressive Mooren's ulcer was made after the exclusion of all systemic and ocular conditions that may possibly cause PUK.

Investigations:

- A meticulous systemic workup was performed, including laboratory investigations like complete

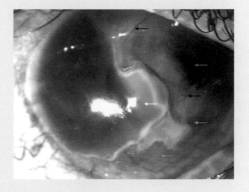

Figure 7.15 Slit lamp photograph of a case of severe Mooren's ulcer in a 22-year-old male presenting as malignant PUK in the right eye. There was severe corneal thinning (yellow arrows) and ulceration in the superior, nasal and inferior cornea along with corneal vascularisation (black arrows) with stromal haze in the involved regions of the cornea (white arrow). The central corneal haze and induced astigmatism was responsible for low presenting visual acuity in this case. Also note the impending perforation (green arrow) seen in the nasal quadrant with iris tissue seen underneath.

haemogram with ESR, viral serology (tests for HIV, hepatitis B and C), VDRL test for syphilis, Mantoux test, chest X-ray, baseline kidney and liver function tests, peripheral blood smear, blood culture and urine routine and microscopic evaluation. Additional tests included RF, serum ANA, antineutrophil cytoplasmic antibodies (cANCA and pANCA), anti-SSA and anti-SSB antibodies, serum calcium and serum ACE. All possible etiological conditions associated with PUK were ruled out.

Treatment:
- Topical prednisolone acetate (1%) drops (started at every two hours

for first week then every six hours for two weeks then tapered slowly according to clinical response), topical antibiotics (moxifloxacin 0.5% QID for two weeks), cycloplegic thrice a day and topical lubricants (carboxymethylcellulose 0.5% every two hours). Oral prednisolone 60 mg was prescribed to be taken in the morning.
- A crescentic corneal patch graft using fibrin glue with amniotic membrane transplantation was planned.

Outcome:
- There was slow and incomplete healing with aBCVA of 6/60 at six weeks after medical management.

CASE 7.7

CLINICAL FEATURES

A 53-year-old male presented with a history of past episodes of recurrent pain and redness in both eyes, lasting for three to four weeks. The last such episode was four months back in the right eye. There was a history of recurrent dyspnoea and nasal bleeds for the past six months for which the patient was on medications. The examination findings and slit lamp appearance are shown in Figure 7.16.

KEY POINTS

Diagnosis:
- The above clinical scenario describes a case of PUK with recurrent necrotising scleritis due to Wegener's granulomatosis (now called granulomatosis with polyangiitis).

Investigations:
- A meticulous systemic workup was performed, including the following laboratory investigations: complete haemogram with ESR, viral serology (tests for HIV, hepatitis B and C), VDRL test for syphilis, Mantoux test, chest X-ray, paranasal sinuses X-ray, baseline kidney and liver function tests, peripheral blood smear, blood culture and urine routine and

microscopic evaluation. Additional tests included RF, serum ANA, antineutrophil cytoplasmic antibodies (cANCA and pANCA), anti-SSA and anti-SSB antibodies, serum calcium and serum ACE.

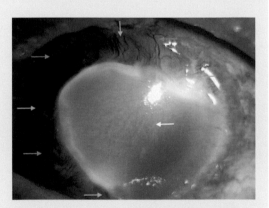

Figure 7.16 Slit lamp photograph of a case of Wegener's granulomatosis showing more than 270 degrees of limbal destruction, seen as stromal thinning and peripheral gutter formation (green arrows), overhanging edges (black arrow), total corneal stromal haze (white arrow), diffuse scleritis and 360 degrees of profuse peripheral corneal vascularisation along with episcleral, and scleral inflammation (grey arrows).

- The chest X-ray showed pulmonary infiltrates bilaterally. Paranasal sinuses and nose X-ray showed maxillary sinusitis and destructive changes in nasal septum cartilage. Urine microscopy showed RBC casts in urine and suggested glomerulonephritis.
- Scleral biopsy specimen from left eye illustrating collagen necrosis, and granulomatous inflammation with lymphocytes, eosinophils, epithelioid cells and multinucleated giant cells.

Treatment:
- Patient was managed on systemic immunosuppression (oral steroids and oral cyclophosphamide) indicated for recurrent scleritis with topical low-potency steroids: fluorometholone (1%) drops (three times for two weeks then tapered slowly according to clinical response), homatropine 2% three times a day, topical antibiotics (moxifloxacin 0.5% four times a day for two weeks) and topical lubricants (carboxymethylcellulose 0.5% every two hours).
- The drug dosage of immunosuppressants was modified to obtain a good therapeutic effect with minimal complications of cytotoxic agents, such as declining leukocyte count in consultation with the rheumatologist.

Outcome:
- Response to therapy and adequate healing was noted with systemic immunosuppression and the ocular lesion healed after six months of therapy.

Supplementary Information and Additional Tips
- Initiation of appropriate and timely immunosuppressive therapy along with ocular management in patients with Wegener's granulomatosis results in the resolution of PUK and accompanying scleritis with eventual scarring and neovascularisation (Figure 7.17).

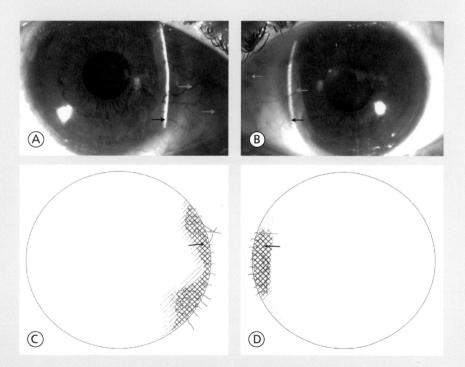

Figure 7.17 Slit lamp photograph of a case of bilateral healed PUK and resolved scleritis in the right (A) and left (B) eye showing bilateral peripheral corneal thinning with opacification (black arrow) seen in thin slit illumination with superficial vascularisation (grey arrow) and patches of non-necrotising scleritis (yellow arrow). Corresponding schematic corneal diagram of the right eye (C) and left eye (D) reveal the same findings.

CASE 7.8

CLINICAL FEATURES

A 48-year-old female with a past medical history of autoimmune hepatitis presented with tearing, pain, foreign body sensation and redness in the left eye for four weeks. The BCVA was 6/36 and 6/9 in the right and left eye, respectively. She did not give any history of similar episodes in the past. She was diagnosed with hepatitis for over 10 years and was on low-dose steroid maintenance therapy for the condition. The examination findings and slit lamp appearance are shown in Figure 7.18.

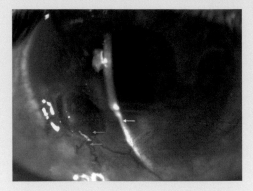

Figure 7.18 Slit lamp photograph of a case of PUK with corneal neovascularisation showing peripheral corneal thinning (white arrow) with uveal tissue prolapse and deep corneal vessels (yellow arrows).

KEY POINTS

Diagnosis:
- The above clinical scenario describes a case of PUK with associated scleritis in a patient with autoimmune hepatitis.

Investigations:
- Meticulous systemic workup was performed. Liver function tests were deranged.

Treatment:
- The patient was managed with oral (1 mg/kg prednisolone) and topical steroids (1% prednisolone acetate drops six times a day and tapered over six to eight weeks) for the autoimmune condition and to halt the immune-mediated keratolysis. Oral doxycycline 100 mg twice a day, prophylactic topical antibiotic drops (moxifloxacin hydrochloride 0.5% four times a day) along with preservative-free lubricants (carboxymethylcellulose 1%) every two hours.
- The patient was treated by the gastroenterologist for management and control of the systemic disease. She was started on oral azathioprine 150 mg and oral prednisolone 60 mg daily.
- A corneal patch graft along with iris repositioning was performed to provide tectonic support and promote healing.

Outcome:
- Adequate healing (anatomical outcome) and aBCVA of 6/12 (functional outcome) were achieved at the completion of six weeks after the surgery.

CASE 7.9

CLINICAL FEATURES

A 64-year-old female presented with pain and redness in the left eye for four weeks. The BCVA was 6/60 and 6/9 in the right and left eye, respectively. She gave a history of a previous episode and was on long-term therapy for dry eye disease. She was a diagnosed case of seropositive rheumatoid arthritis and was in the remission phase. The examination findings and slit lamp appearance are shown in Figure 7.19.

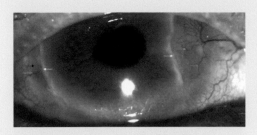

Figure 7.19 Slit lamp photograph of a patient with peripheral ulcerative keratitis with nasal (black arrow) and temporal (yellow arrow) peripheral corneal thinning in a case of rheumatoid arthritis with well-demarcated edges (white arrows) of the ulcer with peripheral corneal vascularisation (grey arrows) along with scleral inflammation.

KEY POINTS

Diagnosis:
- The above clinical scenario describes a case of healing PUK in a patient with rheumatoid arthritis disease.

Investigations:
- A meticulous systemic workup was performed.
- RF was controlled in this case.

Treatment:
- The systemic disease was well controlled on methotrexate (7.5 mg orally every week).
- The patient was managed with crescentic corneal patch graft surgery along with oral (1 mg/kg prednisolone) and topical steroids (1% prednisolone acetate drops six times a day and tapered over six to eight weeks) for the autoimmune condition and to halt the immune-mediated keratolysis.

Outcome:
- Adequate healing (anatomical outcome) and aBCVA of 6/9 (functional outcome) were achieved at the end of three months.

CASE 7.10

CLINICAL FEATURES

A 33-year-old male presented with pain and redness in both eyes for four weeks. He did not give any history of prior similar episodes. The BCVA was 6/60 and 6/9 in the right and left eye, respectively. Ocular adnexa, corneal sensations and dilated fundus examination of both eyes were normal. A systemic workup revealed low CD4 counts and seropositivity for human immunodeficiency virus. The examination findings and slit lamp appearance are shown in Figure 7.20.

KEY POINTS

Diagnosis:
- The above clinical scenario describes a case of bilateral PUK in a patient with HIV infection.

Investigations:
- A meticulous systemic workup was performed.

- The rheumatology opinion showed no clinical evidence of collagen vascular disorder. All blood investigations, Mantoux test (4 mm induration), ESR (15 mm) and chest X-ray were normal.
- ELISA for HIV was reported to be positive.
- Corneal scraping was subjected to Gram and Giemsa stains, KOH mount and culture and sensitivity, and was reported to be negative.
- Impression cytology of the lesion showed inflammatory cells (neutrophils and lymphocytes) suggesting an active disease process.

Treatment:
- The patient was started on anti-retroviral therapy (ART), namely, zidovudine 300 mg BD and lamivudine 150 mg BD.

Outcome:
- The lesion that initially showed worsening after starting ART

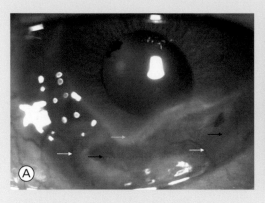

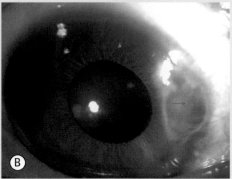

Figure 7.20 Slit lamp photograph of a case of bilateral PUK showing (A) progressive corneal thinning seen as peripheral corneal stromal ulceration (black arrows) of nearly 180-degrees extent and corneal vascularisation (white arrows) with mild reducing stromal haze (yellow arrow) in the left eye. Examination of the other eye revealed (B) a focal area of peripheral ulceration (green arrow) of nearly two clock hours temporally along with vascularisation.

(immune recovery response) showed almost complete resolution over the next four months, with minimal residual subconjunctival scarring and peripheral corneal opacity.

Supplementary Information and Additional Tips

- The eventual outcome in cases of healed PUK after re-epithelialisation and halting of progressive corneal ulceration is corneal opacification with corneal thinning (Figure 7.21).

- In certain cases of PUK with more than six clock hours of involvement, extensive peripheral cornea opacification may result (Figure 7.22) that leads to permanent decrease in visual acuity due to induced astigmatism. Such cases can be effectively managed with refractive correction or fitting of rigid gas-permeable contact lenses.

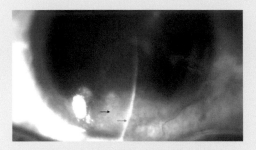

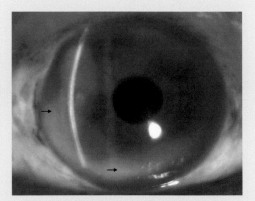

Figure 7.21 Slit lamp photograph of a case of healed PUK, corneal scarring (black arrow) with appreciable localised thinning (grey arrow) and normal surrounding cornea seen in thin slit illumination after resolution of acute inflammation and regression of corneal vessels.

Figure 7.22 Slit lamp photograph of a case of healed PUK in a 50-year-old female, with multiple healed peripheral ulcers (black arrows), eventually leaving behind a peripheral maculo-leucomatous corneal opacity.

REFERENCES

1. Tandon R, Galor A, Sangwan VS, Ray M. *Peripheral Ulcerative Keratitis: A Comprehensive Guide*. Cham, Switzerland AG: Springer International Publishing; 2017.
2. Cao Y, Zhang W, Wu J, Zhang H, Zhou H. Peripheral ulcerative keratitis associated with autoimmune disease: Pathogenesis and treatment. *J Ophthalmol*. 2017; 2017:7298026. doi: 10.1155/2017/7298026. Epub 2017 Jul 13.
3. Squirrell DM, Winfield J, Amos RS. Peripheral ulcerative keratitis 'corneal melt' and rheumatoid arthritis: A case series. *Rheumatology (Oxford)*. 1999; 38(12):1245–1248.

8 Neurotrophic Keratitis

Vipul Singh, Ritika Mukhija, Noopur Gupta

INTRODUCTION

Neurotrophic keratitis is a degenerative corneal epithelial disease and occurs as a result of damage to corneal innervation and consequent corneal hypoesthesia. It is also known as neurotrophic keratopathy; however, it is important to note that the pathology involves varying degrees of associated corneal and adjacent conjunctival inflammation, and, in fact, is classified under ICD10 as neurotrophic keratoconjunctivitis. Epithelial breakdown progresses from punctate keratitis and focal epithelial loss in early stages to persistent non-healing epithelial defects, stromal ulceration and melting in late stages.[1,2] Absence or decrease in corneal sensations can occur due to a variety of causes, such as ocular infections (herpes simplex and herpes zoster keratitis), trigeminal palsy, topical medications, chemical burns, systemic diseases (diabetes mellitus, leprosy, Riley-day syndrome, Moebius syndrome) or iatrogenic causes (contact lens wear, refractive surgery, surgical ablation for neuralgia). Pure neuroparalytic keratitis is secondary to fifth nerve palsy and may occur secondary to damage of the trigeminal nucleus, root, ganglion or any segment of the ophthalmic branch of the fifth nerve.

CASE 8.1

CLINICAL FEATURES

A 35-year-old female presented with redness, watering, foreign body sensation and blurring of vision in the right eye for the past three weeks. The patient gave a history of three similar episodes in the past year and was diagnosed and managed as a case of recurrent herpes simplex virus (HSV) keratitis. On examination, corneal sensations were reduced in the right eye; vision was 6/60 and intraocular pressure was within normal limits. Examination findings and slit lamp appearance are illustrated in Figure 8.1.

KEY POINTS

Diagnosis:
- The above clinical scenario describes a case of post-herpes simplex neurotrophic keratitis.

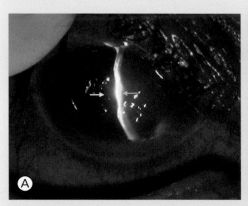
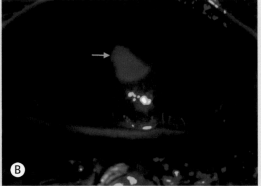

Figure 8.1 Slit lamp photograph of a patient with neurotrophic ulcer in herpes simplex keratitis showing (A) central 2×2 mm punched-out epithelial defect in the central cornea (white arrow) with corneal thinning (green arrow) and surrounding oedema on slit illumination along with conjunctival congestion. A cobalt blue filter with fluorescein stain (B) enhances the epithelial defect as a green defect (grey arrow) and demonstrates the sharp borders of the defect.

Investigations:

- The diagnosis was made primarily on the basis of clinical history and examination findings.
- Corneal scrapings from the edges of the neurotrophic ulcer or the tear fluid can be assessed by indirect immunofluorescent assay via amplification through polymerase chain reaction for detecting HSV.
- It is important to rule out the underlying cause through appropriate investigations for proper management (herpes simplex, herpes zoster, diabetes or stroke).

Treatment:

- The patient was managed with topical lubricants (preservative-free carboxymethylcellulose 1% every two hours), prophylactic topical antibiotic (chloramphenicol 0.5% three times a day) and nighttime taping of lids after instilling lubricating ointment.
- Acyclovir ointment was discontinued as it inhibits re-epithelialisation, especially when given for prolonged periods; similarly, any possible epitheliotoxic medication should be stopped on a case-to-case basis.

Outcome:

- The epithelial defect healed with a nebular corneal opacity in the area of epithelial defect in about three weeks and the best-corrected visual acuity improved to 6/9.

Supplementary Information and Additional Tips

- Oral doxycycline and ascorbate (vitamin C) may also be prescribed as required.
- It is important to note that persistent epithelial defects are common in patients undergoing penetrating keratoplasty for healed herpetic keratitis due to reduced tear film and neurotrophic deficiencies.
- Herpes zoster virus is known to cause more segmental hypoesthesia than HSV (Figure 8.2) and can promote classic neurotrophic lesions, which can even occur without viral epithelial infection.
- Bandage contact lens application after surgery may be considered in most patients; adjunctive therapies like autologous serum eye drops and surgical procedures, such as tarsorrhaphy and amniotic membrane transplantation, may also be necessary in some cases (Figure 8.3).
- The amniotic membrane provides mechanical protection to the epithelial surface and exhibits anti-inflammatory, anti-scarring and pro-regenerative properties.

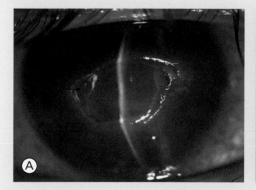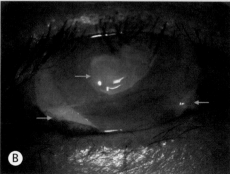

Figure 8.2 Slit lamp photograph of a patient with post-herpes zoster neurotrophic keratitis showing (A) central ulcer with punched-out epithelial defect (black arrow) with surrounding thickened and rolled edges (grey arrow) consisting of unhealthy and heaped-up epithelium. The patient underwent multilayered amniotic membrane grafting (B), with one layer filling up the defect (yellow arrow) and the other acting as an overlying patch sutured with 8,0 vicryl (green arrows).

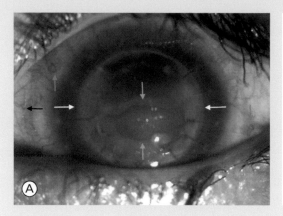 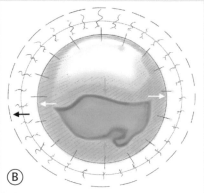

Figure 8.3 Clinical photograph (A) and corresponding corneal diagram (B) of a 4-year-old child with persistent epithelial defect who underwent penetrating keratoplasty for healed viral keratitis; note the punched-out epithelial defect with rolled and thickened edges in the central part of the cornea (yellow arrows) and the surrounding unhealthy epithelium and corneal haze. The graft-host junction (white arrows), remnant vicryl sutures (grey arrows) from previously performed amniotic membrane transplantation and a bandage contact lens in situ (black arrow) can also be appreciated.

- Amniotic membrane transplantation techniques include inlay or graft technique (one or more layers of amniotic membrane are cut to the defect size and placed in the ulcer bed), overlay or patch technique (oversized amniotic membrane covers the entire cornea and limbus area) and the sandwich technique (combination of both inlay and overlay technique).

CASE 8.2

CLINICAL FEATURES

A 30-year-old female presented with a four-week history of blurring of vision in her right eye. She was a known case of acoustic neuroma and had undergone surgery for the same. On examination, visual acuity in the right eye was 6/60 with a normal intraocular pressure. A mild lagophthalmos, probably due to facial nerve involvement, was also noted; however, there was a good Bell's response with no corneal exposure. The examination findings and clinical appearance are illustrated in Figure 8.4.

KEY POINTS

Diagnosis:
- The above clinical scenario describes a case of neuroparalytic keratitis in a patient with trigeminal palsy secondary to acoustic neuroma and/or surgery.

Investigations:
- Corneal sensations as measured by Cochet-Bonnet esthesiometer and reflex tearing (Schirmer I) were markedly reduced.

Treatment:
- The patient was managed with hourly preservative-free lubricants along with a prophylactic topical antibiotic.
- In addition, oral doxycycline 100 mg BD and vitamin A and carbomer gel at bedtime followed by lid taping were advised.
- As the corneal sensations were markedly reduced, a temporary para-median tarsorrhaphy was performed to promoted healing and reduce the risk of subsequent stromal lysis and ulceration.

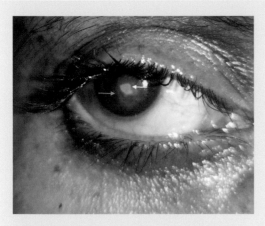

Figure 8.4 Clinical photograph of neuroparalytic keratitis in a patient with trigeminal palsy secondary to acoustic neuroma showing fluorescein-stained epithelial defect (white arrow) with surrounding scarring (yellow arrow). Note that there is no significant congestion and the patient is comfortably opening the eyes indicating reduced ocular surface sensations.

Outcome:

- The epithelial defect healed with formation of a nebulo-macular corneal opacity in about three weeks and the best-corrected visual acuity improved to 6/12.
- Tarsorrhaphy was removed at four weeks and patient was advised to continue life-long lubricants and regular follow-up.

Supplementary Information and Additional Tips

- In this case, the diagnosis was quite straightforward as the patient was already diagnosed with acoustic neuroma; however, it is important to rule out any other cause for fifth nerve palsy in cases with corneal anaesthesia or marked hypoesthesia.
- A meticulous examination for other cranial nerves is also warranted as the presence of other neurologic deficits may help to localise the pathology.

CASE 8.3

CLINICAL FEATURES

A 55-year-old diabetic male presented with complaints of redness, discharge and painful diminution of vision in the left eye for the past two months. He was diagnosed as a case of polymicrobial keratitis and was being treated with fortified antibiotics and antifungals, cycloplegic drops and topical antiglaucoma (timolol 0.5%) for the same. Although a good response was noted in the first one month of treatment, the patient stopped showing signs of improvement thereafter, and was referred to us as a case of non-resolving ulcer. On examination, the vision in the left eye was 1/60 and intraocular pressure was 28 mm Hg; corneal sensations were also reduced. The examination findings and slit lamp appearance are illustrated in Figure 8.5.

KEY POINTS

Diagnosis:

- The above clinical scenario describes a case of a healing polymicrobial keratitis with neurotrophic ulcer in a diabetic patient.

Investigations:

- The diagnosis was based on past clinical records, history and examination findings.
- Corneal scraping for microbiological diagnosis was not needed in this case but may be performed as needed. B-scan ultrasound revealed a normal posterior segment.
- The patient's diabetic status was assessed by fasting and post-prandial blood sugar levels and serum HbA1c, all of which were deranged.

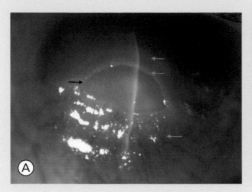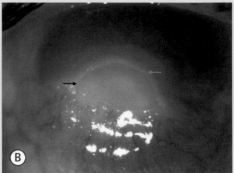

Figure 8.5 Slit lamp photograph showing (A) healing polymicrobial keratitis with neurotrophic ulcer in a diabetic patient; note the punched-out epithelial defect (black arrow) with thickened and rolled edges (grey arrow); surrounding stromal scarring (green arrow) and superficial vascularisation (yellow arrow) indicative of a healing response. Fluorescein staining (B) enhances the epithelial defect (black arrow) and heaped-up epithelium (grey arrow) which are characteristic of neurotrophic keratitis.

Treatment:

- The existing treatment for the patient was modified: fortified antibiotics (cefazolin 5% and tobramycin 1.3%) were replaced with topical fluoroquinolone (gatifloxacin 0.5% every four hours), topical antiglaucoma (timolol maleate) was stopped and oral acetazolamide was prescribed instead.
- Antifungal drops (natamycin 5%) were also reduced in frequency from every two hours to every four hours for a week, followed by every six hours.
- Preservative-free artificial tear drops along with a nighttime lubricating ointment, oral doxycycline (100 mg twice a day) and vitamin C (500 mg BD) were also added to the treatment regimen.
- The patient was also referred to an endocrinologist for adequate management of his diabetes.

Outcome:

- The ulcer healed slowly in about five weeks, leaving behind a residual leucomatous corneal opacity with a best-corrected visual acuity of 6/36.

Supplementary Information and Additional Tips

- Prolonged use of topical antimicrobial drugs can hamper epithelial healing, and therefore, it is important to

titrate the treatment with the clinical response.
- Compaction of infiltrates, development of surrounding corneal scarring and vascularisation, as seen in this case, are signs of healing and the antimicrobial drugs should be tapered accordingly.
- If a neurotrophic ulcer is present without any signs of active infective keratitis (Figure 8.6), withdrawal of all antimicrobial drugs for 24–48 hours cases may be considered to help in confirmation of diagnosis and aid further management.

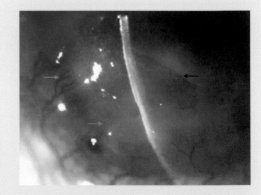

Figure 8.6 Slit lamp photograph showing a case with healed bacterial keratitis with a neurotrophic ulcer showing punched-out epithelial defect (black arrow) with surrounding stromal scarring (grey arrow) and superficial vascularisation (yellow arrow).

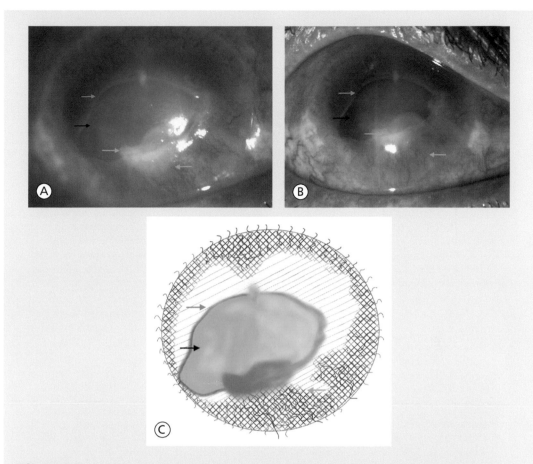

Figure 8.7 Slit lamp photographs (A, B) and corresponding corneal diagram (C) of a patient with rheumatoid arthritis and recurrent sclero-kerato-uveitis demonstrating a large neurotrophic ulcer, which can be visualised clearly, with or without fluorescein stain. The distinct punched-out margins (grey arrow) of the epithelial defect (black arrow) along with heaped-up unhealthy epithelium at the edges, more prominent inferiorly (yellow arrow) and superficial vascularisation (green arrow) are evident.

- Before initiating treatment, a gentle mechanical debridement of the heaped-up loose epithelium (Figure 8.7) can be performed with a cotton swab to promote early healing and smooth centripetal migration of epithelial cells.

CASE 8.4

CLINICAL FEATURES

A 70-year-old male presented with complaints of blurring of vision along with mild redness and pain in his left eye for the past three weeks. The symptoms had increased markedly in the past week. The patient was a known case of primary open-angle glaucoma and intraocular pressure was controlled with three topical medications (timolol maleate 0.5%, brimonidine tartrate 0.2% and latanoprost 0.005%) in both eyes. He had undergone uneventful cataract surgery in both eyes around six months back. The examination findings and slit lamp appearance are illustrated in Figure 8.8.

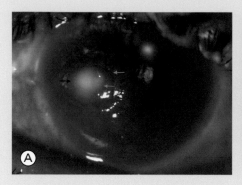 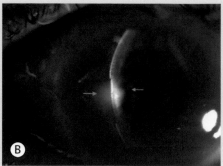

Figure 8.8 Slit lamp photograph of a patient demonstrating neurotrophic keratitis with secondary fungal infection (A); note the punched-out epithelial defect (black arrow) in the paracentral cornea with surrounding thickened and rolled edges (green arrow) and localised white fuzzy stromal infiltrates (grey arrow). Parallelepiped section showing (B) epithelial deep stromal infiltrates (grey arrow) with heaped-up epithelium at the edges of the ulcer (green arrow).

KEY POINTS

Diagnosis:
- The above clinical scenario highlights a case of neurotrophic ulcer with secondary fungal keratitis in a patient with primary open-angle glaucoma.

Investigations:
- The diagnosis was established by classical features of neurotrophic ulcer (clean, well-demarcated, punched-out epithelial defect) along with white fuzzy infiltrates and confirmed by the growth of *Candida albicans* on fungal culture.
- Anterior segment optical coherence tomography revealed focal corneal oedema with Descemet's membrane undulations with an anterior paracentral excavation at the site of the ulcer.

Treatment:
- The patient was treated with topical amphotericin-B (0.15%), initiated as an hourly loading dose for the first 24 hours and every two hours for next 48 hours followed by every four hour frequency.
- A prophylactic topical antibiotic (moxifloxacin hydrochloride 0.5% four times a day), cycloplegic (homatropine hydrobromide 2% three times a day) and lubricants (preservative-free carboxymethylcellulose 0.5% six times a day) were also prescribed.

- Antiglaucoma medications were altered: preservative-free timolol maleate 0.5% was prescribed along with sustained-release oral acetazolamide (500 mg BD) and brimonidine and latanoprost eye drops were temporarily discontinued.
- Oral fluconazole (150 mg BD) and vitamin C were also added to the regimen after one week of initiating treatment.

Outcome:
- The neurotrophic ulcer along with the secondary fungal infection healed completely in about six weeks leaving behind a residual macular corneal opacity.

Supplementary Information and Additional Tips

- Chronic use of topical medications containing preservatives (like benzalkonium chloride) may reduce corneal sensation via nerve damage and affect corneal epithelial healing.
- Increasing age is another risk factor for development of both neurotrophic and fungal keratitis.
- Patients with long-standing pseudophakic corneal decompensation are also at risk of developing neurotrophic keratitis (Figure 8.9); poor ocular surface, recurrent epithelial breakdown and chronic use of topical medications may contribute to the same.

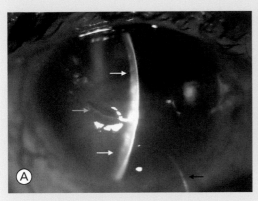
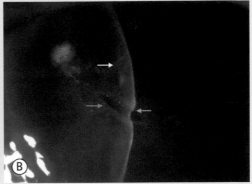

Figure 8.9 Slit lamp photograph showing a small linear neurotrophic ulcer (green arrow) in a patient with long-standing pseudophakic corneal decompensation (A); note the diffuse corneal oedema (white arrows) evident by increased corneal thickness, stromal haze and scarring and Descemet's folds and a single trichiatic cilia (black arrow) that possibly contributed to the epithelial breakdown. Magnified image (B) with parallelepiped clearly reveals the punched-out defect with loss of stromal tissue (yellow arrow) and the unhealthy epithelium at the edge of the defect (grey arrow).

CASE 8.5

A 56-year-old male presented with complaints of redness, watering, foreign body sensation and blurring of vision in the right eye for the past week. He had undergone right eye pars plana vitrectomy with endolaser treatment and silicone oil tamponade for rhegmatogenous retinal detachment six weeks back. On examination, the vision in right eye was 2/60 with a normal intraocular pressure and reduced corneal sensations. The examination findings and slit lamp appearance are illustrated in Figure 8.10.

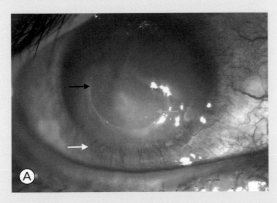
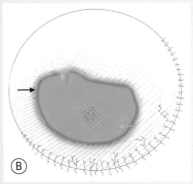

Figure 8.10 Slit lamp photograph (A) and corresponding corneal diagram (B) of a patient showing neurotrophic ulceration after retinal detachment surgery and endolaser treatment that resulted in a punched-out epithelial defect with thickened and rolled edges (black arrow); note the unhealthy appearance of the cornea with stromal oedema and haze (yellow arrow) and superficial vascularisation (white arrow).

KEY POINTS

Diagnosis:

- The above clinical scenario describes a case of iatrogenic neurotrophic ulceration after retinal detachment surgery with endolaser.

Investigations:

- The diagnosis was made primarily on the basis of clinical history and examination findings; a B-scan ultrasound was performed to assess the posterior segment, which was within normal limits.

Treatment:

- The patient's ongoing postoperative treatment was modified by withdrawal of topical steroids, stepping up of preservative-free topical lubricants and continuation of antibiotic eye drops.
- Additionally, vitamin A with carbomer ointment (twice a day) and oral vitamin C were advised.

Outcome:

- The defect healed with mild stromal thinning and scarring over a period of three weeks.

Supplementary Information and Additional Tips

- Heavy confluent retinal laser treatment should be avoided at 3- and 9 o'clock positions in order to prevent long ciliary nerve damage.
- Early recognition and prompt treatment of iatrogenic neurotrophic keratitis is important to minimise the risk for subsequent ulceration and visual loss.
- Cenegermin (Oxervate™), a recombinant human nerve growth factor (rhNGF), is the first approved topical medication for neurotrophic keratitis and may be prescribed in moderate-to-severe cases.[3]

REFERENCES

1. Chang BH, Groos Jr EB. Chapter 87. Neurotrophic keratitis. In: Cornea; Volume 1 – Fundamentals, Diagnosis and Management. 4th ed. USA: Elsevier; 2017; 1035–1042.
2. Weisenthal RW, Daly MK, Freitas D, Feder RS, Orlin SE, Tu EY et al. Structural and exogenous conditions associated with ocular surface disorders. In: Cantor LB, editor. American Academy of Ophthalmology: External Disease and Cornea, 2018–19. USA: American Academy of Ophthalmology/Elsevier. pp. 65–73.
3. Bonini S, Lambiase A, Rama P, Sinigaglia F, Allegretti M, Chao W, et al. Phase II Randomized, Double-Masked, Vehicle-Controlled Trial of Recombinant Human Nerve Growth Factor for Neurotrophic Keratitis. Ophthalmology. 2018 Sep. 125(9):1332–1343.

9 Vernal Keratoconjunctivitis

Ritika Mukhija, T Monikha, Suresh Azimeera, Noopur Gupta

INTRODUCTION

Vernal keratoconjunctivitis (VKC) is a recurrent allergic inflammatory bilateral disease that affects patients primarily in the first and second decades of life. It is more common in warm, dry climates and tropical regions and affects males more often than females. Environmental risk factors include exposure to dust, pollen, smoke and ultraviolet radiation in addition to a systemic allergic predisposition. It is classified as palpebral VKC, limbal VKC and mixed VKC depending on the morphological features and the area of involvement.[1] The diagnosis is essentially clinical and investigations are not routinely indicated. VKC is an important cause of ocular morbidity in young patients, resulting mainly from corneal manifestations, cataract and glaucoma; the last two occur as a result of long-term, inadvertent use of topical steroids prescribed for allergic symptoms.[2] This chapter aims to provide a brief overview of the ocular surface and corneal manifestations arising due to the inflammatory and allergic component of VKC.[3]

CASE 9.1

CLINICAL FEATURES

A 14-year-old male presented with symptoms of itching, foreign body sensation and mild diminution of vision in both eyes for the past three months with the development of photophobia and pain since the past two days in the left eye. He gave a history of similar episodes of itching, profuse watering and redness for the past four years, for which he took intermittent therapy from multiple local practitioners. He did not give any history of other ocular or systemic complaints. The examination findings and slit lamp appearance are illustrated in Figure 9.1. Visual acuity of the child at presentation was 6/24 and was recorded with difficulty as the child could not open his eyes comfortably.

KEY POINTS

Diagnosis:
- The above clinical scenario describes a case of palpebral VKC with multiple giant papillae, imparting a typical cobblestone appearance to the upper

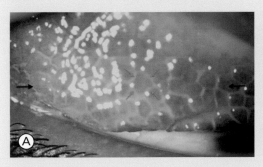
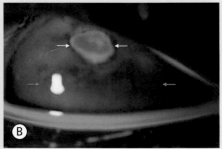

Figure 9.1 Slit lamp photograph of a child with vernal keratoconjunctivitis revealing multiple, diffuse giant papillae (papillae more than 1 mm in size) and intense conjunctival congestion (A) on upper lid eversion (black arrows). The tarsal conjunctiva shows flat-topped, discrete papillae that are clearly delineated and the margins of a single papilla are highlighted by fluorescein stain (grey arrows). Slit lamp examination of the cornea (B) in the child reveals a shield ulcer in the upper half of the cornea (white arrows), the hazy margins of which reveal signs of inflammation and staining of the ulcer bed with fluorescein is evident when examined under cobalt blue filter. Corneal xerosis is noted with the appearance of diffuse punctate keratopathy (grey arrows).

lid. The papillae are well demarcated and flat topped and usually consist of hyperplastic conjunctival epithelium with a fibrovascular core and the presence of inflammatory cells like eosinophils, mast cells and neutrophils on histopathological examination.

■ Shield ulcer is an inflammatory ulcer which may get secondarily infected but usually results due to mechanical abrasion by the papillary outgrowths of the upper lid in severe cases of VKC. The chemical mediators released by eosinophils such as eosinophilic granule major basic protein, among others, are known to be cytotoxic and inhibit healing of the shield ulcer, which worsens if not treated in time.

Investigations:

■ The diagnosis is usually straightforward and based on clinical features; however, upper lid eversion and high clinical suspicion are paramount for prompt and effective management of these cases.

Treatment:

■ The patient was treated with topical antihistamine/mast cell stabilisers (olopatadine hydrochloride 0.1% twice a day), topical antibiotic (moxifloxacin hydrochloride 0.5% four times a day), cycloplegic (homatropine hydrobromide 2% twice a day) and lubricants (preservative-free carboxymethylcellulose 0.5% six times a day). Antibiotic ointment was prescribed at night.

■ In addition, a short tapering course of low-potency topical steroids (topical fluorometholone 0.1%) was also given as the ulcer is caused as a result of inflammation.

■ Intermittent patching to aid in epithelial healing, debridement in case of plaque formation, use of a bandage contact lens and an amniotic membrane graft in chronic severe cases may also be useful.

Outcome:

■ The lesion responded to treatment and healed without a scar in around ten days.

■ Long-term anti-allergic therapy, allergen avoidance, if any, cold compresses and ocular support in the form of lubricants were continued.

■ Cycloplegic refraction was performed in this case after complete healing of the ulcer and the patient improved to 6/6 with refractive correction.

Supplementary Information and Additional Tips

■ Corneal changes present as punctate epithelial erosions in the initial stage which progress to coarse epitheliopathy and macroerosions if not treated promptly and contribute to formation of a shield ulcer.

CASE 9.2

CLINICAL FEATURES

A 10-year-old male presented with symptoms of intense itching, mild redness, watering and history of ropy discharge in the morning for the past month. He did not report any similar episodes in the past. He did not give any history of other ocular or systemic complaints. The examination findings and slit lamp appearance are illustrated in Figure 9.2. Visual acuity of the child at presentation was 6/9.

KEY POINTS

Diagnosis:

■ The above clinical scenario describes a case of a mixed variety of VKC with diffuse papillary conjunctivitis of the upper tarsal conjunctiva with limbal involvement seen in the form of gelatinous, elevated, globular limbal papillae arranged in a concentric fashion at the upper limbus.

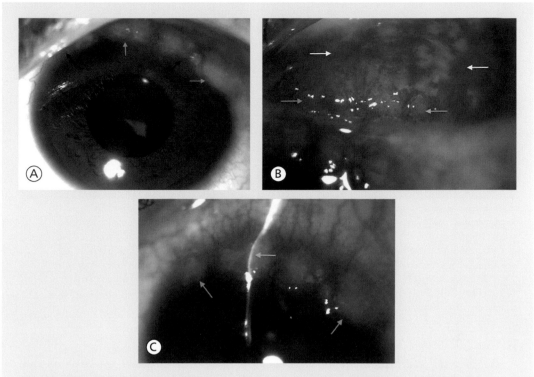

Figure 9.2 Slit lamp examination showing a case of VKC with mixed presentation, so that both the upper tarsal conjunctiva and limbus are involved in the disease process. Gelatinous, globular limbal papillae (grey arrows) with fuzzy margins (A) and active inflammation with intervening superficial vascularisation (black arrows) are seen on the upper limbal area. Superficial perilimbal vascularisation is evident in all clock hours. The palpebral component of VKC (B) is evident by the intense conjunctival injection and diffuse velvety papillary hypertrophy (white arrows) along with few distinguishable larger-sized papillae (green arrows) in the upper tarsal conjunctiva. A magnified slit-illumination view (C) of the upper limbus in the child revealed raised limbal papillae (yellow arrow), profuse peripheral vascularisation (black arrow) and multiple upper limbal nodules (grey arrows) due to active VKC.

- The presence of conjunctival hyperaemia is a sign of clinical activity.

Investigations:
- The diagnosis is based on clinical features; however, if the papillae are excised, histopathology of excised tissue and the tear fluid analysis in active cases reveals eosinophils and inflammatory cytokines in the acute stage.

Treatment:
- The patient was treated with topical and systemic antihistamine/mast cell stabilisers (olopatadine hydrochloride 0.1% twice a day), and lubricants (preservative-free carboxymethylcellulose 0.5% six times a day). Cold compresses were advised twice a day and the child was categorically advised not to rub their eyes to reduce the risk of developing secondary corneal ectasia.
- The lesions usually respond to treatment; if, however, a partial response is noted with anti-allergic and palliative therapy, a short course of low-potency topical steroids (topical fluorometholone 0.1%) may be prescribed for early resolution of acute signs.

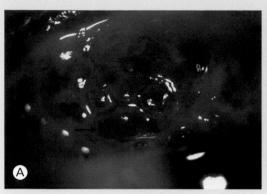
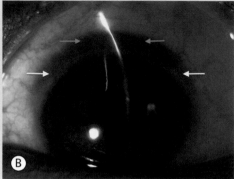

Figure 9.3 Slit lamp photograph of a case with long-standing VKC (A) that revealed giant papillae with characteristic pigmentary changes in the upper tarsal conjunctiva (black arrow) noted on lid eversion. In the same patient, an upper paralimbal band of superficial scarring, seen (B) as a greyish-white lipid deposition commonly known as pseudogerontoxon (white arrows) was evident on slit lamp examination as a result of recurrent limbal disease. Also note the dense brown upper limbal pigmentation (green arrows) from 10 to 2 o'clock.

Outcome:

- The acute stage usually responds to anti-allergic and topical steroid therapy. The treating ophthalmologist needs to ensure strict follow up and compliance to therapy to reduce recurrences and monitor for long-term complications of steroid therapy like cataract and glaucoma and should also assess corneal topography at regular intervals to pick up any subtle signs of keratoconus.
- Long-term anti-allergic therapy, allergen avoidance, if any, cold compresses and ocular support in the form of lubricants were continued.

a size of 6 mm or more, in which case, they may need to be excised and amniotic membrane grafting may be required to cover the raw surface of the upper tarsal conjunctiva after excision.

- Alternatively, supratarsal triamcinolone acetonide injection may also be administered in cases at low risk of developing steroid-induced glaucoma.

Supplementary Information and Additional Tips

- The hallmark of VKC is papillary hyperplasia that predominantly involves the upper tarsus and limbus, as was seen this case. Clinically, papillae are variable in size from 0.1 to 5 mm and may become pigmented in certain cases (Figure 9.3).
- With long-standing, severe VKC, the papillae may become enlarged and pendulous (Figure 9.4), even assuming

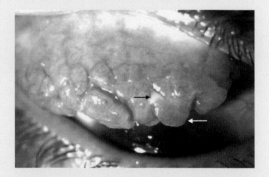

Figure 9.4 Slit lamp photograph of a patient with chronic palpebral VKC showing multiple, pendulous, giant papillae on the upper tarsal conjunctiva. Note the mucous discharge (black arrow) plugged between the grooves of the large overhanging papillae (white arrow).

CASE 9.3

CLINICAL FEATURES

A 13-year-old female living in rural North India presented with recurrent symptoms of mild itching, redness and watering for the past two years. The acute red eye was associated with systemic symptoms of rhinorrhea, mild fever and excessive sneezing. Her daily routine involved spending most of the time outdoors in the sun with her parents, who were farmers by profession. There was no other history of other ocular or systemic disease. The examination findings and slit lamp appearance are illustrated in Figure 9.5. Visual acuity at presentation was 6/9.

KEY POINTS

Diagnosis:
- The above clinical scenario describes a case of mild to moderate VKC with perilimbal pigmentation and the presence of conjunctival hyperaemia and papillary conjunctivitis. The presence of risk factors such as exposure to a dusty and dry tropical climate along with systemic allergic features clinches the diagnosis in these cases.

Treatment:
- The patient was treated with topical and systemic antihistamine/ mast cell stabilisers (olopatadine hydrochloride 0.1% twice a day), and lubricants (preservative-free carboxymethylcellulose 0.5% six times a day). Cold compresses were advised twice a day.
- Paediatric consultation for systemic control of allergy is essential to control the recurrences and avoidance of ultraviolet exposure helps markedly in all such presentations of VKC.

Outcome:
- The acute stage usually responds to anti-allergic and topical steroid therapy.
- Long-term anti-allergic therapy, allergen avoidance, if any, cold compresses and ocular support in the form of lubricants were continued.

Supplementary Information and Additional Tips

- Paediatric consultation and reducing exposure to exacerbating factors improve outcomes by reducing long-term morbidity and recurrence rates.

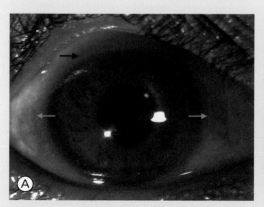 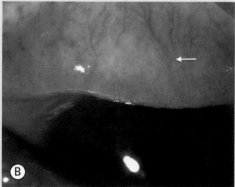

Figure 9.5 Slit lamp examination of a patient with VKC (A) presenting with muddy discoloration (A) of the conjunctiva (grey arrows) and superficial vascularisation (black arrows). On upper lid eversion (B), inflamed and boggy conjunctiva with diffuse hyperaemia and hypertrophy (white arrow) in the upper tarsal conjunctiva were seen.

CASE 9.4

CLINICAL FEATURES

A 28-year-old male patient presented with symptoms of itching, burning, redness and watering for the past two years. There was no other history of other ocular or systemic disease. The examination findings and slit lamp appearance are illustrated in Figure 9.6. Best corrected visual acuity at presentation was 6/6 and he had suffered from compound myopic astigmatism for the past 14 years.

KEY POINTS

Diagnosis:
- The above clinical scenario describes a case of limbal VKC with active limbitis, peripheral corneal vascularisation and inflammation with asymmetric involvement in the two eyes.

Treatment:
- The patient was treated with topical and systemic antihistamine/mast cell stabilisers (bepotastine besilate 1.5% once a day), topical tacrolimus 0.03% ointment twice daily and lubricants (preservative-free carboxymethylcellulose 0.5% six times a day). Cold compresses were advised twice a day.

Outcome:
- The acute stage usually responds to anti-allergic and topical steroid therapy.

Supplementary Information and Additional Tip

- Limbal VKC is characterised by the presence of gelatinous confluent limbal papillae as seen in this patient.
- The use of immunomodulators like cyclosporine and tacrolimus has been found to be safe and well tolerated for the treatment of severe allergic conjunctivitis, especially in long-standing chronic cases due to their steroid-sparing advantage.
- Chronic cases may progress to intense peripheral corneal neovascularisation, corneal scarring (Figure 9.7), irregular astigmatism and visual impairment. Limbal stem cell deficiency (LSCD) is known to be associated with prolonged VKC. The various factors responsible for damage to the limbal stem cells include chronic limbal inflammation, change in the microenvironment of limbal stem cell niche and cytotoxic damage by eosinophils and other inflammatory chemokines.

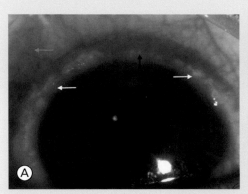
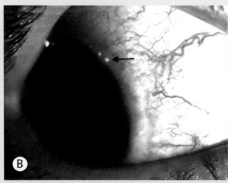

Figure 9.6 Slit lamp examination of a patient with a limbal form of VKC (A) demonstrating diffuse limbal conjunctival papillae (white arrows) along with a few Horner-Trantas dots (black arrow). Note the diffuse congestion of the bulbar conjunctiva (grey arrow) denoting activity of the disease. The limbal papillae are topped with chalky white excrescences made of eosinophils and epithelial cells, commonly called Horner-Trantas spots (black arrow), are more prominent (B) in the other eye of the patient showing relatively lesser limbal inflammation.

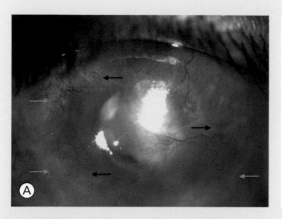 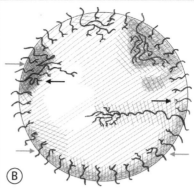

Figure 9.7 Slit lamp photograph of a patient with severe chronic VKC and long-term sequalae is shown. Limbal stem cell deficiency (LSCD) in the form of conjunctivalisation of the cornea (A) due to chronic inflammatory processes in VKC with evidence of diffuse superficial corneal vessels (black arrows) and scarring of corneal layers with loss of corneal transparency (grey arrows) is evident. There is a loss of limbal stem cells (Palisades of Vogt) as a result of severe recurrent episodes of inflammation. The corresponding schematic representation (B) of the eye with LSCD is depicted.

CASE 9.5

CLINICAL FEATURES

A 33-year-old male patient presented with mild itching and significant foreign body sensation and decreased vision for the past six months. He gave a history of similar episodes of itching, profuse watering and redness in childhood which resolved when he was 24 years old. He remained symptom free for nearly a decade with only mild episodes of intermittent itching on using computers or doing excessive near work. There was no other history of other ocular or systemic disease. The examination findings and slit lamp appearance are illustrated in Figure 9.8. Visual acuity at presentation was 6/18 in right eye and 6/24 in left eye.

KEY POINTS

Diagnosis:
- The above clinical scenario describes a case of chronic VKC and allergic conjunctivitis with superior pannus and development of secondary Salzmann nodular degeneration (SND).

Treatment:
- The patient was treated with topical and systemic antihistamine/mast cell stabilisers (olopatadine hydrochloride 0.1% twice a day), and lubricants (preservative-free carboxymethylcellulose 0.5% six times a day). Cold compresses were advised twice a day.

Outcome:
- Refractive correction led to an improvement of visual acuity to 6/9 bilaterally. Contact lenses are not recommended due to ongoing allergic conjunctivitis.
- The likelihood of developing SND in a patient of VKC is low. Refractive correction due to the induced astigmatism with control of allergy and ocular surface xerosis helps in most cases. Superficial keratectomy may be planned in advanced cases for visual rehabilitation or for symptomatic improvement in cases with significant foreign body sensation due to the elevated nodules.

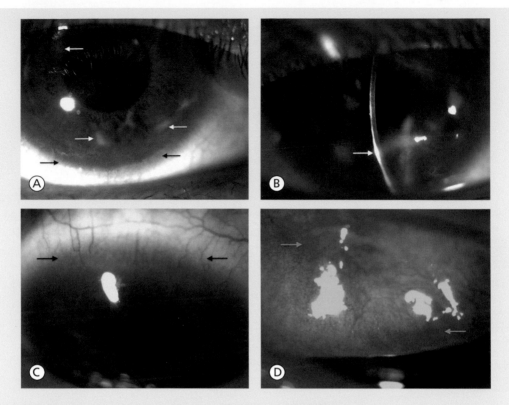

Figure 9.8 Slit lamp photograph of a patient of chronic VKC with secondary Salzman nodular degeneration. The characteristic grey-white superficial raised nodules (A) are seen in the mid-periphery and peripheral cornea (white arrows) along with diffuse superficial limbal vascularisation (black arrows). Slit-illumination view of the other eye (B) of same patient with similar nodules (white arrow) and loss of corneal transparency is evident. Superior limbus (C) shows diffuse superficial limbal vascularisation (black arrows) and eversion of the upper lid (D) reveals diffuse hyperaemia and inflamed conjunctiva (grey arrows) due to chronic allergy in VKC.

Supplementary Information and Additional Tips

■ SND in VKC results due to poor ocular surface due to induced dry eye in cases with chronic allergic conjunctivitis and chronic irritation or mechanical disruption of the epithelial-stromal barrier during rubbing in acute exacerbation of the allergy.

CASE 9.6

CLINICAL FEATURES

A 17-year-old male presented with photophobia, pain, profuse watering and inability to open eyes since the past week. He gave a history of episodes of itching, watering and redness for the past four years, for which he took treatment but was not compliant as the symptoms were recurrent. He did not give any history of other ocular or systemic complaints. The examination findings and slit lamp appearance are illustrated in Figure 9.9. Visual acuity of the patient at presentation was 6/18 in the right eye and 6/9 in the left eye.

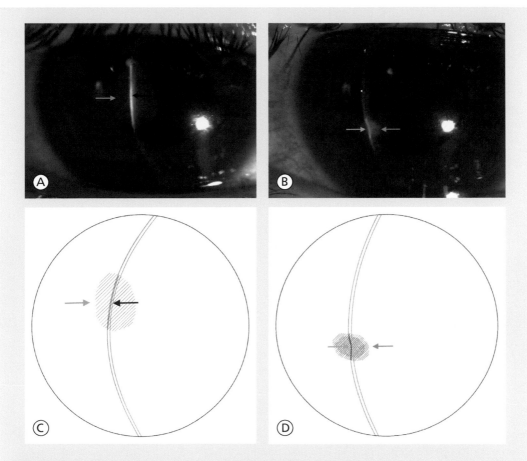

Figure 9.9 Slit lamp photographs of bilateral healing shield ulcers (grey arrow) occurring as a result of corneal involvement in a case of VKC. Superficial corneal scarring (black arrow) in the right eye (A) is evident in the pupillary area. The left eye (B) reveals significant stromal thinning (yellow arrow) with dense scar formation (grey arrow) following resolution of the shield ulcer. The corresponding schematic pictures of the right (C) and left eyes (D) demonstrate the key findings of the healing shield ulcers in the two eyes.

KEY POINTS

Diagnosis:

- The above clinical scenario describes a case of bilateral shield ulcers occurring as a result of corneal involvement in case of VKC.

Investigations:

- The diagnosis is usually straightforward and based on clinical features; however, upper lid eversion and high clinical suspicion are paramount for prompt and effective management of these cases.

Treatment:

- The patient was treated with topical antihistamine/mast cell stabilisers (olopatadine hydrochloride 0.1% twice a day), topical antibiotic (moxifloxacin hydrochloride 0.5% four times a day), cycloplegic (homatropine hydrobromide 2% twice a day) and lubricants (preservative-free carboxymethylcellulose 0.5% six times a day). Vitamin A ointment was prescribed at night.
- In addition, a short tapering course of low-potency topical steroids (topical fluorometholone 0.1%) was also given as the ulcer was caused as a result of inflammation.

Outcome:

- The lesion responded to treatment and healed with a scar in around two weeks. Dense corneal scarring with stromal thinning was evident after the ulcer resolved with treatment.

- Long-term anti-allergic therapy, allergen avoidance, if any, cold compresses and ocular support in the form of lubricants were continued.
- Cycloplegic refraction was performed in this case after complete healing of the ulcer and the patient improved to 6/6 with refractive correction.

Supplementary Information and Additional Tips

- In certain cases, dense plaque formation with neovascularisation may occur in the acute stage due to deposition of fibrin and mucous over the ulcer (Figure 9.10) that inhibits corneal re-epithelialisation. This may need surgical removal/peeling along with the placement of an amniotic patch graft secured with sutures or fibrin glue to promote healing.

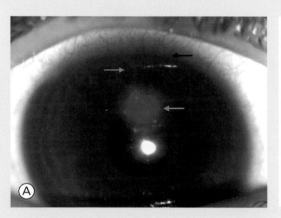
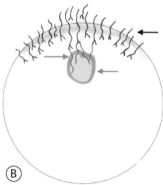

Figure 9.10 Slit lamp photograph of a patient with chronic VKC and a long-standing shield ulcer (A) reveals deposition of fibrin and mucous over the ulcer in the form of a plaque (grey arrow) that inhibits corneal re-epithelialisation and promotes corneal neovascularisation (green arrow). Superior limbal vascularisation (black arrow) and vessels invading the cornea to reach the area of the ulcer suggest the chronicity of the disease. The corresponding schematic diagram of the clinical picture is also depicted (B).

REFERENCES

1. Singhal D, Sahay P, Maharana PK, Raj N, Sharma N, Titiyal JS. Vernal Keratoconjunctivitis. Surv Ophthalmol. 2019; 64(3):289–311.
2. Mantelli F, Santos MS, Petitti T, et al. Systematic review and meta-analysis of randomised clinical trials on topical treatments for vernal keratoconjunctivitis. Br J Ophthalmol. 2007; 91(12):1656–61.
3. Barney NP. Chapter 47. Vernal and Atopic Keratoconjunctivitis. In: Cornea; Volume 1 – Fundamentals, Diagnosis and Management. 4th ed. USA: Elsevier; 533–42.

10 Ocular Surface Disorders

Rashmi Singh, Ritika Mukhija, Alisha Kishore, Noopur Gupta, M Vanathi

INTRODUCTION

The ocular surface is comprised of the cornea, conjunctiva, eyelids and the lacrimal glands. Any alteration in the delicate balance of these structures can result in ocular surface disease (OSD). OSD is a spectrum of conditions that occur due to the disruption in the external and internal milieu of the ocular surface and includes dry eye disease, blepharitis, meibomian gland dysfunction and may occur secondary to allergic eye disease, Stevens-Johnson syndrome (SJS) and chemical and thermal burns that result in limbal stem cell deficiency. OSD can affect vision, hamper the quality of life and can even cause blindness in severe cases.[1-4]

CASE 10.1

CLINICAL FEATURES

A 36-year-old female presented with complaints of watering, foreign body sensation and congestion in both eyes for the past month. The symptoms were more severe in the right eye. There was no history of trauma or contact lens wear and no known systemic illness. The vision in both eyes was 6/12 with normal intraocular pressure. Examination findings and slit lamp appearance are shown in Figure 10.1.

KEY POINTS

Diagnosis:
- The above clinical scenario is a case of bilateral severe dry eye with right eye filamentary keratitis.

Investigations:
- Ocular investigations for assessing severity of dry eye were performed.
- Tear film break-up time (TBUT) was instantaneous. Schirmer's test was 5 mm in the right eye and 8 mm in the left eye.

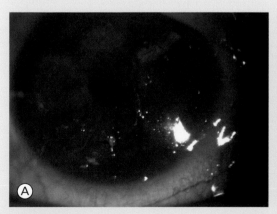
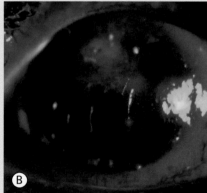

Figure 10.1 Slit lamp photograph of a patient with filamentary keratitis demonstrating (A) mild congestion, poor ocular surface, surface irregularity and corneal xerosis with several filaments (black arrow) which are degenerated epithelial cells surrounding a mucus core along with dry ocular surface. Fluorescein staining (B) enhances the filaments when examined under cobalt blue filter (black arrow). Note the poor surface wettability and irregular corneal surface due to non-uniform distribution of the tear film.

- Any underlying cause (keratoconjunctivitis sicca, excessive contact lens wear, corneal epithelial instability, bullous keratopathy and neurotrophic keratopathy) was ruled out.
- Systemic workup was done to rule out any autoimmune disorder.

Treatment:
- The patient was treated with copious, preservative-free lubricants (carboxy methylcellulose 1% every two hours and hydroxy propyl methylcellulose 0.3% gel three times a day).
- Topical N-acetyl cysteine 10% (mucolytic) was given four times a day for four weeks.
- A low potency steroid loteprednol etabonate 0.5% four times a day was given in tapering dose over the next three weeks.

Outcome:
- The symptoms resolved in two weeks and the visual acuity in both eyes improved to 6/6.
- Additionally, the patient was prescribed long-term application of topical lubricants and advised regular follow-up for the dry eye disease.

Supplementary Information and Additional Tips

- Occasionally, large filaments can be seen which do not respond to topical therapy. These may be removed using McPherson forceps on the slit lamp after instilling proparacaine 0.5% eyedrops to provide symptomatic relief (Figure 10.2).

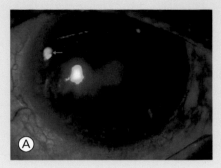

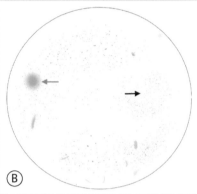

Figure 10.2 Slit lamp photograph revealing (A) instantaneous break-up of the tear film, filamentary keratitis, fine punctate staining (black arrow) with a large filament (grey arrow) when examined under cobalt blue filter after instilling fluorescein dye in the lower cul-de-sac. The corresponding diagram (B) highlights the same findings.

- Hypertonic saline (5% drops and 6% ointment) can also be given as it encourages the adhesion of loose epithelium. Bandage contact lens (BCL) may protect the cornea from the shearing action of the lids.

CASE 10.2

CLINICAL FEATURES

A 24-year-old female with a history of undergoing corneal refractive surgery one month prior presented with complaints of foreign body sensation, burning and itching in both eyes. On examination, the vision was 6/9 with normal intraocular pressure in both eyes. Examination findings and slit lamp appearance are illustrated in Figure 10.3.

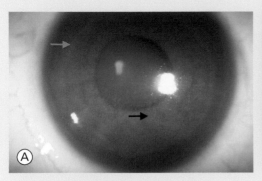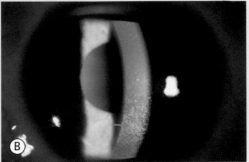

Figure 10.3 Slit lamp photograph showing (A) post-LASIK (laser in situ keratomileusis) dry eye disease in the form of punctate opacities (black arrow) and the LASIK flap (grey arrow) under diffuse illumination. Broad slit illumination (B) reveals multiple punctate opacities in the inferior part of the cornea (grey arrow) suggestive of corneal xerosis and dry eye disease.

KEY POINTS

Diagnosis:
- The above clinical scenario describes a case of post-LASIK (laser in situ keratomileusis) dry eye disease.

Investigations:
- Investigations for assessing ocular surface health were performed. TBUT was two seconds and Schirmer's test was 8 mm in both eyes.

Treatment:
- The patient was managed with frequent instillation of preservative-free lubricants (carboxy methylcellulose 1% every two hours and hydroxyl propyl methylcellulose 0.3% gel at nighttime).

- Further, advice on decreasing digital screen time was given.

Outcome:
- The symptoms decreased gradually over a month of using the medications and the vision improved to 6/6 in both eyes; thereafter, the patient was kept on lubricants to control dry eye disease.

Supplementary Information and Additional Tips

- It is important to look for compromised ocular surface in all patients undergoing refractive surgery. Dry eye may be aggravated following refractive surgery due to transection of corneal nerves during creation of the LASIK flap.

CASE 10.3

CLINICAL FEATURES

A 40-year-old female presented with complaints of foreign body sensation, irritation and watering for the past six months. The patient was a known case of thyroid carcinoma and had received radiation therapy one year back. On examination, visual acuity was 6/9 in the right eye and 6/6 in the left eye. Intraocular pressure was normal in both eyes. Lid and adnexal structures were within normal limits. Examination findings and slit lamp appearance are illustrated in Figure 10.4.

KEY POINTS

Diagnosis:
- Based on clinical features and examination, a diagnosis of post-radiation dry eye disease was made.

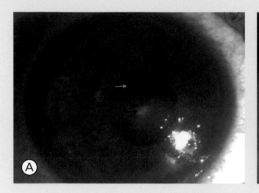
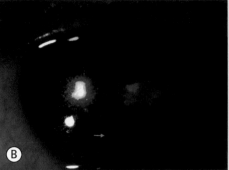

Figure 10.4 Slit lamp photograph of a patient with features of post-radiation dry eye disease showing (A) poor ocular surface, mild conjunctival congestion, central corneal opacity (black arrow), corneal xerosis and diffuse, superficial punctate opacities (grey arrow) suggestive of an uneven distribution of the tear film. On fluorescein staining (B), coarse (black arrow) and fine (grey arrow) punctate staining may be appreciated on examination under cobalt blue filter.

Investigations:

- Schirmer's test was less than 5 mm with an instantaneous TBUT in both eyes; ocular surface staining scores were also outside normal limits.

Treatment:

- The patient was started on preservative-free lubricants (carboxy methylcellulose 1% every two hours and hydroxyl propyl methylcellulose 0.3% gel thrice a day) along with topical cyclosporine 0.05% twice a day.
- In addition, oral capsules containing omega-3 fatty acids were prescribed.

Outcome:

- At one month follow-up the patient reported decrease in symptoms and an improvement in the signs of dry eye disease with improved comfort.

CASE 10.4

CLINICAL FEATURES

A 38-year-old female presented with dryness, foreign body sensation and blurring of vision in both eyes, more so in the left eye for the past three months with associated symptoms of dry mouth. On examination, the vision in the right eye was 6/9 and 6/18 in left eye. The intraocular pressure was within the normal limit in both eyes. Examination findings and slit lamp appearance are shown in Figure 10.5.

KEY POINTS

Diagnosis:

- The above clinical scenario describes a case of Sjögren's syndrome with chronic dry eyes and dellen formation.

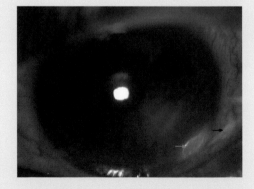

Figure 10.5 Slit lamp photograph of patient with Sjögren's syndrome showing an oval-shaped epithelial defect at the inferotemporal limbus (grey arrow) with surrounding inflamed conjunctiva (black arrow) and tear film instability suggestive of dry eye.

Investigations:

- A baseline ocular surface assessment and systemic workup, including complete blood count, ESR and liver and kidney function tests were performed.
- A referral was made to the rheumatology department, where a detailed workup and the presence of anti-nuclear antibodies led to the diagnosis of Sjögren's syndrome.

Treatment:

- This case was managed using topical, preservative-free lubricants (carboxy methylcellulose 1% given every two hours and hydroxyl propyl methylcellulose 0.3% three times a day) along with antibiotic (moxifloxacin 0.5%) for one week.

- The underlying Sjögren's syndrome was treated by the rheumatologist with oral pilocarpine.

Outcome:

- The dellen resolved in two weeks and the vision improved to 6/9 in both the eyes. The patient continued instilling lubricants as per prescription and was advised to follow up regularly with the ophthalmologist and rheumatologist.

Supplementary Information and Additional Tips

- In cases of dellen, other underlying causes, such as pinguecula, inflamed conjunctiva or focal tear film deficiency, should also be ruled out and treated accordingly.

CASE 10.5

CLINICAL FEATURES

A 55-year-old female presented with complaints of foreign body sensation, redness and grittiness in both her eyes. The patient was a known case of rheumatoid arthritis and on treatment for the same. Visual acuity was hand movements close to face (HMCF) with accurate projection of rays (PR) in both eyes. Intraocular pressure was normal. Examination findings and slit lamp appearance are illustrated in Figure 10.6.

KEY POINTS

Diagnosis:

- Based on history and examination, a diagnosis of bilateral severe dry eye was made in the setting of rheumatoid arthritis.

Investigations:

- Ocular surface assessment revealed severe dry eye with Schirmer's test of 2 mm and instantaneous tear break-up time in both the eyes.
- Ultrasonography (USG) B-scan for posterior segment did not reveal any abnormality.

Treatment:

- The patient was started on preservative-free lubricants, carboxymethyl cellulose 0.5% once every hour and sodium hyaluronate 0.1% four times a day. Cyclosporine 0.1% twice a day was started in both eyes.
- The patient underwent bilateral mucous membrane grafting (MMG) of the lower lid for lid margin keratinisation.

Outcome:

- On follow-up, patient showed a decrease in symptoms in both eyes. MMG uptake was good and an improvement in ocular surface and wettability was observed.

Supplementary Information and Additional Tips

- Severe keratinisation of the cornea and conjunctiva can be seen in severe dry eye disease (Figure 10.7).
- Minor salivary gland transplantation (MSGT) may be performed to improve ocular surface wettability in cases with long-standing severe dry eye

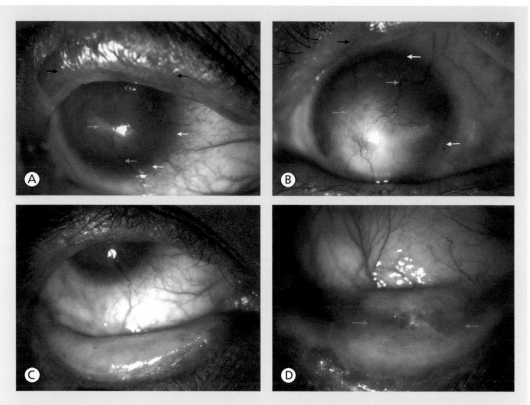

Figure 10.6 Slit lamp photograph of a patient with bilateral severe dry eye showing (A) diffuse nebulo-macular corneal opacity (yellow arrow) with superficial corneal vascularisation (grey arrow), 360° limbal stem cell deficiency (white arrows) and upper lid scarring with lid margin keratinisation (black arrows) with a similar picture (B) in the other eye, revealing upper lid scarring (black arrow), 360° limbal stem cell deficiency (white arrows) with leucomatous corneal opacity (yellow arrow) with superficial vascularisation (grey arrow). The patient underwent mucous membrane grafting (blue arrows) for lower lid margin keratinisation, in right (C) and left eyes (D) sequentially to stabilise the ocular surface.

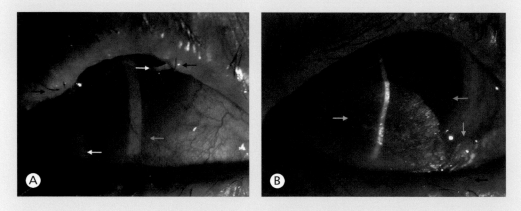

Figure 10.7 Slit lamp photograph of a patient with chronic dry eye disease showing (A) limbal stem cell deficiency (grey arrow), mucoid discharge (white arrows) and metaplastic lashes (black arrows). The fellow eye exhibited (B) extensive keratinisation over the cornea as well as conjunctiva (yellow arrows) along with corneal opacification with vascularisation (grey arrow).

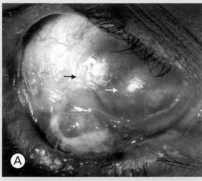

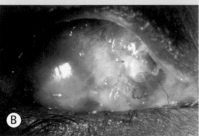

Figure 10.8 Slit lamp photograph demonstrating (A) a vascularised corneal opacity (white arrow), keratinisation (black arrow) with transplanted minor salivary glands (yellow arrow) with overlying amniotic membrane graft (grey arrow) in inferior and (B) superior quadrant with absorbable 8-0 vicryl sutures (green arrow) in a case of operated minor salivary gland transplantation (MSGT) for treating severe dry eye.

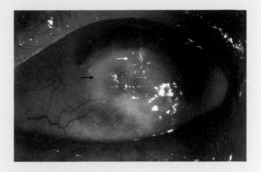

Figure 10.9 Slit lamp photograph of a patient with chronic ocular surface disease showing spheroidal degeneration (white arrow), leucomatous corneal opacity (black arrow) with corneal vascularisation (grey arrow). Note the corneal ulceration (yellow arrow) with thinning (green arrows) and surface irregularity.

cases that are refractory to medical therapy (Figure 10.8).

■ Cases with severe dry eye disease are prone to secondary infection and, if left untreated, may develop secondary keratitis with corneal thinning (Figure 10.9). These cases then require surgical management in the form of cyanoacrylate glue with BCL, patch graft or tectonic keratoplasty.

CASE 10.6

CLINICAL FEATURES

A 20-year-old male presented with diminution of vision, foreign body sensation, watering and discomfort for the past one year in his right eye. There was history of chemical injury with 'chuna' (calcium hydroxide) particle one year back. On examination, the visual acuity in the right eye was 6/36 with a raised intraocular pressure. Examination findings and slit lamp appearance are illustrated in Figure 10.10.

KEY POINTS

Diagnosis:
■ The above clinical scenario describes a case of unilateral chemical injury sequelae (post-alkali burn) with dry eye disease and limbal stem cell deficiency (LSCD).

Investigations:
■ Ocular surface assessment, including Schirmer's test, TBUT and staining scores, revealed moderate dry eye.

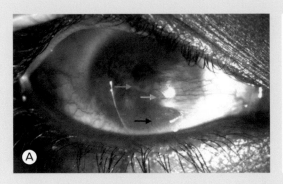
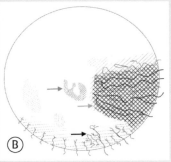

Figure 10.10   Slit lamp photograph of a patient with ocular chemical injury sequelae showing (A) partial limbal stem cell deficiency with formation of a pseudopterygium (yellow arrow), diffuse nebulo-macular corneal opacity (grey arrow) with superficial vascularisation (black arrow). The corresponding schematic picture (B) depicts the same clinical features.

- Impression cytology from the right eye revealed goblet cells in three quadrants of the cornea suggestive of partial LSCD.
- Anterior segment ocular coherence tomography revealed that the corneal opacity was limited mainly to the anterior half of the stroma.

Treatment:
- The patient was treated symptomatically with frequent preservative-free lubricants (carboxy methylcellulose 1% given once every hour and hydroxyl propyl methylcellulose 0.3% gel three times a day).
- The intraocular pressure was controlled using topical antiglaucoma medications (timolol 0.5% and brimonidine 0.2% given twice daily).

Outcome:
- The patient showed good response to conservative management, with control of inflammation and stabilisation of the ocular surface.
- Surgical intervention was not performed in this case as the central visual axis was partially clear, there was no restriction of extra-ocular movements and an acceptable best spectacle corrected visual acuity of 6/12 was achieved after one month of treatment.

Supplementary Information and Additional Tips
- In chemical injury sequelae, the primary aim is to control the inflammation; subsequently stem cell transplantation may be performed to stabilise the ocular surface, followed by keratoplasty for the residual corneal opacity and visual rehabilitation as required.
- In cases with unilateral chemical injury sequelae and partial LSCD, pannus excision with limbal stem cell transplant (LSCT) from the fellow normal eye is usually sufficient without the need for lamellar keratoplasty. LSCT from the fellow normal eye can be done in the form of simple limbal epithelial transplantation (SLET) or cultivated limbal epithelial transplantation (CLET), wherein the limbal stem cells from the fellow eye are grown and propagated in vitro on a biological substrate like amniotic membrane, then transplanted in the affected eye (Figure 10.11).

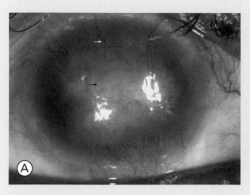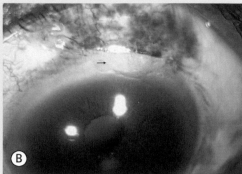

Figure 10.11 Slit lamp photograph of a patient with ocular chemical injury sequelae showing (A) extensive corneal opacification (black arrow) with spheroidal degeneration (grey arrow) and corneal vascularisation (white arrow) suggestive of limbal stem cell deficiency (yellow arrow). The fellow normal eye reveals (B) the donor site for limbal stem cells to be utilised for cultivated limbal epithelial transplant (black arrow).

■ Corneal transplantation can be either in the form of manual lamellar keratoplasty following limbal lenticule transplantation (Figure 10.12) or deep anterior lamellar transplantation following SLET (Figure 10.13) for treating LSCD and is performed only when there is no evidence of LSCD on impression cytology.

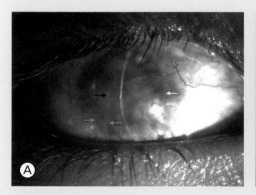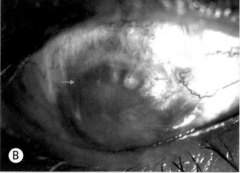

Figure 10.12 Slit lamp photograph of a child who had sustained ocular chemical injury sequelae and had undergone operated manual anterior lamellar keratoplasty with limbal stem cell transplantation (limbal lenticule from fellow normal eye). Clinical features noted were (A) diffuse nebulo-macular haze in the graft (black arrow) consequent to resolved graft infection with few buried 10-0 monofilament nylon sutures (yellow arrow). Note the conjunctival vasculature (white arrow) invading the cornea. On downgaze (B), same clinical features are seen along with well-apposed graft-host junction (green arrows) and degrading nylon sutures.

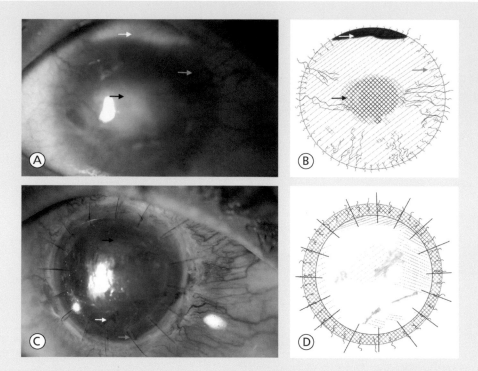

Figure 10.13 Slit lamp photograph of a 10-year-old child with ocular chemical injury sequelae showing (A) corneal opacity (black arrow) with corneal vascularisation (grey arrow) with lipid deposition superiorly (white arrow). Corresponding schematic diagram of the preoperative presentation (B) reveals the same findings. The patient underwent simple limbal epithelial transplantation followed by manual deep anterior lamellar keratoplasty and the clinical picture reveals (C) a clear graft (black arrow), well-apposed graft-host junction (yellow arrow), fine blood debris in the interface (white arrow) and well-buried interrupted 10-0 monofilament nylon sutures (grey arrow). Corresponding schematic diagram of the postoperative presentation (D) reveals the same findings.

CASE 10.7

CLINICAL FEATURES

A 33-year-old male patient presented with significant foreign body sensation and decreased vision for the past year with sudden development of pain in left eye. He gave a history of similar episodes of itching, profuse watering and redness since childhood, which continued in adulthood, more so, on using computers or doing excessive near work. There was no other history of other ocular or systemic disease. The examination findings and slit lamp appearance are illustrated in Figure 10.14. Visual acuity at presentation was 6/18 in the right eye and finger counting close to face (FCCF) in left eye with accurate PR.

KEY POINTS

Diagnosis:
- The above clinical scenario describes a case of bilateral chronic allergic conjunctivitis with LSCD and left chronic OSD with secondary corneal thinning and ulceration.

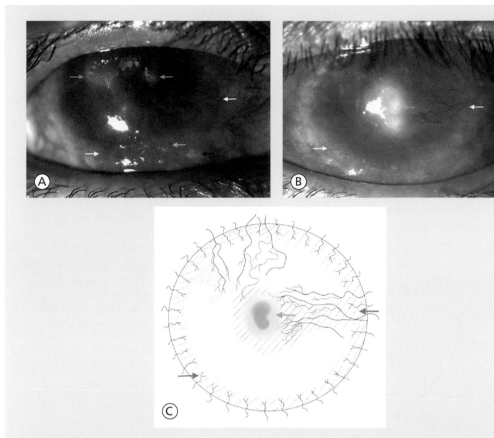

Figure 10.14 Slit lamp photograph of a patient with chronic allergic conjunctivitis and limbal stem cell deficiency showing (A) diffuse conjunctival congestion, limbal inflammation and nodules (black arrow) with corneal opacification (grey arrows) and vascularisation (white arrows) and eventual limbal stem cell deficiency (green arrow). The other eye reveals (B) diffuse conjunctival congestion with corneal opacification, thinning and ulceration (yellow arrow). The corresponding schematic corneal diagram of the left eye (C) depicts the salient clinical findings.

Investigations:
- Baseline ocular surface assessment for the right eye and corneal scarping and posterior segment B-scan USG were performed for the left eye.

Treatment:
- The patient was treated with topical and systemic antihistamine/mast cell stabilisers (olopatadine hydrochloride 0.1% twice a day), and lubricants (preservative-free carboxymethylcellulose 0.5% six times a day and ointment carbomer with vitamin A at night).
- Cold compresses were advised twice a day and patient was advised to avoid rubbing and exposure to dust.

- The left eye was treated with topical moxifloxacin 0.5% and fortified tobramycin 1.3% every two hours, which were tapered gradually as per clinical response, along with homatropine hydrobromide 2% thrice a day and timolol maleate.
- The patient was also started on topical immunosuppressants (cyclosporine drops) in both eyes after the left corneal ulcer healed.

Outcome:
- Refractive correction led to improvement of visual acuity to 6/9 in the right eye, while the left eye healed with a residual corneal opacity and best-corrected visual acuity of 6/24.

CASE 10.8

CLINICAL FEATURES

A 50-year-old male reported diminution of vision, dryness, foreign body sensation and discomfort in both eyes for the past one year. There was a history of allergic reaction after drug intake for fever (possibly ibuprofen), and the symptoms of ocular pain and redness occurred after the onset of fever. On examination, the vision in both the eyes was HMCF with accurate PR. The intraocular pressure was within normal limits. Examination findings and slit lamp appearance are illustrated in Figure 10.15.

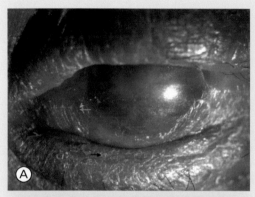

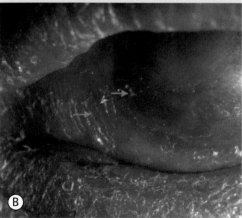

Figure 10.15 Slit lamp photograph of bilateral end stage chronic Stevens-Johnson syndrome sequelae (A) showing severe keratinisation of the lid margin (black arrow) and the conjunctiva (grey arrow), corneal opacification, loss of lashes and parch dry ocular surface, better appreciated on (B) higher magnification.

KEY POINTS

Diagnosis:
- The above clinical scenario describes a case of chronic SJS sequelae.

Investigations:
- The diagnosis was primarily based on thorough history and examination findings. A skin biopsy may help to establish the diagnosis but is rarely necessary.
- USG B-scan for posterior segment did not show any abnormality.

Treatment:
- This patient was managed medically to maintain wettability of the ocular surface and control inflammation; topical, preservative-free lubricants (carboxy methylcellulose 1% given once every hour and D-Panthenol 5% gel three times a day) and topical cyclosporine 0.05% twice a day were prescribed.
- Punctal occlusion can be tried if the medical treatment fails.

Outcome:
- The patient showed symptomatic improvement and gained some ambulatory vision with conservative management. He was prescribed long-term use of topical lubricants and advised regular follow-up.

Supplementary Information and Additional Tips

- In the acute stage of SJS, the patient presents with haemorrhagic crusting of the lid margins and conjunctivitis (Figure 10.16) along with ocular surface inflammation and xerosis.
- In the chronic stage, eyelid complications including cicatricial entropion, loss of eyelashes, metaplastic lashes (Figure 10.17), fibrosis of lacrimal puncta and ankyloblepharon (Figure 10.18) are frequently seen.
- The management is different for acute and chronic SJS. In acute SJS, preservative-free lubricants are given; topical steroids (for iritis and inflammation) and cycloplegics

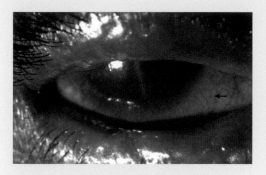

Figure 10.16 Slit lamp photograph of a patient presenting with acute stage of Stevens-Johnson syndrome showing conjunctivitis, ocular discharge, inflamed and thickened lid margins along with diffuse conjunctival congestion due to inflamed conjunctiva (black arrow). Mild corneal xerosis is evident.

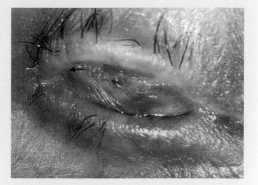

Figure 10.18 External photograph of a patient with chronic sequelae of Stevens-Johnson syndrome showing cicatricial entropion with metaplastic lashes (grey arrow), extensive keratinisation and ankyloblepharon (black arrow).

may improve comfort. Lysis of symblepharon is important in the early stages to prevent eventual ankyloblepharon which can be done by using an antibiotic-coated glass rod or inserting a scleral ring.

- Surgical intervention in the form of mucosal membrane transplantation (MMT) with amniotic membrane transplantation (AMT) and MSGT for keratinisation of the conjunctiva can be done.

- In severe and long-standing cases of SJS, osteo-odontokeratoprosthesis (OOKP) is the last option for visual rehabilitation (Figure 10.19). Retro-prosthetic membrane is the most common cause for decreased vision in postoperative period and might need surgical membranectomy if significant drop in vision is noticed.

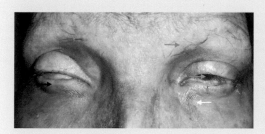

Figure 10.17 External photograph of a patient of chronic Stevens-Johnson syndrome showing bilateral lid changes in the form of skin excoriation and fibrosis (white arrow), loss of eyebrows (grey arrow), eyelid complications including loss of eyelashes (black arrow) and metaplastic eyelashes (yellow arrow). Note the conjunctival congestion and reduced opening of the palpebral aperture due to ankyloblepharon and extensive symblepharon.

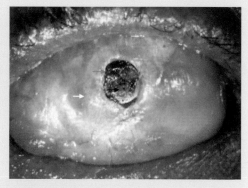

Figure 10.19 Slit lamp photograph showing a case of operated osteo-odontokeratoprosthesis (OOKP) showing the optical cylinder (grey arrow) with retro-prosthesis membrane (black arrow) held in place and straddled by the conjunctiva and buccal mucosal graft (white arrow) of the patient.

CASE 10.9

CLINICAL FEATURES

A 25-year-old female presented with complaints of diminution of vision, watering and photophobia in both eyes for the last six months. The patient had a history of developing severe allergic reaction after taking some medicine for fever one year ago. On examination, patient had a visual acuity of 6/36 in the right eye and 2/60 in the left eye. Examination findings and slit lamp appearance are illustrated in Figure 10.20.

KEY POINTS

Diagnosis:
- Based on the history and clinical features, a diagnosis of chronic SJS sequelae was made.

Investigations:
- Schirmer's test was 8 mm with instantaneous tear break-up time in both eyes.

- Anterior segment optical coherence tomography (ASOCT) was done which showed the depth of corneal opacity up to the mid-stromal level.

Treatment:
- The patient was started on topical, preservative-free lubricants; carboxy methyl cellulose 0.5% every two hours, cyclosporine 0.05% TDS and D-Panthenol ointment at night.
- Oral omega-3 fatty acids capsules 500 mg were prescribed twice a day.
- The right eye underwent cultivated oral mucosal epithelial transplantation (COMET) and the left eye was planned for COMET followed by manual anterior lamellar keratoplasty as there was significant corneal opacity in the visual axis.

Outcome:
- There was a significant improvement in the ocular surface as well as visual acuity.

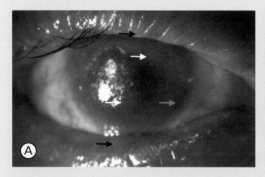 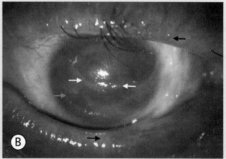

Figure 10.20 Slit lamp photograph of a patient with bilateral chronic Stevens-Johnson syndrome showing (A) loss of eyelashes (black arrows) with 360° limbal stem cell deficiency with nebulo-macular corneal opacity (white arrow) with corneal vascularisation (grey arrow). Similar findings (B) were seen in the left eye with keratinisation of the corneal surface.

CASE 10.10

CLINICAL FEATURES

A 60-year-old female presented with complaints of gradually progressive diminution of vision in both eyes for last five years. The patient had an episode of allergic drug reaction six years ago when she had developed skin lesions along with pain, redness and watering in both eyes which was managed medically with topical eye drops. Even though the pain and watering subsided gradually, the patient continued to have progressive loss of vision.

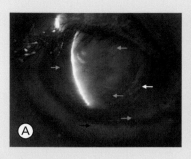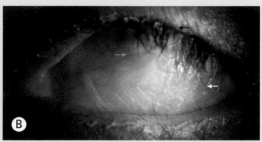

Figure 10.21 Slit lamp photograph of a case of severe bilateral chronic Stevens-Johnson syndrome showing (A) lower lid ectropion (black arrow) with shortening of inferior fornix (grey arrow), peripheral conjunctivalisation of the cornea with pannus formation (yellow arrows) and keratinisation (white arrow). Similar findings were observed in the other eye (B) revealing upper lid entropion (black arrow) with lower lid distichiasis (grey arrow) and corneal vascularisation (yellow arrow) with keratinised surface (white arrow).

On examination, visual acuity in both eyes was HMCF with accurate PR in all four quadrants. Intraocular pressure was within normal limits in both eyes. Examination findings and slit lamp appearance are illustrated in Figure 10.21.

KEY POINTS

Diagnosis:
- Based on the history and clinical examination, a diagnosis of severe case of bilateral chronic Stevens-Johnson sequelae was made.

Investigations:
- Schirmer's test was zero with instantaneous tear break-up time in both eyes. ASOCT was done to evaluate the corneal thickness and regularity.

- USG B-scan did not show any abnormality. Visually evoked response (VER) was performed to establish the visual potential and was within normal limits.

Treatment:
- The patient was prescribed round-the-clock preservative-free lubricants along with ointment at bedtime.
- Ectropion correction surgery was planned for the right eye and a keratoprosthesis implant was planned for the left eye.

Outcome:
- The patient gained some useful vision in the left eye after keratoprosthesis surgery and has been on regular follow-up.

CASE 10.11

CLINICAL FEATURES

A 36-year-old male presented with complaints of redness, pain and watering in both eyes for the previous two weeks. The patient was a diagnosed case of SJS and had complaints of foreign body sensation, irritation and low vision for the past year. Examination findings and slit lamp appearance at presentation and follow-up are illustrated in Figure 10.22.

KEY POINTS

Diagnosis:
- Based on clinical features and examination findings, the patient was diagnosed to have bilateral chronic SJS with secondary keratitis with impending corneal perforation.

Investigations:
- Corneal scraping was not performed in view of the impending perforation;

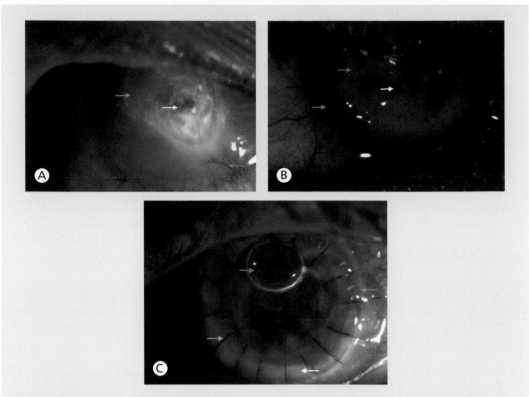

Figure 10.22   Slit lamp photograph of a patient with bilateral chronic Stevens-Johnson syndrome with secondary corneal thinning and ulceration showing (A) conjunctival congestion (black arrow) and corneal ulcer (yellow arrow) with central perforation (white arrow) with inferonasal vascularisation (grey arrow). Examination of the left eye revealed (B) conjunctival congestion (black arrow), corneal opacification and ulceration (yellow arrow) with perforation (white arrow) and corneal vascularisation (grey arrow). The patient underwent tectonic keratoplasty (C) in the left eye which resulted in a clear graft (black arrow) secured, with interrupted 10-0 monofilament nylon sutures (green arrow) and minimal inflammatory hypopyon (white arrow) with an air bubble superiorly (grey arrow) that was seen postoperatively.

a B-scan USG was carefully performed and revealed a normal posterior segment.

Treatment:
- Patient was started on fortified antibiotics (topical cefazolin 5% and tobramycin 1.3%), topical antifungal (natamycin 5%), homatropine 2% thrice a day and timolol 0.5% twice a day in the right eye.
- Due to the impending perforation, cyanoacrylate glue with a BCL was applied to the right eye.
- Tectonic keratoplasty was performed in the left eye to restore globe integrity and postoperatively the patient was

prescribed topical antibiotics, steroids and lubricants.

Outcome:
- On postoperative day 1, the graft was clear with well-apposed graft-host junction (GHJ); anterior chamber was well formed with mild anterior chamber inflammation and a small hypopyon.
- On further follow-up visits, hypopyon disappeared and patient attained a visual acuity of 6/36.
- The right eye keratitis resolved with a central adherent leucoma; however, the rest of the anterior chamber was well formed.

CASE 10.12

CLINICAL FEATURES

A 37-year-old male presented with complaints of diminution of vision, foreign body sensation, irritation, redness and photophobia in both eyes for the previous year. The patient had a history of allergic reaction after intake of an oral sulfamethoxazole-trimethoprim combination for fever and urinary tract infection. Patient had a visual acuity of HMCF in the right eye and 1/60 in the left eye with accurate PR in all four quadrants. Examination findings and slit lamp appearance are illustrated in Figure 10.23.

KEY POINTS

Diagnosis:
- The above clinical scenario depicts a case of bilateral SJS sequelae with OSD and left eye descemetocele.

Investigations:
- Ocular surface assessment was performed for both eyes. Schirmer's test was less than 2 mm and TBUT was less than five seconds in the right eye.
- Fluorescein staining revealed diffuse punctate staining over the cornea in both eyes; Seidel's test was negative in the left eye.

- ASOCT demonstrated localised thinning of the cornea in the left eye confirming the diagnosis of descemetocele.

Treatment:
- Fibrin-aprotinin glue application with BCL insertion was performed under topical anaesthesia for the left eye. Topical, preservative-free drops of carboxymethyl cellulose 0.5% every hour, sodium hyaluronate 0.1% four times a day, moxifloxacin 0.5% thrice a day, homatropine 2% thrice a day and timolol 0.5% twice a day were administered postoperatively.
- Oral doxycycline 100 mg twice a day and vitamin C 500 mg twice a day were also started and the patient was advised to take a diet rich in omega-3 fatty acids.

Outcome:
- On follow-up, patient showed improvement in symptoms, along with a decrease in congestion and photophobia.

Supplementary Information and Additional Tips

- Cases with chronic SJS with descemetocele may heal with formation of a corneal opacity with surface keratinisation (Figure 10.24) over the cornea.

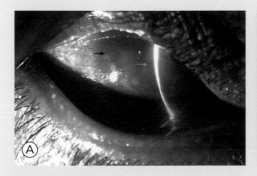 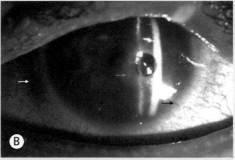

Figure 10.23 Slit lamp photograph of a patient with bilateral Stevens-Johnson syndrome sequelae and extensive ocular surface disease showing (A) nebulo-macular corneal opacity (grey arrow) with corneal vascularisation (black arrow) and xerosis in the right eye while the other eye reveals (B) conjunctival congestion (white arrow), paracentral descemetocele (green arrow) with surrounding corneal haze and oedema (grey arrow) and well-formed anterior chamber. Note the peripheral corneal vascularisation (black arrow) due to limbal stem cell deficiency.

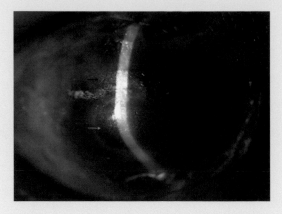

Figure 10.24 Slit lamp photograph of a patient with chronic stage Stevens-Johnson syndrome showing dry and keratinised ocular surface, keratinisation over the cornea (black arrow) with a well-healed descemetocele (grey arrow).

CASE 10.13

CLINICAL FEATURES

A 60-year-old female presented with decrease in vision, redness, watering and foreign body sensation for the past six months in both the eyes. There was a history of eruption of subepidermal blisters in the oral mucosa that was diagnosed as a case of ocular cicatricial pemphigoid. On examination, visual acuity in both eyes was 6/60 with a normal intraocular pressure. Examination findings and slit lamp appearance are illustrated in Figure 10.25.

KEY POINTS

Diagnosis:
- The above clinical scenario describes a case of ocular cicatricial pemphigoid.

Investigations:
- The disease is primarily clinical; however, conjunctival biopsy or mucus membrane biopsy can be considered for immunofluorescence studies.

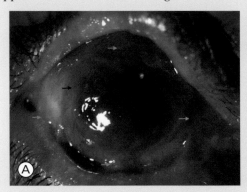
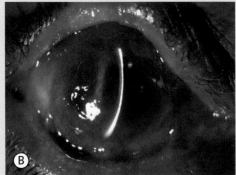

Figure 10.25 Slit lamp photograph of a patient with ocular cicatricial pemphigoid showing (A) diffuse conjunctival congestion (yellow arrow), superior pannus (green arrow), superficial corneal vascularisation (black arrow) and inferior symblepharon (grey arrow) formation along with (B) corneal thinning and melting seen in the superior part (black arrow) of the cornea, as seen on slit illumination.

- Systemic evaluation in consultation with physician and dermatologist is warranted.

Treatment:

- The patient was managed on topical, preservative-free lubricants (carboxy methylcellulose 1% given every hour and hydroxyl propyl methylcellulose 0.3% gel three times a day) and topical cyclosporine 0.05% twice a day along with a prophylactic antibiotic (moxifloxacin 0.5%).
- Systemic treatment is the mainstay of management. The patient was started on oral dapsone after dermatology opinion.
- Reconstructive surgery for lids, ocular surface and cornea can be considered once the active disease is under control.

Outcome:

- The acute exacerbation was controlled in three weeks and the patient was kept on lubricants and frequent follow-up. The uncorrected visual acuity improved to 6/18 in both eyes.

Supplementary Information and Additional Tips

- Patients with ocular cicatricial pemphigoid may present with asymmetric involvement of the two eyes with LSCD, distinct keratinisation of the ocular surface or fornix foreshortening with congested, vascularised and oedematous ocular surface due to ocular surface squamous neoplasia with acute inflammation (Figure 10.26); both entities may occur together due to a proposed common pathophysiology of immune dysfunction and chronic inflammation, leading to eventual oncogenesis in the latter.

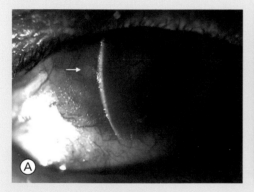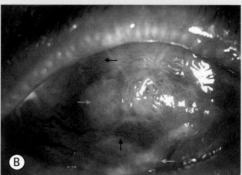

Figure 10.26 Slit lamp photograph of a 51-year-old patient with bilateral ocular cicatricial pemphigoid showing (A) limbal stem cell deficiency with consequent corneal opacification (white arrow), keratinisation (blue arrow) and 360° corneal vascularisation (black arrows). Examination of the left eye (B) shows conjunctival and corneal vascularisation (black arrows), mucoid discharge (yellow arrow) and a congested, vascularised mass (grey arrow) due to ocular surface squamous neoplasia. Note the poor ocular surface and pooling of mucus and debris due to impaired blinking and shrinkage of the fornices.

CASE 10.14

CLINICAL FEATURES

A 25-year-old patient presented with complaints of diminution of vision, watering, photophobia, foreign body sensation in both eyes for the previous year. On examination, the visual acuity was 6/12 in the right eye and 6/18 in the left eye with normal intraocular pressure.

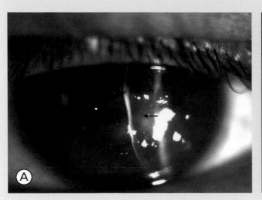 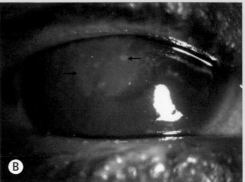

Figure 10.27 Slit lamp photograph of a patient with gelatinous, drop-like corneal dystrophy showing (A) gelatinous waxy nodules (black arrow) involving pupillary axis along with corneal thinning, dirty tear film and ocular surface disease. The other eye (B) shows corneal surface irregularity and xerosis with meibomian gland dysfunction in the form of blockage and capping of the meibomian orifices with meibum (green arrow).

The examination findings and slit lamp appearance are shown in Figure 10.27.

KEY POINTS

Diagnosis:
- Based on clinical features and examination, a diagnosis of OSD with meibomian gland dysfunction (MGD) was made in a patient with gelatinous drop-like dystrophy (GDLD).

Investigations:
- Schirmer's test was more than 25 mm in both eyes, probably due to reflex tearing; TBUT was instantaneous in both eyes.
- Infrared meibography revealed 48% and 53% meibomian gland loss in the right and left eye, respectively.

Treatment:
- The patient was started on topical carboxy methyl cellulose 0.5% every two hours. Oral doxycycline 100 mg twice a day was prescribed for MGD. Antibiotic ointment was prescribed at night along with lid massage with warm compresses.
- The patient was also advised to have one teaspoon of roasted and powdered flax seeds.

- Anterior lamellar therapeutic keratoplasty was planned for the left eye as there was a significant opacity in the visual axis.

Outcome:
- Patient showed symptomatic improvement in both eyes; the visual acuity improving to 6/9 in the right eye.

Supplementary Information and Additional Tips

- MGD and recurrent erosions with surface irregularity is a common feature in patients with GDLD.
- MGD, an important cause of evaporative dry eye, is a chronic, diffuse abnormality of the Meibomian glands, commonly characterised by terminal duct obstruction and/or qualitative/quantitative changes in the glandular secretion that manifests as Meibomian orifice plugging, eyelid margin foaminess, blepharitis, hyperaemia/telangiectasias, hyper-keratinisation and changes in orifice position with respect to the muco-cutaneous junction (Figure 10.28).

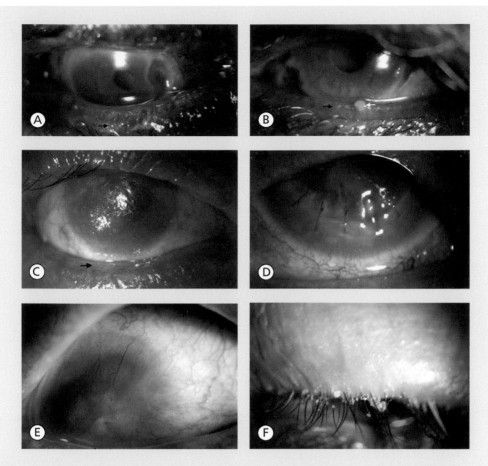

Figure 10.28 Slit lamp photographs demonstrating morphological characteristics of meibomian gland dysfunction (MGD) with (A) eyelid margin foaminess and frothing (black arrow), (B) meibomian duct obstruction (black arrow), capped meibomian orifices with meibomian gland cyst (white arrow), (C) complications of MGD-like gland atrophy (black arrow), (D) lid margin hyperaemia and telangiectasia (black arrow), (E) lid margin keratinisation (black arrow) and (F) blepharitis demonstrated by extensive lid margin contamination (white arrow).

CASE 10.15

CLINICAL FEATURES

A 27-year-old male presented with blurring of vision in both eyes which was slowly progressive over the previous year. The patient had a history of recurrent episodes of pain, redness and watering in both eyes for the last few years. The patient had a visual acuity of HMCF and finger counting close to face with accurate PR in the right and left eye, respectively. The patient had decreased corneal sensations in both eyes. Examination findings and slit lamp appearance are illustrated in Figure 10.29.

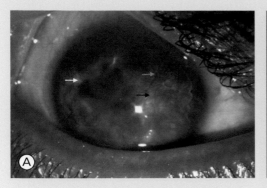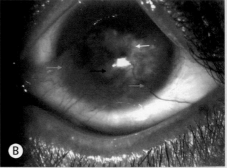

Figure 10.29 Slit lamp photograph of a patient with showing bilateral healed viral keratitis showing (A) nebulo-macular corneal opacity (black arrow) along with corneal vascularisation (grey arrow) with intrastromal lipid deposition (white arrow). The other eye (B) shows localised limbal stem cell deficiency infero-nasally, overlying pannus (yellow arrow) with nebulo-macular corneal opacity (black arrow) and vascularisation (grey arrow) along with intrastromal lipid deposits (white arrow).

KEY POINTS

Diagnosis:
- Based on clinical features and examination, the clinical picture was that of a case of bilateral healed viral keratitis with bilateral LSCD.

Investigations:
- Ocular surface assessment revealed Schirmer's test of more than 15 mm and TBUT of more than ten seconds in both the eyes.
- ASOCT was done to see the depth of the corneal opacity and differential thinning; global pachymetry was also noted.

- USG B-scan showed no obvious abnormality.

Treatment:
- The patient was prescribed lubricating eye drops and ointment and planned for anterior lamellar keratoplasty in the right eye.
- Prophylactic oral acyclovir (400 mg BD) was started before the surgery and continued thereafter.

Outcome:
- Patient showed symptomatic improvement in both eyes; the uncorrected visual acuity improved to 6/24 at one month postoperative follow-up in the right eye.

CASE 10.16

CLINICAL FEATURES

A 65-year-old male with bilateral healed viral keratitis underwent right eye optical penetrating keratoplasty. In the postoperative period, the graft was clear with a well apposed GHJ. Soon after, the patient presented with intense pain and photophobia. Visual acuity was 6/36. Intraocular pressure was normal. Examination findings and slit lamp appearance are illustrated in Figure 10.30.

KEY POINTS

Diagnosis:
- A diagnosis of post-keratoplasty persistent epithelial defect (PED) (an epithelial defect which persists even after two weeks of surgery) was made.

Investigations:
- Serial clinical pictures were taken to note the healing of epithelial defect.

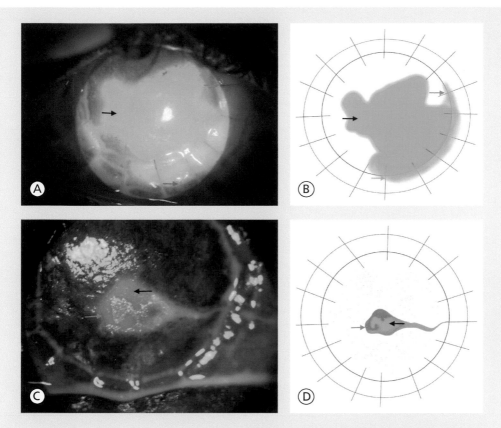

Figure 10.30 Slit lamp photograph of a patient who had undergone penetrating keratoplasty and developed (A) persistent epithelial defect (PED) measuring 6×7 mm (black arrow) involving inferonasal graft-host junction (yellow arrow) secured with interrupted 10-0 monofilament nylon sutures (grey arrow). After two weeks of treatment (C), the epithelial defect reduced in size to 2×3 mm (black arrow) with heaped-up edges (green arrow). The corresponding schematic diagrams of pretreatment (B) and posttreatment (D) clinical presentation highlight the salient findings in the case.

- ASOCT through the GHJ in the quadrant of the epithelial defect was done to rule out graft overriding.

Treatment:

- The preservative-free lubricating eye drops were increased in frequency to promote early healing of the PED.
- Topical antiglaucoma drugs were changed to oral medications to decrease preservative toxicity on the ocular surface.
- After no significant response for about a week, the edges of the PED were debrided so as to remove the heaped-up edges that prevent

epithelisation and the patient was additionally prescribed autologous serum eye drops (20%) four times a day.

- Oral doxycycline 100 mg BD and an omega-3 fatty acid capsule were also added to the treatment regimen.

Outcome:

- After initiating treatment with autologous serum, the patient started responding with a decrease in the size of the epithelial defect, which completely healed in two more weeks.

CASE 10.17

CLINICAL FEATURES

A 55-year-old female presented with blurring of vision, watering, irritation and foreign body sensation in the left eye for last three months. The patient had a history of recurrent episodes of watering in the left eye followed by Dacryocystorhinostomy (DCR) six months back. The patient initially showed mild improvement after surgery followed by recurrence of symptoms. Examination findings and slit lamp appearance are illustrated in Figure 10.31.

KEY POINTS

Diagnosis:
- Based on the history and clinical examination, a diagnosis of failed DCR with epitheliopathy was made.

Investigations:
- A Schirmer test more than 15 mm and TBUT more than ten seconds was noted. A syringing and probing test revealed nasal lacrimal duct obstruction suggestive of failed DCR.

Treatment:
- Patient was started on carboxymethylcellulose 0.5% and loteprednol four times a day and advised for a repeat DCR.

Outcome:
- The patient underwent a successful repeat DCR with an improvement in the ocular surface.

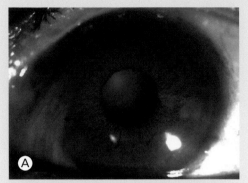
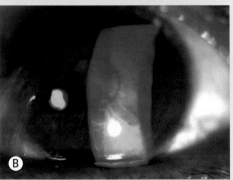

Figure 10.31 Slit lamp photograph in a case with a failed Dacryocystorhinostomy showing (A) a nasal pseudo-pterygium (black arrow). Fluorescein staining and examination under cobalt blue filter revealed (B) the nasal pseudo-pterygium (black arrow) and strands of heaped-up epithelium in the inferior cornea (grey arrow) due to tear film stasis.

CASE 10.18

CLINICAL FEATURES

A 40-year-old male presented with gradually progressive diminution of vision in both eyes for the past six months; prior to this, he gave a history of bilateral ocular pain, redness, foreign body sensation and photophobia. He was a known case of chronic kidney disease (CKD) and had undergone renal transplant one year back. At the initial presentation he was diagnosed as a case of bilateral ocular graft-versus-host disease (oGVHD) with marginal keratitis in the right eye and corneal perforation in the left eye. He was managed conservatively in the right eye with topical antibiotics, steroids and lubricants, following which there was symptomatic improvement. A tectonic patch graft was performed in the left eye and the patient gained some vision following the surgery; however, gradual deterioration was noted thereafter. The examination findings and slit lamp appearance are illustrated in Figure 10.32.

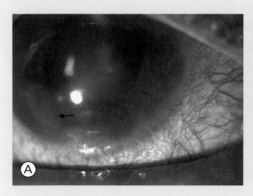 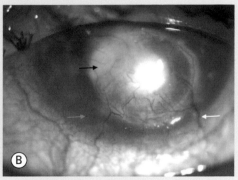

Figure 10.32 Slit lamp photograph of a patient with bilateral chronic ocular graft-versus-host disease (oGVHD) showing (A) healed keratitis with limbal stem cell deficiency in the right eye; note the mild conjunctival congestion, inferior nebular corneal opacity (grey arrow) and corneal vascularisation (black arrow). Examination of the left eye revealed (B) opacified tectonic patch graft (black arrow) with superficial corneal vascularisation (grey arrow) and deep vascularisation involving the graft (white arrow).

KEY POINTS

Diagnosis:

- The above clinical scenario highlights a case of chronic oGVHD with healed marginal keratitis in one eye and a failed graft with vascularised corneal opacity in the other.

Investigations:

- Baseline ocular surface, including Schirmer's test, TBUT and surface staining scores were performed; a subjective refraction for visual rehabilitation was also performed.

Treatment:

- Patient was managed with lubricating eye drops and ointment along with long-term topical immunosuppression (cyclosporine eye drops).
- As the patient had acceptable best-corrected visual acuity in the right eye, no surgical intervention was planned for the left eye.

Outcome:

- Patient maintained good visual acuity in the right eye and was kept on regular follow-up.

Supplementary Information and Additional Tips

- oGVHD occurs as a complication following haematopoietic stem cell transplantation; it can occur as conjunctival hyperaemia or chemosis,

pseudomembranous or membranous conjunctivitis, kerato-conjunctivitis sicca, corneal epithelial sloughing, persistent corneal epitheliopathy and corneal ulceration (Figure 10.33).

- Limbal stem cell transplantation and penetrating keratoplasty are not commonly performed in oGVHD owing to the poor prognosis for graft survival because of severe pre-existing inflammation.
- Keratoprosthesis may be considered for visual rehabilitation in severe cases with bilateral blindness.

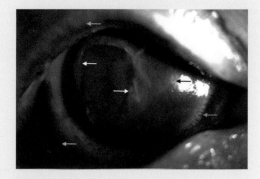

Figure 10.33 Slit lamp photograph of a patient with acute oGVHD showing conjunctival hyperaemia and chemosis (green arrow), lid margin oedema and congestion (yellow arrow), corneal epitheliopathy (black arrow) with epithelial sloughing (white arrows) and early corneal neovascularisation (grey arrow).

REFERENCES

1. Bohm KJ, Djalilian AR, Pflugfelder SC, Starr CE. Dry Eye. In: Cornea; Volume 1 – Fundamentals, Diagnosis and Management. 4th ed. USA: Elsevier; 377–96.
2. Valenzuela FA, Perez VL. Mucous Membrane Pemphigoid. In: Cornea; Volume 1 – Fundamentals, Diagnosis and Management. 4th ed. USA: Elsevier; 549–58.
3. Gregory DG, Holland EJ. Erythema Multiforme, Stevens-Johnson Syndrome and Toxic Epidermal Necrolysis. In: Cornea; Volume 1 – Fundamentals, Diagnosis and Management. 4th ed. USA: Elsevier; 558–73.
4. McGhee CNJ, Crawford AZ, Meyer JJ, Patel DV. CHAPTER 94. Chemical and Thermal Injuries of the Eye. In: Cornea; Volume 1 – Fundamentals, Diagnosis and Management. 4th ed. USA: Elsevier; 2017; 1106–19.

11 Trachoma

Shubhi Jain, Ritika Mukhija, Praveen Vashist, Noopur Gupta

INTRODUCTION

Trachoma is a chronic keratoconjunctivitis primarily affecting the superficial epithelium of the conjunctiva and cornea simultaneously presenting as a mixed follicular and papillary response of the conjunctival tissue. The disease is characterised by recurrent or persistent inflammation of the conjunctivae after many repeated infections with an intracellular, obligatory bacterium *Chlamydia trachomatis* serotypes A, B, Ba and C. This leads to conjunctival scarring and entropion, trichiasis and altered ocular surface that ensue in some individuals to cause corneal abrasions, secondary infections and corneal opacity.[1,2] It is still one of the leading infective causes of blindness in the world.[3] Clinical presentations may vary from mild ocular surface disease and conjunctival inflammation to more severe infections, corneal perforations and eventual corneal opacification causing blindness that are amenable to both full-thickness and lamellar corneal transplantation.

CASE 11.1

CLINICAL FEATURES

A 68-year-old female patient presented to our outpatient department with symptoms of pain, itching and foreign body sensation on the inside of the upper eyelids and diminution of vision over the last four years. She gave a history of eyelashes turning in and rubbing the surface of the eye, for which she underwent eyelid surgery three years back. Visual acuity at presentation was 6/36 and hand movements close to face in the right and left eye, respectively. Clinical findings and slit lamp appearance of the cornea and everted upper tarsal conjunctiva are illustrated in Figures 11.1 and 11.2.

KEY POINTS

Diagnosis:
- The clinical picture describes a case of trachomatous keratopathy with a history of upper eyelid entropion surgery. Signs of repeated trachomatous infections and resultant chronic sequelae like subconjunctival upper lid scarring, pannus, Herbert pits and concretions on the upper palpebral conjunctiva were noted.

Investigations:
- Ocular surface assessment revealed reduced Schirmer's test (6 mm in five minutes) and tear film break-up time of five seconds. The conjunctival and corneal fluorescein staining scores of 7/18 and 11/15, respectively, were recorded. Meibomian gland dysfunction was noted on meibography and slit lamp examination. Meibomian gland loss was noted to be 55% on ocular surface assessment through the ocular surface analyser. There was no evidence of posterior segment pathology on B-scan ultrasonography.

Treatment:
- The patient was managed with hot compresses thrice a day along with lid hygiene, topical gatifloxacin 0.3% thrice daily, carboxymethylcellulose 1% six times a day and antibiotic ointment at night. Oral azithromycin 1g single dose was also prescribed.
- Patient underwent right penetrating keratoplasty for visual rehabilitation in the left eye and had undergone cataract surgery two years back in the right eye with paracentral corneal opacity that developed after corneal perforation following infective keratitis.

Outcome:
- The patient demonstrated a significant improvement in the left eye with a best corrected visual acuity (BCVA) of (6/12) after keratoplasty with a clear graft and a mean total corneal thickness of 507 microns.

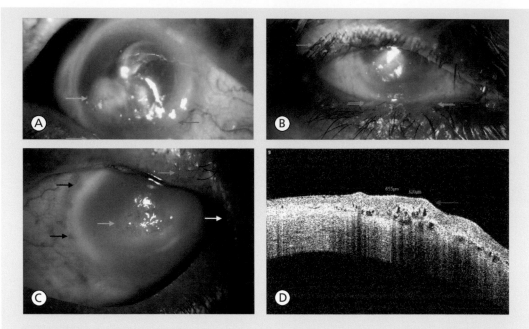

Figure 11.1 Slit lamp photograph of a patient with trachomatous keratopathy (A) with paracentral adherent leucoma (green arrow) secondary to healed keratitis along with thick arcus senilis (blue arrow), meibomian gland dysfunction (grey arrows) and pseudophakia. (B) Poor ocular surface with matting of eyelashes due to poor lid hygiene, frothing at lid margins and features of meibomian gland dysfunction like gland blockage (grey arrows), lid thickening and hyperemia were evident. (C) The other eye demonstrated metaplastic eyelashes and thickened upper eyelid margin (grey arrow) with ankyloblepharon (white arrow), Herbert's pits (black arrows) at the superior limbus, diffuse corneal haze with central corneal opacity and extensive yellow-amber granular deposits of spheroidal degeneration (yellow arrow), that is well illustrated on (D) anterior segment optical coherence tomography that reveals cystic spaces, increased corneal thickness with elevation of the corneal epithelium (red arrow) and disruption of the Bowman's membrane due to the deposited spherules.

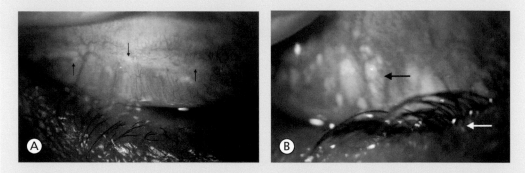

Figure 11.2 Slit lamp photograph of patients with trachomatous sequelae demonstrating on upper lid eversion (A) tarsal conjunctival scarring with few concretions (grey arrow) and a faint Arlt's line with fibrotic scars (black arrows) and (B) multiple upper lid concretions (black arrow), inflamed tarsal conjunctiva and lower lid trichiasis (white arrow).

Supplementary Information and Additional Tips

- The WHO FISTO classification (F = follicles, I = intense inflammation, S = conjunctival scarring, T = trichiasis, O = corneal opacity) is the most commonly followed grading system to classify into active disease and chronic sequelae of trachoma (Figures 11.3–11.6).[3]
- When inflammation is severe, an intense papillary reaction on the tarsal conjunctiva is associated with a diffuse thickening of the conjunctiva, obscuration of the deep tarsal vessels and, sometimes, eyelid oedema (Figure 11.7).
- Treatment of entropion (tarsal fracture performed in this case) and trichiatic cilia, control of inflammation and ocular surface disease including meibomian gland dysfunction are

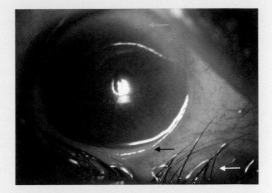

Figure 11.4 Slit lamp photograph of a patient with features of trachoma sequelae demonstrating lower lid entropion with inward turning of eyelashes (white arrow), regressed superior pannus (yellow arrow) and conjunctivochalasis (black arrow).

critical for obtaining good outcomes with corneal transplantation for trachomatous keratopathy.
- Cataract surgery in cases with paracentral corneal opacities sparing the visual axis demonstrates promising outcomes without the need for corneal grafting.

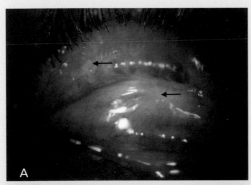

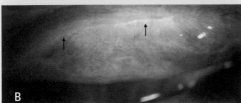

Figure 11.3 Slit lamp photographs (A and B) of patients demonstrating chronic sequelae of trachoma infection in the form of trachomatous scarring (TS) clearly seen as fibrotic scars and a thick Arlt's line (black arrows) with lid thickening; note that complete eversion of the upper lid is difficult due to tylosis.

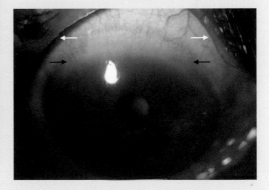

Figure 11.5 Slit lamp photograph of a patient demonstrating signs of trachomatous sequelae in the form of regressed pannus (black arrows) and irregular posterior lid margin with meibomian gland plugging suggestive of meibomian gland dysfunction (white arrows).

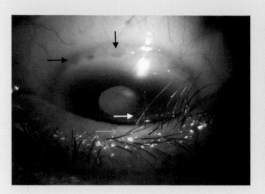

Figure 11.6 Slit lamp photograph demonstrating signs in a patient with chronic trachomatous sequelae such as lower lid entropion, trichiatic and metaplastic cilia (white arrow) eyelid discharge (yellow arrow) with lid margin telangiectasia and multiple Herbert's pits (black arrows) along with limbal scarring.

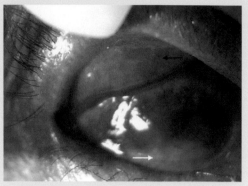

Figure 11.7 Slit lamp photograph showing intense inflammation (TI) in a patient with trachomatous sequelae in the form of vascularised corneal opacity (white arrow). Note that the everted upper lid shows an intense papillary reaction on the tarsal conjunctiva with diffuse thickening of the conjunctiva (black arrow), difficult lid eversion and obscuration of the deep tarsal vessels with eyelid oedema.

CASE 11.2

CLINICAL FEATURES

A 64-year-old male patient, resident of Faridabad, Haryana, India, and farmer by occupation, presented to us with painless, progressive diminution of vision, itching, yellow deposits and foreign body sensation in the right eye over the last four months. He gave a history of frequent epilation of eyelashes of the upper lid. Best corrected visual acuity achieved with refractive correction in the right eye was 4/60. Examination findings and slit lamp appearance are illustrated in Figure 11.8.

KEY POINTS

Diagnosis:
■ The above clinical scenario describes a case of anterior corneal involvement due to trachomatous

corneal opacity along with spheroidal degeneration.
■ Other signs of trachoma sequelae like Herbert's pits, upper tarsal fibrosis, regressive pannus at the upper limbus and trichiasis were also present.

Investigations:
■ Anterior segment optical coherence tomography revealed corneal opacification up to 245 microns depth of the cornea.

Treatment:
■ The patient was managed with topical antibiotic (moxifloxacin hydrochloride 0.5%, three times a day), Tab doxycycline 100 mg twice a day for two weeks, polyethylene glycol 0.4% + propylene glycol 0.3% four times a day and antibiotic ointment at night.

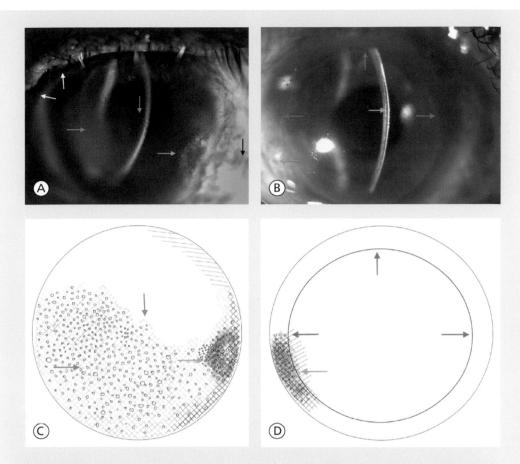

Figure 11.8 Slit lamp photograph of a patient with bilateral trachomatous keratopathy with left eye (A) spheroidal degeneration (grey arrows), which is more advanced in the peripheral cornea (yellow arrow). Also note the lipoid degeneration in the bulbar conjunctiva (black arrow) and trichiatic and metaplastic cilia in the upper lid along with irregular lid margin (white arrows). The patient underwent sutureless hemi-automated anterior lamellar keratoplasty (HALK) in his right eye (B) for optical rehabilitation. Note the well-apposed graft-host junction (blue arrows) and the clear interface (green arrow) and peripheral spheroidal degeneration (yellow arrow). The corresponding schematic diagrams of the left (C) and right eye (D) depicts the same findings.

- The patient finally underwent fibrin glue assisted, sutureless hemi-automated anterior lamellar keratoplasty (HALK) under peribulbar anaesthesia.

Outcome:
- The donor cornea remained clear on follow-up with good morphological outcome following lamellar keratoplasty with no interface haze.
- The patient underwent conventional rigid gas-permeable (RGP) contact lens trial (postoperatively) and finally attained the BCVA of 6/6.

CASE 11.3

CLINICAL FEATURES

A 70-year-old female patient presented with painless, progressive loss of vision in both eyes over the last two years. She did not give any history of epilation or entropion surgery. There was no history of any past episodes of painful red eye suggestive of infective keratitis. Examination findings and slit lamp appearance are illustrated in Figure 11.9.

KEY POINTS

Diagnosis:

- The above clinical scenario describes a case with atypical corneal involvement due to trachoma and secondary amyloidosis. Diffuse corneal haze was present due to amyloid deposition in subepithelial and stromal layers of the cornea occurring secondary to chronic ocular disorders like trachoma, trichiasis, spheroidal degeneration etc.

Investigations:

- Confocal microscopic images revealed hyper-reflective, needle-shaped crystalline deposits at the level of mid- to deep stroma, consistent with amyloidosis, that was confirmed on histopathological examination that demonstrated Congo red positive amyloid deposits.

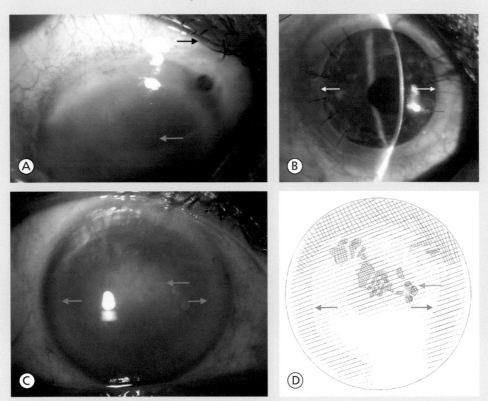

Figure 11.9 Slit lamp photograph of a patient with trachomatous keratopathy (A) with diffuse corneal haze (grey arrow) with regressed superior pannus (yellow arrow) and few, peripheral metaplastic lashes in the upper lid (black arrow). The patient underwent penetrating keratoplasty for optical rehabilitation (B) following which histopathological examination of the host cornea revealed secondary amyloidosis. A clear graft with peripheral suture marks (blue arrow) and well-apposed graft-host junction can be seen (white arrows). Examination of the other eye revealed (C) patchy central corneal opacities (green arrow) with intervening haze along with a thick peripheral arcus senilis (grey arrows), as has also been depicted in the schematic diagram (D).

Treatment:

- The patient underwent optical penetrating keratoplasty with cataract surgery for visual rehabilitation in the right eye.

Outcome:

- BCVA of 6/18 was achieved at the six-month follow-up visit.

Supplementary Information and Additional Tips

- It is important to recognise that there is a wide spectrum of post-trachoma corneal sequelae ranging from mild corneal scarring without severe adnexal disease to end-stage corneal scarring and vascularisation associated with severe ankyloblepharon and symblepharon, and that the prognosis may vary accordingly.
- Judicious selection of cases, prior and appropriate management of eyelid abnormalities, such as trichiasis and entropion, and aggressive treatment of ocular surface disease may help in achieving a better prognosis for graft survival and good visual outcomes following keratoplasty.

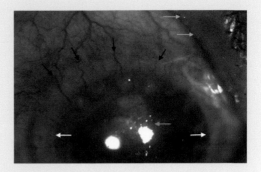

Figure 11.10 Slit lamp photograph of a patient with trachomatous keratopathy who underwent optical penetrating keratoplasty six months back showing multiple areas of suture-site vascularisation (black arrows), well-apposed graft-host junction (white arrows) and mild corneal haze (grey arrow) in the graft. Poor ocular surface and meibomian gland dysfunction (green arrows) can also be seen.

- Following keratoplasty, patients of trachoma may develop suture-related problems like suture erosions and graft melting, suture infiltrates, suture infection or suture vascularisation (Figure 11.10) due to the ongoing ocular surface disease and inflammation.

CASE 11.4

CLINICAL FEATURES

A 75-year-old male patient presented to the cornea clinic of our tertiary care hospital with symptoms of pain, redness, itching and irritation of the eyes, diminution of vision and eyelash rubbing against the eyeball over the last five years. He reported a sudden drop in vision in the right eye over the last five days. Visual acuity in the right eye was presence of perception of light with inaccurate projection of rays and appreciation of hand movements close to face in the left eye. Examination findings and slit lamp appearance of the two eyes are illustrated in Figures 11.11 and 11.12.

KEY POINTS

Diagnosis:

- The above clinical scenario describes a case with central perforated corneal ulcer with trachomatous keratopathy, uveal tissue prolapse, flat anterior chamber with infiltrates and trichiatic lashes with inflammatory lid changes.
- The other eye was diagnosed to have trachomatous keratopathy with diffuse pannus, central corneal opacity following repeated episodes of infective keratitis along with spheroidal degeneration.

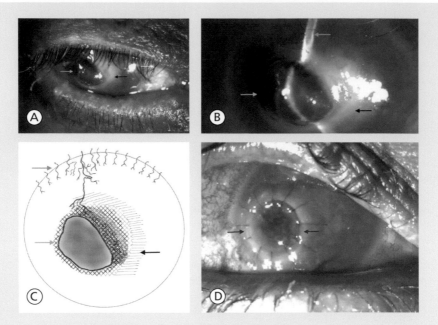

Figure 11.11   Clinical photographs of a patient with trachomatous keratopathy demonstrating (A) features of meibomian gland dysfunction and gland blockage (blue arrow) with infective keratitis that eventually developed into a large central perforated corneal ulcer with uveal tissue prolapse (yellow arrow). Note the flat anterior chamber (green arrow) as seen on the (B) magnified corneal slit view, corneal opacification (black arrow), superficial corneal vascularisation (grey arrow) at the superior limbus and upper lid trichiatic lashes (white arrow) rubbing the cornea. The corresponding schematic diagram (C) highlights these clinical findings. The patient underwent electrolysis of the metaplastic and trichiatic lashes before tectonic penetrating keratoplasty (patch graft) with iris abscission (D) in the right eye with successful postoperative outcome with restored globe integrity and well-apposed graft-host junction (red arrows).

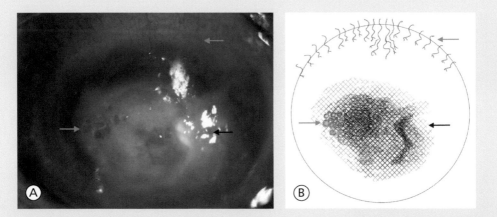

Figure 11.12   Slit lamp photograph of the left eye of Case 4 with trachomatous keratopathy demonstrating features of (A) central corneal opacity secondary to healed keratitis. Note the hypertrophic scar (black arrow) with multiple epithelial bullae (green arrow) and superficial corneal vascularisation (grey arrow), depicted in the clinical photograph and the schematic diagram (B).

Investigations:
- B-scan ultrasonography was within normal limits in both eyes.

Treatment:
- The patient was managed with topical antibiotic (moxifloxacin hydrochloride 0.5%) four times a day, cycloplegic (homatropine hydrobromide 2%), oral vitamin C (250 mg four times a day), preservative-free carboxymethylcellulose 1% along with oral and topical antiglaucoma medication to control the increased intraocular pressure.
- Electrolysis of the metaplastic and trichiatic lashes was performed before corneal grafting.
- Tectonic penetrating keratoplasty (patch graft) was performed for the right eye in view of the large central perforation.

Outcome:
- Globe integrity was maintained and patient gained a visual acuity of 6/60 with accurate projection of rays in the right eye postoperatively. Optical penetrating keratoplasty in the left eye was planned for visual rehabilitation.

Supplementary Information and Additional Tips

- Ocular surface disease and frank meibomian gland disease in patients with trachoma can lead to corneal thinning, descemetocele formation (Figure 11.13) and sterile corneal melting. The chronic state of severe desiccation, tear film instability, repeated microtrauma due to trichiatic lashes and increased immune activation in trachomatous dry eye along with lacrimal gland infiltration may contribute to corneal thinning. It needs to be effectively treated and all underlying causative factors need to be controlled to halt the process of corneal melting.

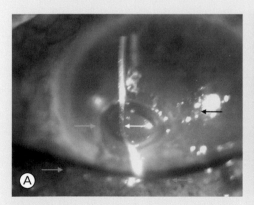
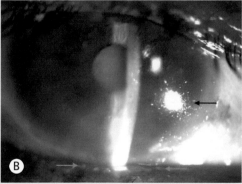

Figure 11.13 Slit lamp photograph of a patient with (A) ocular surface disease with corneal opacification (black arrow) due to trachomatous sequelae and formation of a punched-out descemetocele (yellow arrow) in the inferonasal quadrant of the left eye of the patient. Iris tissue could be visualised clearly from the thin remaining intact Descemet's membrane (white arrow). Ocular surface disease and frank meibomian gland disease (grey arrows) contributed to corneal thinning and descemetocele formation in this case. Examination of the other eye (B) revealed significant corneal xerosis, dirty tear film (black arrow), mild corneal haze and frank meibomian gland disease (grey arrows).

CASE 11.5

CLINICAL FEATURES

A 73-year-old male patient presented to our outpatient department with diminution of vision over the past two years. He had lost vision in the other eye at 40 years of age following an episode of infective keratitis. He gave a history of eyelashes rubbing the surface of the eyes with episodes of photophobia, foreign body sensation, pain and redness in that eye. Visual acuity was 2/60 and absent perception of light in right and left eye, respectively. The examination findings and slit lamp appearance are illustrated in Figure 11.14.

KEY POINTS

Diagnosis:
- The above clinical scenario describes a case of anterior corneal involvement due to trachomatous corneal opacity in right eye and chronic trachoma sequelae with phthisis bulbi as a result of long-standing infective keratitis and secondary glaucoma in the other eye.
- Other signs of trachoma sequelae like Herbert's pits, upper tarsal fibrosis, regressive pannus at the upper limbus, trichiasis and meibomian gland dysfunction were also present.

Investigations:
- Anterior segment optical coherence tomography of revealed corneal opacification up to 200 microns depth of the cornea.

Treatment:
- The patient was managed with topical antibiotic (moxifloxacin hydrochloride 0.5%, three times a day), Tab doxycycline 100 mg twice a day for two weeks, polyethylene glycol 0.4% + propylene glycol 0.3% four times a day and antibiotic ointment at night.
- The patient underwent intraoperative optical coherence tomography guided anterior lamellar therapeutic keratoplasty (ALTK) under peribulbar anaesthesia.

Outcome:
- The donor cornea remained clear on follow-up with good morphological outcome following lamellar keratoplasty.
- The patient had unaided visual acuity of 6/12 three months after surgery.

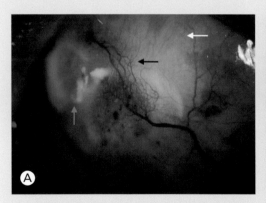
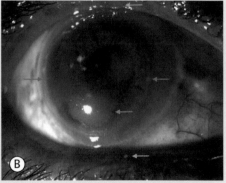

Figure 11.14 Slit lamp photograph of a patient with (A) phthisis bulbi as a result of long-standing infective keratitis occurring in an eye with trichiasis and chronic trachoma sequelae. Note the indistinguishable limbus (white arrow) with calcification (grey arrow) and dense vascularisation (black arrow). The other eye of the same patient (B) underwent sutureless lamellar keratoplasty for corneal opacification limited to anterior two-thirds of the corneal thickness. Note the clear donor graft, well-apposed graft-host junction (blue arrows) and residual fibrin glue (green arrow) at the graft-host interface. Meibomian glad plugging (yellow arrow) was also evident.

CASE 11.6

CLINICAL FEATURES

A 64-year-old male patient, resident of Etawah, Uttar Pradesh, India, presented to our tertiary eye care hospital with painless, progressive diminution of vision and foreign body sensation in the right eye for two years. He gave a history of frequent epilation of eyelashes of the upper lid. The left eye had no vision for the past five years and was diagnosed to have healed keratitis with secondary glaucoma as per hospital records. BCVA was perception of light with inaccurate projection of rays in the right eye and finger counting close to face with accurate projection of rays in the left eye. Examination findings and slit lamp appearance are illustrated in Figure 11.15.

KEY POINTS

Diagnosis:
- The above clinical scenario describes a case of trachomatous corneal opacification in the left eye and healed keratitis with corneal thinning and secondary glaucoma in the right eye.
- Other signs of trachoma sequelae like Herbert's pits, upper tarsal fibrosis, regressive pannus at the upper limbus and trichiasis were also present.

Investigations:
- B-scan ultrasonography of the left eye revealed optic nerve head cupping, suggesting the possibility of glaucoma in the left eye.

Treatment:
- The patient was managed with topical antibiotic (moxifloxacin hydrochloride 0.5%, three times a day), Tab doxycycline 100 mg twice a day for two weeks, polyethylene glycol 0.4% + propylene glycol 0.3% four times a day and antibiotic ointment at night.
- The patient underwent optical penetrating keratoplasty in the left eye under peribulbar anaesthesia.

Outcome:
- The patient had a clear graft at one-year follow-up but gained suboptimal visual acuity of 5/60 with accurate projection of rays due to glaucomatous optic nerve head damage.
- On follow-up, mucoid discharge was noted at the site of the 6 o'clock suture (Figure 11.15B), which needs to be managed in a timely manner to prevent future complications like suture infections and eventual graft rejection and graft failure.

Supplementary Information and Additional Tips

- Due to concomitant ocular surface disease, poor hygiene and ongoing inflammation in patients of trachoma, frequent follow-up to pick up early suture-related problems is advisable.

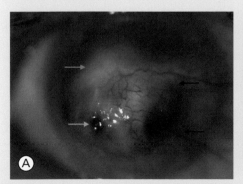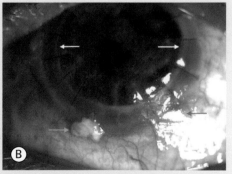

Figure 11.15 Slit lamp photograph of a patient with long-standing trachomatous corneal opacification due to healed keratitis demonstrating (A) central leucomatous corneal opacity (grey arrow) with dense vascularisation (black arrows) along with corneal thinning (green arrow). The patient underwent optical penetrating keratoplasty in the left eye for adherent leukoma and attained a clear graft (B) with well-apposed graft-host junction (white arrows). Note the mucoid discharge at the site of the 6 o'clock suture (yellow arrow), and corneal xerosis (blue arrow).

CASE 11.7

CLINICAL FEATURES

A 66-year-old male patient presented to us with sudden onset pain, redness, watering and foreign body sensation in the right eye over the past month. He had lost vision in the right eye three years back following repeated episodes of pain and redness. A history of frequent epilation of eyelashes of the upper lid was also elicited. Visual acuity recorded was finger counting close to face and 6/18 in the right and left eye, respectively. Examination findings and slit lamp appearance are illustrated in Figure 11.16.

KEY POINTS

Diagnosis:
- The above clinical scenario describes a case of infective keratitis occurring secondary to abrasions caused by inturned eyelashes in trachoma. Vascularised corneal opacity, a chronic sequela of recurrent trachomatous infection and inflammation, was present.
- Other signs of trachoma sequelae like Herbert's pits, upper tarsal fibrosis, regressive pannus at the upper limbus and trichiasis were also present bilaterally.

Investigations:
- Microbiological investigations were performed from corneal scrapings: Gram stain, Giemsa stain, calcofluor white stain, KOH mount, bacterial culture on blood agar, fungal culture on Sabouraud dextrose agar and thioglycollate broth, and drug sensitivity testing. A bacterial corneal ulcer was established as the laboratory diagnosis for this patient, due to *Staphylococcus epidermidis* growth in culture media.
- B-scan ultrasonography of left eye was anechoic.

Treatment:
- As the ulcer was small and superficial and the patient ensured compliance to treatment and follow-up, he was started on topical moxifloxacin hydrochloride 0.5% and cycloplegics. The antibiotic was prescribed hourly for first 24 hours, then every two hours for 48 hours (round the clock), then given every four hours for one week, then every six hours for a week and then tapered.
- Additionally, the patient was also prescribed Tab doxycycline 100 mg twice a day for two weeks,

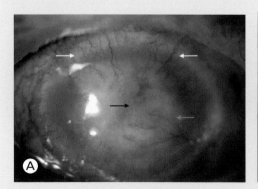
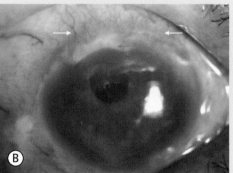

Figure 11.16 Slit lamp photograph of a patient (A) with total vascularised corneal opacity (grey arrow) with secondary infective keratitis (black arrow) occurring secondary to abrasions caused by inturned eyelashes in trachoma. Note the peripheral corneal vascularisation (white arrows), a chronic sequela of recurrent trachomatous infection and inflammation. Examination of the other eye (B) revealed Herbert's pits, superior pannus (white arrows), fibrous ingrowth scar (grey arrow) occurring post-cataract surgery and few paracentral nebulo-macular corneal opacities.

polyethylene glycol 0.4% + propylene glycol 0.3% four times a day and antibiotic ointment twice a day.

Outcome:

- The infiltrates were noted to resolve with treatment on follow-up. The signs of resolution noted were healing of the epithelial defect, decrease in size and density of infiltrates, decreasing conjunctival injection and reduced surrounding corneal oedema.
- The other eye gained useful vison with cataract surgery.

Supplementary Information and Additional Tips

- In patients with chronic trachomatous sequelae, blindness is caused by corneal opacification through the traumatic effect of entropion and/ or trichiasis and possibly secondary bacterial infection.
- Corneal scarring with vascularisation occurs due to repeated abrasions damaging the Bowman's membrane and secondary infections occur in patients with trachoma due to the inturned lashes that abrade the cornea in these individuals.
- Bacterial pathogens colonising the scarred conjunctiva may predispose to the development of corneal ulcers and the presence of dry and abraded epithelium secondary to lowered ocular defence mechanisms along with lid problems and blinking abnormalities add to the problem, thus contributing to the increased incidence of infective keratitis in patients with trachoma.

REFERENCES

1. Gupta V, Gupta N, Senjam S, Vashist P. Trachoma. In: Singh S. (eds) Neglected Tropical Diseases – South Asia. Cham: Springer; 2017.
2. Gambhir M, Basanez MG, Burton MJ, Solomon AW, Bailey RL, Holland MJ, et al. The development of an age-structured model for trachoma transmission dynamics, pathogenesis and control. PLoS Negl Trop Dis. 2009; 3(6):e462.
3. Taylor HR, Burton MJ, Haddad D, West S, Wright H. Trachoma. Lancet. 2014, 384(9960):2142–52.

12 Exposure Keratopathy

Vipul Singh, Ritika Mukhija, Radhika Tandon

INTRODUCTION

Exposure keratopathy results from persistent exposure of the ocular surface to the external environment, with drying of the cornea despite normal tear production due to abnormalities in lid closure and blinking mechanism. It results in epithelial breakdown and various complications like infective keratitis, perforation, extensive scarring and even visual loss.[1] The causative factors can be broadly classified as neurological and those occurring as a result of malposition of eyelids; the latter is usually caused by any pathology resulting in either proptosis or lagophthalmos.[2] The management of exposure keratopathy revolves around treating the underlying disorder and supportive therapy to prevent ocular damage and secondary complications.[3]

CASE 12.1

CLINICAL FEATURES

A 42-year-old female, a known case of thyroid disorder, presented with protrusion of the left eye along with redness, pain and blurring of vision for the past two weeks. There was no history of any preceding trauma. On, examination, the vision in the left eye was 1/60. Abaxial proptosis with periocular erythema, lid oedema, ptosis and incomplete left-eye closure along with exposed cornea and purulent discharge were evident. There was no restriction of extraocular movements and pupillary reactions were within normal limits. Examination findings and slit lamp appearance are illustrated in Figure 12.1.

KEY POINTS

Diagnosis:
- The above clinical scenario describes a case of thyroid eye disease (TED), left eye abaxial proptosis, exposure keratopathy and secondary infective keratitis.

Investigations:
- Investigations were done to isolate the causative organism (corneal scraping for microbiological diagnosis) and to rule out underlying causes of proptosis. The latter included complete blood count, erythrocyte sedimentation rate and thyroid function tests, which were severely deranged.
- Contrast-enhanced computed tomography of the orbit and paranasal sinus was performed to look for the extent of the pathology and to rule out orbital cellulitis; the findings were suggestive of TED.

Treatment:
- The patient was treated with fortified antibiotics (vancomycin 5% and tobramycin 1.3%) started every hour round the clock and tapered gradually as per response, along with

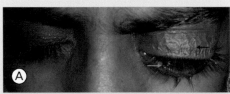
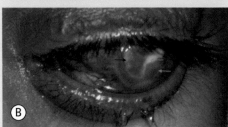

Figure 12.1 External photograph of a patient with thyroid eye disease (A) showing abaxial proptosis (black arrow) with incomplete left eye closure (yellow arrow). Ocular examination of the same eye (B) revealing infective keratitis with epithelial defect (black arrow), infiltrates (yellow arrow), hypopyon and vascularisation (grey arrow).

cycloplegic (homatropine 2%) and antiglaucoma medications.

- A cover ointment of gatifloxacin 0.3% twice a day along with preservative-free lubricants was also given.
- Patient was referred to the endocrinology department for management of acute thyroid storm.

Outcome:
- The infective keratitis responded to medical management and the ulcer healed, leaving a residual macular corneal opacity, in around six weeks.

Supplementary Information and Additional Tips

- TED is the most common cause of proptosis, bilateral or unilateral, in the adult age group. Other causes are orbital tumours, neurofibromatosis, carotid-cavernous sinus fistulae, arachnoid cysts, craniosynostosis syndromes, Cushing syndrome and ocular trauma.
- Although TED usually has a slowly progressive clinical course, acute-on-chronic presentations may occur, as in the current case.
- Proptosis may limit complete eye closure in some cases, leading to exposure keratopathy; supportive management in the form of lubrication and eyelid closure as appropriate is important to prevent drastic complications like infective keratitis and orbital cellulitis.

CASE 12.2

CLINICAL FEATURES

A 70-year-old female presented with redness, watering and foreign body sensation in the left eye for the past four weeks. She underwent left-eye cataract surgery 15 years ago. Examination findings and slit lamp appearance are illustrated in Figure 12.2.

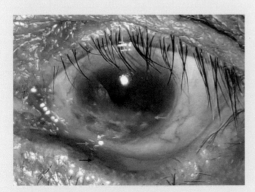

Figure 12.2 External photograph of a patient with left eye lower lid ectropion showing loss of lower lid-globe apposition (black arrow), inferior conjunctival congestion, pooling of fluorescein dye in inferior fornix (grey arrow) and fluorescein stained epithelial breakdown in inferior third of the cornea (yellow arrow).

KEY POINTS

Diagnosis:
- The above clinical scenario describes a case of left eye lower lid senile ectropion with exposure keratopathy.

Investigations:
- The diagnosis is based on clinical history and examination findings; baseline tests for ocular surface health (Schirmer's, tear break-up time and surface staining scores) along with a detailed workup for ectropion, including assessment of lid laxity, canthal tendon laxity and lower lid retractors, were performed.

Treatment:
- The patient was managed on preservative-free topical lubricants every two hours (carboxymethylcellulose 1%) and topical antibiotic (moxifloxacin hydrochloride 0.5%) four times a day to prevent secondary bacterial infection.
- Ointment vitamin A with carbomer at night followed by lid taping during sleeping was advised till ectropion surgery was planned. Subsequently, lazy-T ectropion repair was done for lower lid involutional ectropion.

Outcome:

- Lid-globe contact was regained and the epithelial defect healed with the appearance of a peripheral corneal opacity.

Supplementary Information and Additional Tips

- Senile ectropion may be associated with lagophthalmos and exposure keratitis (Figure 12.3). Conservative management and supportive care for corneal exposure are important in such cases; even surgical correction of lid position may be required in some cases.

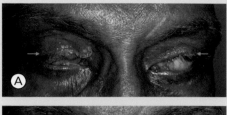
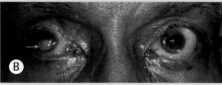

Figure 12.3 External photograph of a patient with bilateral lower lid ectropion and significant lagophthalmos (A) demonstrating inability to fully close both eyes (yellow arrows) and inferior conjunctival congestion (grey arrow) in the right eye. On opening the eyes (B), exposure keratopathy with inferior corneal opacity (yellow arrows) is evident in both eyes.

CASE 12.3

CLINICAL FEATURES

A 65-year-old male presented with complaints of appearance of white patch in his right eye, along with redness and blurring of vision for the past one week. He had a history of a stroke three months back, following which he developed right-sided hemiplegia and facial nerve palsy. He was hospitalised for about three weeks and was advised lubricating eye drops and nighttime eye taping to prevent exposure keratopathy in the right eye by the ophthalmologist on discharge. Examination findings and slit lamp appearance are illustrated in Figure 12.4.

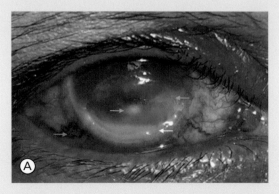
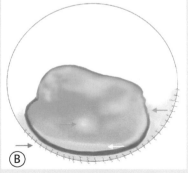

Figure 12.4 Slit lamp photograph (A) and corresponding corneal diagram (B) of a case of exposure keratopathy with secondary infective keratitis in a patient with facial nerve palsy. Note the large epithelial defect (green arrow), few stromal infiltrates (yellow arrow), hypopyon (white arrow) and ciliary congestion (grey arrow).

KEY POINTS

Diagnosis:

- The above clinical scenario describes a case of exposure keratopathy with secondary infective keratitis and hypopyon in a patient with facial nerve palsy.
- He was unable to close the right eye completely with significant lagophthalmos and a poor Bell's response resulting in exposure of the inferior half of cornea.

Investigations:

- The diagnosis was based on clinical history and examination findings; however, corneal scraping was sent for microbiological investigations to identify the causative organism.

Treatment:

- Patient was treated with fortified antibiotics, cycloplegic drops, preservative-free lubricants and nighttime antibiotic ointment followed by taping of the eye lid.
- As the infiltrates resolved, antibiotics were decreased in frequency and lubricants stepped up, which were continued even after the ulcer healed.

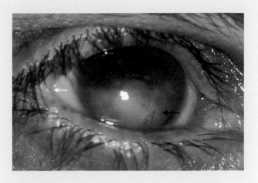

Figure 12.5 Slit lamp photograph of a patient demonstrating exposure keratopathy sequelae (secondary to facial nerve palsy) in the form of inferior vascularised corneal opacity in the right eye (black arrow), that occurred consequent to infective keratitis. Note the lateral tarsorrhaphy (white arrow) in situ.

Outcome:

- Patient showed reasonable response to treatment, and the ulcer healed with formations of nebular corneal opacity in about four weeks of treatment.
- More severe cases of keratitis may result in a denser corneal opacity (Figure 12.5) and may benefit with a temporary or permanent tarsorrhaphy.

REFERENCES

1. Bernard H. Clinical Approach to Ocular Surface Disorders. BCSC series: Pediatric Ophthalmology and Strabismus. USA: American Academy of Ophthalmology; 2017.
2. Kersten Robert C. Chapter 30 – Lagophthalmos and Other Malpositions of the Lid. In: Cornea; Volume 1 – Fundamentals and Medical Aspects of Cornea and External Disease. 3rd ed. USA: Elsevier; 2011.
3. Kousha O, Kousha Z, Paddle J. Exposure keratopathy: incidence, risk factors and impact of protocolised care on exposure keratopathy in critically ill adults. J Crit Care. 2018 Apr; 44:413–8.

POSTSURGICAL INFECTION AND INFLAMMATION

13 Post-Keratoplasty Corneal Infection and Inflammation

Aishwarya Rathod, Pooja Kumari, T Monikha, M Vanathi, Radhika Tandon

INTRODUCTION

Corneal transplantation is an effective mode of therapy for visual rehabilitation of people blind from corneal diseases. Infectious keratitis after penetrating keratoplasty can be devastating to the survival of the graft and consequently, affect the final visual outcome. The precipitating factors for development of infection after any corneal transplant include compromised ocular surface, persistent epithelial defect, suture-related problems, use of bandage contact lenses, trichiasis, dry eye and lid abnormalities along with systemic immunocompromised state.[1] Appropriate preventive measures need to be implemented along with close monitoring of the corneal graft after the surgical procedure to ensure long-term success following keratoplasty. It is imperative to be aware of such complications and risk factors in patients with lamellar or full-thickness corneal transplants to improve their prognostic outcome.[2,3]

Corneal graft rejection, another important cause of graft failure, refers to a specific immunological response of the host to the donor corneal transplant tissue, demonstrating findings like keratic precipitates with or without corneal oedema (total or differential) and anterior chamber cell and flare after the initial resolution of perioperative inflammation. It should be distinguished from other non-immune mediated causes of corneal graft failure. The incidence of graft rejection is greatest in the first year-and-a-half following transplant but can occur up to 20 years or more after surgery.[4]

CASE 13.1

CLINICAL FEATURES

A 60-year-old female presented with sudden onset pain, redness and diminution of vision of the right eye for the past two weeks. She gave a history of undergoing corneal transplantation in the same eye one month back for healed viral keratitis. Her visual acuity was 6/60 with accurate projection of rays in all quadrants. Examination findings and slit lamp appearance are illustrated in Figure 13.1.

KEY POINTS

Diagnosis:
- The above clinical scenario describes a case of corneal abscess following optical penetrating keratoplasty (PKP).

Investigations:
- Microbiological investigations were performed from corneal scrapings. The diagnosis was confirmed on KOH mount of the specimen obtained

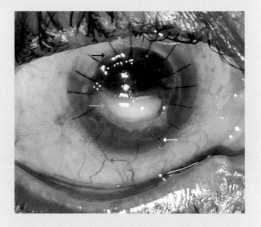

Figure 13.1 Slit lamp photograph of a patient who underwent optical penetrating keratoplasty for adherent leucoma and developed infective keratitis with formation of a corneal abscess (yellow arrow) in the donor cornea one month after the keratoplasty with a well-apposed graft-host junction (black arrow). Note the loose suture (white arrow) at the 4 o'clock position with surrounding corneal vascularisation (grey arrow).

through corneal scraping. Culture on Sabouraud dextrose agar and thioglycollate broth demonstrated colonies of filamentous fungi, *Aspergillus* species.
- Corneal sensation was reduced.
- Ultrasound B-scan was anechoic and did not reveal any posterior segment abnormality.

Treatment:
- The patient was treated with natamycin ophthalmic suspension (5%) every hour for 48 hours followed by tapering the frequency based on the clinical response, prophylactic topical antibiotic (moxifloxacin hydrochloride 0.5% four times a day), cycloplegic (homatropine hydrobromide 2% three times a day) and lubricants (preservative-free carboxymethylcellulose 0.5% six times a day). A two-week course of oral ketoconazole (200 mg two times a day) was added.
- Oral acyclovir 400 mg five times a day for two weeks followed by 400 mg twice a day for one year was prescribed on regular monitoring of her liver and renal function tests.

Outcome:
- The infiltrates were noted to resolve with treatment on follow-up. The lesion responded to treatment and healed within a month of starting therapy with a residual corneal opacity.

Supplementary Information and Additional Tips
- Predisposing factors for development of infective keratitis after optical PKP are persistent epithelial defects, use of contact lens, dry eye and poor ocular surface and suture-related problems. Other pre-existing conditions such as meibomitis, dacryocystitis and blepharitis can also lead to graft tissue infections.
- Poor ocular surface and a previous history of viral keratitis can lead to epithelial disruption and invasion by fungal organisms in the use of topical steroids that are part of the routine postoperative regimen (Figure 13.2).
- Loose sutures and partially removed sutures at the graft-host junction serve as nidus of infection and lead to complications like graft infection and early appearance of focal corneal infiltrates (Figure 13.3).

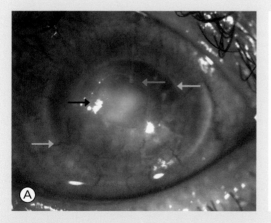
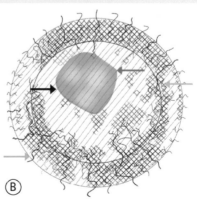

Figure 13.2 Slit lamp photograph of a patient with operated penetrating keratoplasty demonstrating (A) a fungal corneal ulcer of the graft cornea (black arrow) with well-defined margins (grey arrow) following overuse of topical steroids. Patient was operated on for optical penetrating keratoplasty for corneal opacity with poor ocular surface. Note the well-apposed graft-host junction (green arrow) and 360° corneal neovascularisation (yellow arrow). The corresponding corneal diagram (B) depicts the same findings.

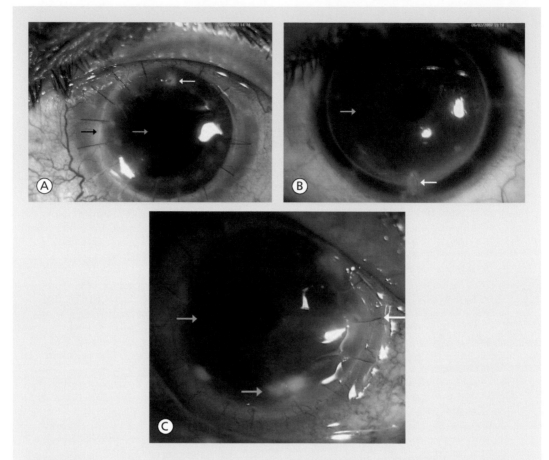

Figure 13.3 Slit lamp photographs demonstrating (A) a broken suture (white arrow) in a case of operated optical keratoplasty showing an optically clear graft (yellow arrow) and healed graft-host junction (black arrow), (B) a loose suture at the 6 o'clock position (white arrow) and intact graft-host junction (black arrow) in an optically clear graft (yellow arrow), and (C) shows multiple loose sutures (white arrow) associated with corneal infiltrates (blue arrow) with clear graft (yellow arrow) in the superior aspect.

- Late graft infections can occur in eyes with poor ocular surface even in the absence of sutures and present as hypopyon corneal ulcers (Figure 13.4).
- In patients with poor ocular surface with ongoing meibomian gland dysfunction, especially in cases with chronic trachomatous inflammation, corneal grafting may be complicated by poor epithelial healing and sterile corneal stromal lysis, especially at the graft-host junction (Figure 13.5).
- Suture-related graft infection may lead to subsequent episodes of graft rejection seen initially as focal corneal oedema and Descemet's membrane folds (Figure 13.6), an important cause of graft failure in developing countries.

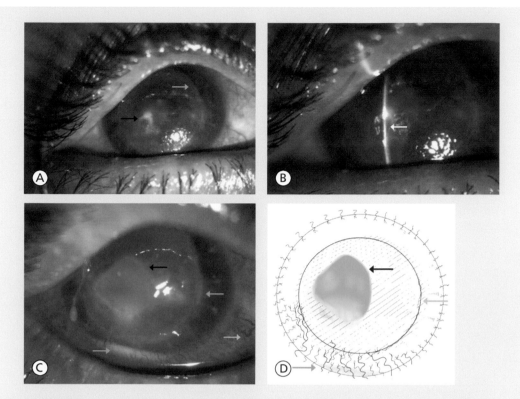

Figure 13.4 Slit lamp photograph of a patient who underwent penetrating keratoplasty ten years ago demonstrating (A) corneal infiltrates (black arrow) in the graft with well-apposed graft-host junction (yellow arrow). On slit illumination (B) corneal thinning (white arrow) and ulceration can be seen. The ulcer progressed (C) to a larger corneal ulcer (black arrow) with hypopyon (blue arrow). Note the well-apposed graft-host junction (yellow arrow) with surrounding conjunctival congestion (green arrow). The corresponding corneal findings (D) are illustrated in a schematic diagram.

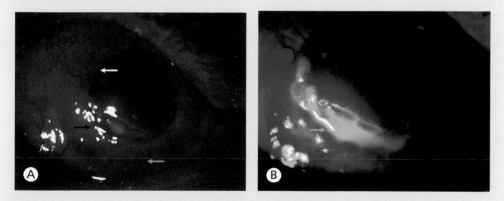

Figure 13.5 Slit lamp photograph of a patient with operated penetrating keratoplasty with poor ocular surface demonstrating (A) a peripheral corneal ulcer (black arrow) in the inferotemporal quadrant near the graft-host junction with 360° of superficial vascularisation (green arrow) with intact graft-host junction (white arrow). Examination under cobalt blue filter after fluorescein staining (B) demonstrated corneal thinning and melting at the graft-host junction, highlighting the circumferential epithelial defect (yellow arrow).

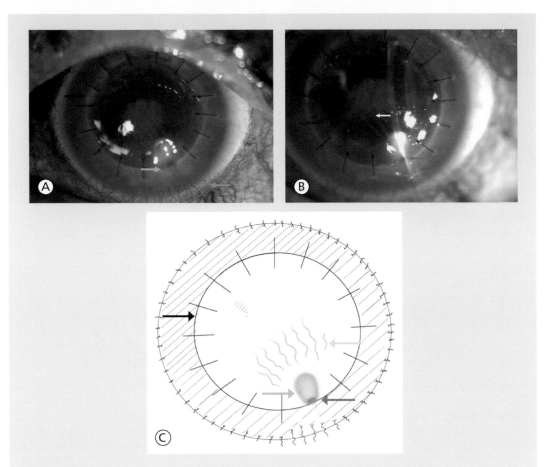

Figure 13.6 Slit lamp photograph of a patient who underwent optical penetrating keratoplasty for macular corneal dystrophy shows (A) well-apposed graft-host junction (black arrow) along with intact and buried sutures. Suture-induced keratitis (yellow arrow) with circumcorneal congestion (green arrow) can be seen. The magnified view (B) focusses on the surrounding corneal infiltrate along with corneal thinning (grey arrow) with Descemet's membrane folds (white arrow). The corresponding schematic diagram (C) highlights the salient features.

CASE 13.2

CLINICAL FEATURES

A 41-year-old female with a history of right eye bullous keratopathy with keratoconjunctivitis sicca underwent optical PKP five months ago. She presented with symptoms of mild photophobia, redness, watering and diminution of vision in the right eye over the past six days. Examination findings and slit lamp appearance at presentation and follow-up are illustrated in Figure 13.7.

KEY POINTS

Diagnosis:
- The above clinical scenario describes a case of corneal graft rejection following PKP.

Investigations:
- In most of the cases, the diagnosis is based on clinical features. Fluorescein staining did not reveal any epithelial defect.

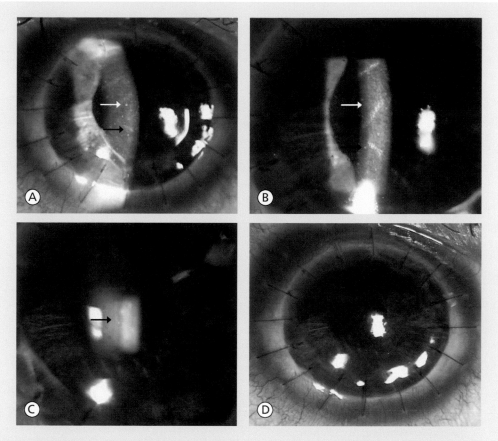

Figure 13.7 Slit lamp photographs (A) and (B) of a patient who underwent penetrating keratoplasty five months ago demonstrating a corneal graft with differential oedema (black arrow) and fresh keratic precipitates (white arrow) indicating graft rejection when examined under slit illumination. The sutures are all buried and intact and the graft clarity is 3+ in the centre. The graft-host junction appears healthy. Slit lamp photograph (C) shows the narrow slit demonstrating the anterior chamber flare in this case of graft rejection. On follow-up (D), the patient responded to therapy with minimal to nil keratic precipitates and resolved corneal oedema (black arrow).

- Anterior segment optical coherence tomography (AS-OCT) revealed a central corneal thickness of 604 microns.

Treatment:
- The patient was treated with intravenous methylprednisolone 1 mg/kg as per body weight for three days, and then put on oral corticosteroids for two weeks.
- Topical prednisolone (1%) every hour was prescribed for three days and was tapered to six times a day after the corneal oedema and keratic precipitates subsided. Additionally,

a topical antibiotic (moxifloxacin hydrochloride 0.5% four times a day) and cycloplegic (homatropine hydrobromide 2% three times a day) was also prescribed.
- Lubricants (carboxymethylcellulose 1% four times a day) and topical timolol maleate 0.5% twice a day were continued as before.

Outcome:
- Corneal oedema and keratic precipitates reduced significantly within a week of therapy, and the visual acuity improved to 6/12.

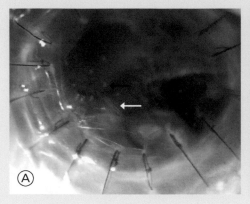
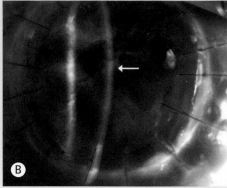

Figure 13.8 Slit lamp photograph of a patient showing (A) features of graft rejection in the form of keratic precipitates (black arrow) and corneal oedema (white arrow). Posterior synechiae and an irregular pupil (B) can also be seen with corneal oedema (white arrow) in another patient who underwent therapeutic keratoplasty for infective keratitis.

Supplementary Information and Additional Tips

- Graft rejection can occur after therapeutic PKP for infective keratitis (Figure 13.8) or as a consequence of graft infection post-PKP (Figure 13.9).
- The risk factors for graft rejection post-PKP include preoperative inflammation, deep corneal neovascularisation (more than two quadrants), peripheral anterior synechiae, large grafts, prior ocular surgery or use of glaucoma medication, prior rejection episode, loose sutures (Figure 13.10), suture track infection and recurrent herpetic infection.
- Endothelial rejection is the most common form of graft rejection, seen as a rejection line named the Khodadoust line (Figure 13.11) that starts in the periphery of the graft, associated with segmental corneal oedema.
- The presence of Descemet's folds can be an early marker of rejection before the development of frank stromal oedema (Figure 13.12).

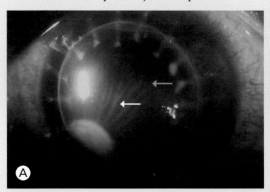
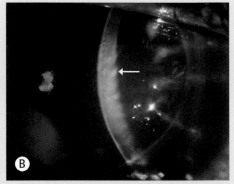

Figure 13.9 Slit lamp photograph of a patient who developed suture-related keratitis following optical penetrating keratoplasty showing (A) corneal infiltrates inferotemporally (black arrow) with localised vascularisation and stromal oedema with prominent Descemet's folds (white arrow). A prominent Khodadoust line (blue arrow), an endothelial rejection line that separates the immunologically damaged endothelium from the clear cornea superiorly, can clearly be seen. Slit illumination demonstrates (B) significant corneal oedema (white arrow) due to graft rejection precipitated by graft infection (black arrow).

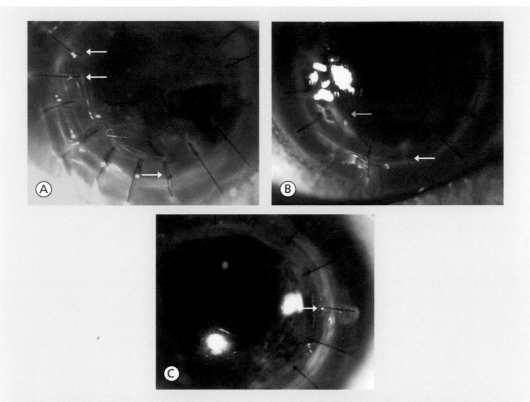

Figure 13.10 Slit lamp photographs (A–C) of three different patients showing penetrating keratoplasty grafts with loose sutures (white arrows) and keratic precipitates (black arrow) and stromal oedema (yellow arrow), suggesting episodes of graft rejection associated with the occurrence and removal of loose sutures in some of these corneal grafts.

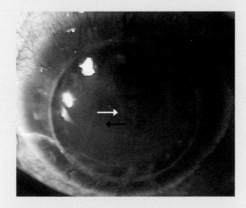

Figure 13.11 Slit lamp photograph showing corneal graft rejection in a patient with operated penetrating keratoplasty. The graft clarity is impaired because of the corneal oedema (white arrow). The rejection line (Khodadoust line) is visible passing near the centre of the graft (black arrow). All the sutures have been removed and corneal vascularisation has set in.

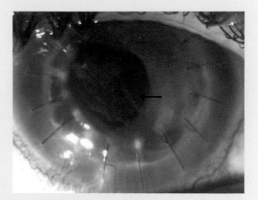

Figure 13.12 Slit lamp photograph of a patient who underwent optical penetrating keratoplasty showing almost minimal to nil keratic precipitates and mild corneal oedema but significant Descemet's folds (black arrow) indicating an early case of graft rejection.

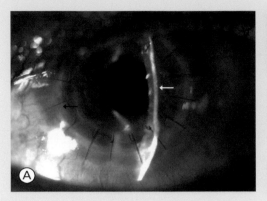
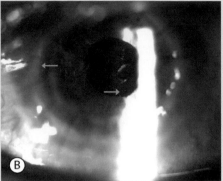

Figure 13.13 Slit lamp photograph of a patient who developed recurrence of viral keratitis following optical penetrating keratoplasty for healed viral keratitis showing (A) graft oedema (white arrow) with Descemet's folds, more so in the host cornea and buried sutures (black arrow). Slit illumination demonstrates (B) the cells in the anterior chamber (blue arrow), signifying inflammation due to an acute episode of viral keratitis along with a well-apposed graft-host junction (yellow arrow).

- Sequential recording of corneal pachymetry can serve as a useful marker to assess response to therapy of rejection in cases of acute corneal graft rejection.
- An important differential diagnosis of corneal graft rejection is recurrence of viral keratitis in a graft. The point to differentiate between the two is that graft rejection involves the donor cornea while recurrence of viral keratitis is seen as anterior segment inflammation and graft oedema involving the host cornea in the initial stages (Figure 13.13).

CASE 13.3

CLINICAL FEATURES

A 49-year-old male with a history of Fuchs' endothelial corneal dystrophy and open-angle glaucoma underwent Descemet's stripping automated endothelial keratoplasty (DSAEK) in the left eye eight months ago. He currently presented with symptoms of mild photophobia, pain, watering and diminution of vision for three days. He had been prescribed topical steroids postoperatively but had not been compliant with the same. Examination findings and slit lamp appearance are illustrated in Figure 13.14.

KEY POINTS

Diagnosis:
- The above clinical scenario describes a case of corneal graft rejection following DSAEK.

Treatment:
- The patient was treated with intravenous pulse therapy of methylprednisolone 1 mg/kg as per body weight for three consecutive days and then shifted to oral corticosteroids (60 mg once daily) for two weeks.
- The patient was also started on topical prednisolone 1% one hourly for two days and was tapered to six times a day from the third day. The patient was also treated with a short course of topical antibiotic (moxifloxacin 0.5% four times a day), cycloplegic (homatropine 2% thrice a day), glaucoma medication (combination of timolol maleate 0.5% and brimonidine tartrate 0.2% twice a day) and preservative-free lubricants.

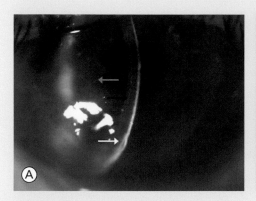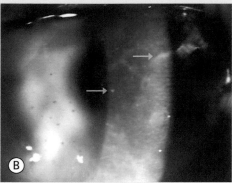

Figure 13.14 Slit lamp photograph of a patient who underwent Descemet's stripping automated endothelial keratoplasty (DSAEK) for pseudophakic corneal decompensation showing (A) features of graft rejection in the form of corneal oedema (grey arrow) and subepithelial oedema (white arrow). Note the interface between the DSAEK graft and the host cornea on the narrow slit (black arrow). The magnified view under slit illumination demonstrates (B) corneal oedema and Descemet's membrane folds (grey arrow) along with keratic precipitates (blue arrow).

Outcome:

- The oedema and the keratic precipitates responded to treatment and the visual acuity gradually improved to that before this episode. The intraocular pressure was controlled on the prescribed drugs on follow-up.
- The patient was counselled regarding the need for compliance to these medications to prevent further such episodes.

Supplementary Information and Additional Tips

- The oedema can be used to monitor the response to treatment and can be easily seen on retro-illumination (Figure 13.15) during slit lamp biomicroscopy or quantitatively measured via pachymetry on AS-OCT.

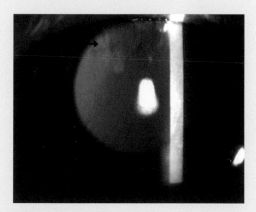

Figure 13.15 Slit lamp photograph showing a patient with acute graft rejection showing corneal oedema superiorly (black arrow), enhanced on retro-illumination as an area filled with fluid.

CASE 13.4

CLINICAL FEATURES

A 63-year-old male patient presented to the outpatient department with symptoms of pain, redness, watering and diminution of vision in the right eye for the previous 15 days. Previous treatment records from elsewhere revealed that the patient had undergone therapeutic keratoplasty of his right eye one month ago and was

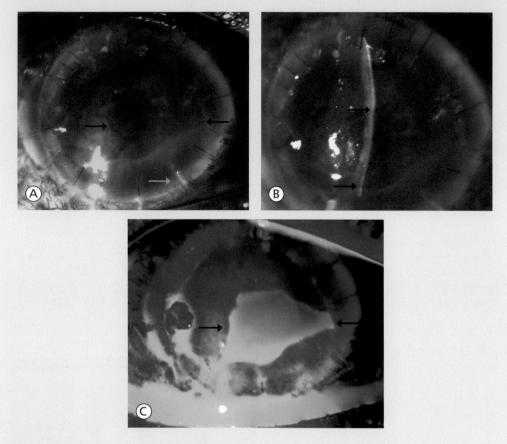

Figure 13.16 Slit lamp photograph of a patient who underwent large graft therapeutic keratoplasty revealing (A) loose and broken sutures (blue arrow) along with central epithelial defect with well-defined horizontal margins (black arrows) and (B) vertical margins (black arrows) with diffuse corneal oedema. Examination under cobalt blue filter after fluorescein staining (C) reveals a 6×4 mm epithelial defect (black arrows) on the corneal graft due to poor ocular surface.

receiving only topical antibiotics for the same. Examination findings and slit lamp appearance are illustrated in Figure 13.16.

KEY POINTS

Diagnosis:
- The above clinical scenario describes a case of right eye surface epithelial keratopathy post-PKP.

Investigations:
- The diagnosis is straightforward and based on clinical features. Fluorescein staining revealed an epithelial defect measuring 6×4 mm.

Treatment:
- This patient was managed with amniotic membrane transplantation and a bandage contact lens (BCL) was placed at the end of the procedure.
- The patient was also started on frequent preservative-free lubricants (carboxymethylcellulose 1%), carbomer and vitamin A ointment at night and preservative-free antibiotics.

Outcome:
- The epithelial defect responded to the treatment and healed without any scar in three weeks. The BCL was removed at four weeks.

Supplementary Information and Additional Tips

- Persistent corneal epithelial defects (PEDs) are defined as a full-thickness loss of epithelial cells that fail to show healing during a given time course of usually two weeks. These disorders cause prolonged inflammation of the ocular surface, which might alter limbal stem cells (LSCs) and the epithelial basement membrane.
- The standard therapies in the treatment of PEDs include artificial lubrication, discontinuation of toxic medications, lacrimal punctal closure, BCL, debridement and tarsorrhaphy (Figure 13.17). The newer therapies consist of amniotic membrane grafting, autologous serum, whole blood-derived products, LSC transplantation and scleral contact lenses.

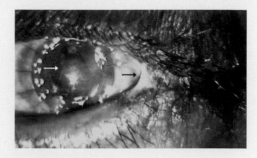

Figure 13.17 Slit lamp photograph of a patient who underwent lateral tarsorrhaphy (black arrow) for non-healing persistent epithelial defect following penetrating keratoplasty; now shows nebulo-macular corneal opacity (white arrow) with no evidence of epithelial defect.

CASE 13.5

CLINICAL FEATURES

A 47-year-old male presented with history of trauma to left eye with an iron nail while working in a factory. He presented to the local hospital for sudden onset pain, redness and discharge. Subsequently, he developed infective keratitis and underwent therapeutic keratoplasty. Two weeks after the surgery, he again presented with pain and discharge. Examination findings and slit lamp appearance are illustrated in Figure 13.18.

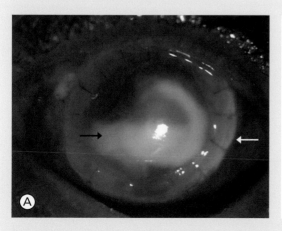
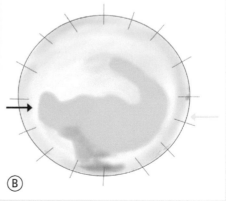

Figure 13.18 Slit lamp photograph of a patient demonstrating (A) anterior chamber exudates (black arrow) two weeks after therapeutic penetrating keratoplasty. Note the oedematous donor cornea with intact sutures and well-apposed graft-host junction (white arrow) at the limbus. The corresponding schematic diagram (B) illustrates the same findings.

KEY POINTS

Diagnosis:
- The above clinical scenario describes a case of post-therapeutic keratoplasty reinfection.

Investigations:
- In this case, a loose suture was removed and sent for bacterial and fungal culture sensitivity. However, the smear and culture reports turned out to be negative in view of previous use of antibiotics and antifungals following therapeutic keratoplasty.
- The host cornea was sent for microbiological investigations at the time of therapeutic keratoplasty. The diagnosis was confirmed by a fungal culture that grew colonies of *Aspergillus flavus* and histopathological

assessment of the host corneal button that demonstrated filamentous fungi.

Treatment:
- The patient was managed with topical and systemic antifungals along with intracameral voriconazole (50 μg/0.1 ml).

Outcome:
- The lesion responded to medical management and subsequently the graft failed on follow-up.

Supplementary Information and Additional Tips
- Poor compliance to antifungal therapy following therapeutic keratoplasty may lead to graft infections with corneal melting (Figure 13.19). Hence

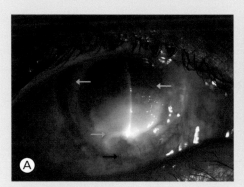
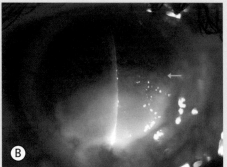
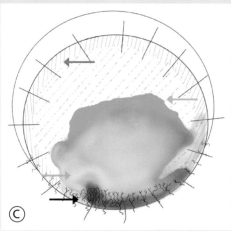

Figure 13.19 Slit lamp photograph of a patient with graft reinfection demonstrating (A) corneal melting (yellow arrow) with loose sutures at 6 o'clock position (black arrow), overlying epithelial defect (green arrow) and intact graft-host junction (grey arrow). The magnified view (B) shows the same findings with well-defined margins of the overlying epithelial defect (green arrow). The corresponding schematic diagram (C) shows the same findings.

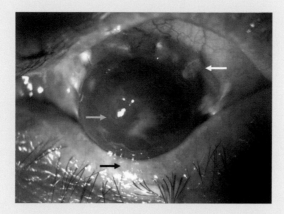

Figure 13.20 Slit lamp photograph of a patient who underwent therapeutic keratoplasty three months prior and presented with total graft melt, iris prolapse and formation of anterior staphyloma (yellow arrow). Multiple loose sutures at the limbus with a small area of host cornea (white arrow) along with indentation of the lower eyelid (black arrow) due to the bulging staphyloma are also noted.

strict drug compliance and control of systemic co-morbidities are very critical in post-therapeutic PK cases for effective management and outcomes.

■ In certain cases, total graft melt with consequent iris prolapse and formation of anterior staphyloma (Figure 13.20) may be observed, especially in cases infected with highly virulent organisms.

CASE 13.6

CLINICAL FEATURES

A 30-year-old female presented with sudden onset redness, pain and diminution of vision of the left eye following deep anterior lamellar keratoplasty (DALK) for advanced keratoconus. A few weeks after the surgery she noticed diminution of vision, watering and redness. Due to the pandemic and lockdown, she was unable to procure medications and hence could not comply with the prescribed postoperative treatment. Examination findings and slit lamp appearance at presentation and follow-up are illustrated in Figure 13.21.

KEY POINTS

Diagnosis:
■ The above clinical scenario describes a case of post-DALK interface infective keratitis.

Investigations:
■ In this case, loose sutures were removed and sent for microbiological evaluation and culture sensitivity which showed *Staphylococcus epidermidis* which was sensitive to moxifloxacin, vancomycin and tobramycin.

Treatment:
■ The patient was managed with topical fortified antibiotics (cefazolin 5% and tobramycin 1.3%) every two hours for two days and was tapered to six times a day from the third day. The patient was also treated with cycloplegic (homatropine 2% thrice a day), glaucoma medication (combination of timolol maleate 0.5% and brimonidine tartrate 0.2% twice a day) and preservative-free lubricants. Gatifloxacin ointment 0.3% was applied at night.

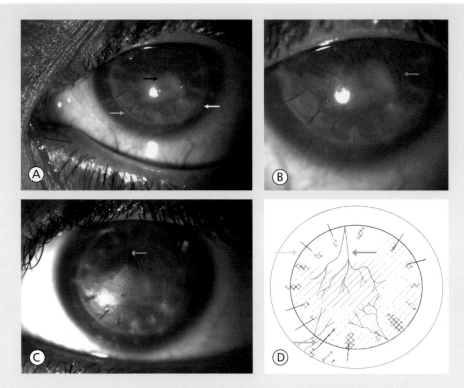

Figure 13.21 Slit lamp photograph of a patient who developed interface keratitis following deep anterior lamellar keratoplasty (DALK) for keratoconus showing (A) exudates with vascularisation in the interface (black arrow) with well-apposed graft-host junction (white arrow) and residual intact sutures (yellow arrow). On higher magnification (B) corneal striae (grey arrow) and infective exudates with deep vascularisation, are seen clearly. The interface keratitis resolved within three months of therapy showing (C) a clear graft, residual sutures and deep vessels in the interface (blue arrow), well illustrated in (D) the corresponding schematic diagram.

Outcome:

- The lesion responded to treatment and on follow-up after three months, the keratitis had resolved, the graft had cleared up with residual haze inferiorly and vascularisation was noted in the interface due to the healing process.

Supplementary Information and Additional Tips

- Patients with poor ocular surface, as occurs with chemical injury and consequent 360° limbal stem cell deficiency (LSCD) treated with simple limbal epithelium transplant (SLET) are prone to develop graft infections (Figure 13.22) after DALK for visual rehabilitation.
- Graft replacement in these patients with post-DALK infective keratitis is the eventual treatment option (Figure 13.23).
- In severe cases of LSCD and ongoing inflammation, extensive conjunctivalisation and graft failure may occur after lamellar keratoplasty (Figure 13.24).

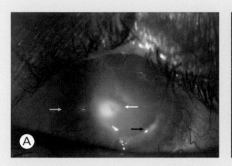
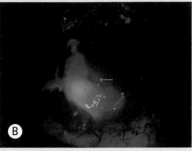

Figure 13.22 Slit lamp photograph of a patient who underwent deep anterior lamellar keratoplasty (DALK) following simple limbal epithelium transplant (SLET) for limbal stem cell deficiency demonstrating (A) infective keratitis (white arrow) with necrotic ulcer margin (black arrow) and loose sutures (yellow arrow). Fluorescein-stained cornea reveals (B) the epithelial defect (grey arrow) on cobalt blue filter with superficial vascularisation (red arrow).

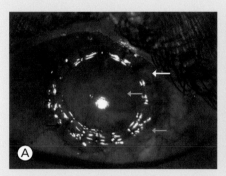
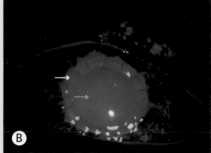

Figure 13.23 Slit lamp photograph of a patient who underwent graft replacement following post-DALK infective keratitis demonstrating (A) hazy graft with no evidence of infection, well-apposed graft-host junction (white arrow), intact sutures (black arrow) along with 360° limbal stem cell deficiency (green arrow). Note the vascularised posterior corneal bed of the host cornea due to LSCD. The total corneal epithelial defect of the donor cornea (yellow arrow) on cobalt blue filter (B) with well-apposed graft-host junction (white arrow) is evident on fluorescein staining.

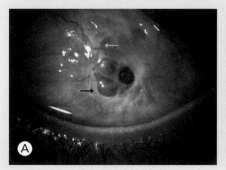
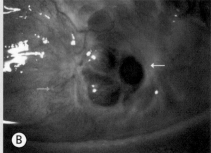

Figure 13.24 Slit lamp photograph of a child who underwent manual lamellar keratoplasty demonstrating (A) conjunctivalisation and limbal stem cell deficiency (green arrow) with total corneal melt and exposed uveal tissue (black arrow). The magnified view reveals (B) deeply buried sutures (yellow arrow) of the previous surgery and scarred fibrous tissue (white arrow) with central corneal thinning.

CASE 13.7

CLINICAL FEATURES

A 75-year-old female presented with sudden onset redness, pain and discharge of the left eye following DSAEK surgery for decompensated cornea. Intraoperatively, the unhealthy epithelium was debrided for better visualisation. Surgery was uneventful and a BCL was placed at the end of the surgery. Visual acuity at presentation was appreciation of hand movements close to face with accurate projection of rays. Examination findings and slit lamp appearance at presentation and follow-up are illustrated in Figure 13.25.

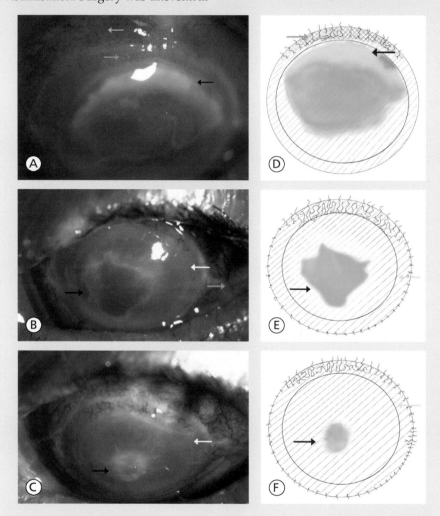

Figure 13.25 Slit lamp photograph of an elderly female who underwent Descemet's stripping automated endothelial keratoplasty (DSAEK) and developed infective keratitis showing (A) tissue necrosis, epithelial defect and infiltrates (black arrow), surrounding congestion (green arrow) with superficial corneal vascularisation (blue arrow). The patient responded to therapy (B) and the corneal infiltrates reduced in size (black arrow) by the end of two weeks. The peripheral margin of the posterior donor lenticule (white arrow) and conjunctival congestion (green arrow) are evident. After four weeks of therapy (C), the epithelial defect reduced in size and measured 2×2 mm (black arrow). The donor corneal graft (white arrow) was clearly seen. The corresponding schematic diagrams at presentation (D), and after two (E) and four weeks (F) of therapy illustrate the salient findings.

KEY POINTS

Diagnosis:

- The above clinical scenario describes a case of infective keratitis following DSAEK.

Investigations:

- The BCL was sent for microbiological evaluation.
- The corneal scraping specimens were inoculated onto culture and showed growth of *Pseudomonas aeruginosa* which was sensitive to Polymyxin B, piperacillin, tazobactam and resistant to all other available antibiotics.

Treatment:

- The patient was started on topical fortified Polymyxin B and topical piperacillin/tazobactam eye drops round the clock and tapered based on the response after 48 hours after confirming the organism on bacterial culture sensitivity.

Outcome:

- As the treatment was initiated early, with the strong possibility of hospital-acquired infection, the infiltrates reduced within a week of treatment and completely healed with a residual macular corneal opacity.
- Eventually, the donor endothelial graft failed due to postoperative insult of infection and the patient underwent PKP for visual restoration.

Supplementary Information and Additional Tips

- In patients with sutured surgical wounds and poor ocular hygiene, suture-related total graft infection may occur following DSAEK that necessitates surgical intervention for control of infection in the form of large graft therapeutic keratoplasty (Figure 13.26).
- Diabetic patients undergoing DSAEK are prone to develop endophthalmitis (Figure 13.27).

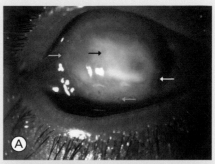

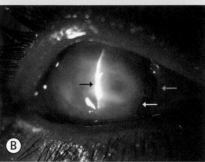

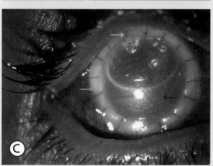

Figure 13.26 Slit lamp photograph of a patient presenting with total graft infection following Descemet's stripping automated endothelial keratoplasty (DSAEK) showing (A) corneal infiltrates (black arrow) involving the donor lenticule (white arrow) along with superficial vascularisation (green arrow) and loose suture (yellow arrow) securing the entry wound of the previous surgery. Slit illumination (B) shows corneal thinning (black arrow) and surrounding vascularisation (green arrow) with the visible peripheral edge of the donor lenticule (white arrow). The patient underwent therapeutic penetrating keratoplasty in view of graft infection that shows (C) well-apposed graft-host junction (blue arrow) and intact sutures (yellow arrow). Note the air bubble inside the anterior chamber (grey arrow) and Descemet's membrane folds in the non-optical grade donor corneal tissue (red arrow).

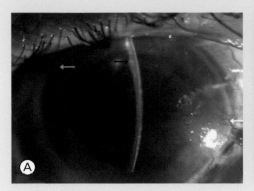
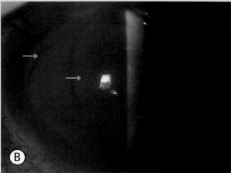

Figure 13.27 Slit lamp photograph of a patient who developed endophthalmitis following Descemet's stripping automated endothelial keratoplasty (DSAEK) showing (A) superficial corneal vascularisation (white arrow) and graft oedema (black arrow) with the posterior layers including the donor cornea being affected to a larger extent, along with intact sutures (green arrow) securing the surgical wound. On retro-illumination (B), note the inflammatory membranes (blue arrow) in the anterior camber, dull fundus glow and foldable intraocular lens in situ (yellow arrow).

CASE 13.8

CLINICAL FEATURES

A 38-year-old male patient, a known case of right eye operated Type I Boston Keratoprosthesis, presented with complains of insidious onset and progressive diminution of vision in the right eye for the previous three months, which was associated with watering and mild pain. He was diagnosed as a case of peri-optic sterile corneal melt and was planned for an emergency repair with keratoprosthesis explant and tectonic keratoplasty, as a substitute keratoprosthesis device was not immediately available for exchange. However, on finding healthy corneal tissue all around the melt, a lamellar corneal overlay procedure with sectoral tuck in was performed instead. This was done primarily to avoid an extensive intraocular surgery or removal of prosthesis. Examination findings and slit lamp appearance are illustrated in Figure 13.28.

KEY POINTS

Diagnosis:
- The above clinical scenario describes a case of Type I post-Boston Keratoprosthesis infective keratitis with corneal melt.

Investigations:
- Ultrasound B-scan was within normal limits.
- Corneal scrapings were sent for bacterial and fungal culture sensitivity. However, the smear and culture reports turned out to be negative.

Treatment:
- The patient was initially treated with topical antibiotics according to the bacterial and fungal culture sensitivity reports. Patient was managed with topical antibiotics (moxifloxacin 0.5% four times a day for two weeks) and topical lubricants (carboxymethylcellulose 0.5% every two hours). A crescentic corneal patch graft was performed.

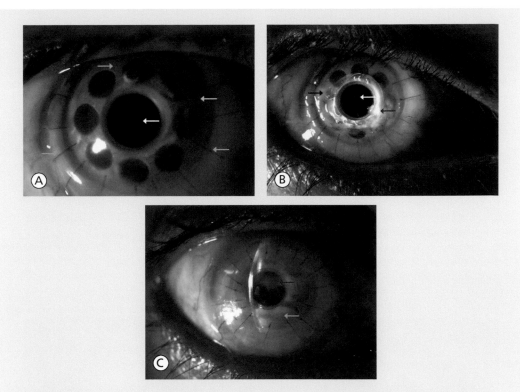

Figure 13.28 Slit lamp photograph of a patient with implanted Boston keratoprosthesis for graft failure demonstrating (A) intact optic (white arrow) and titanium backplate (blue arrow) mounted on the peripheral skirt of the donor cornea (green arrow), secured in place with 10-0 monofilament nylon sutures (yellow arrows). The patient developed (B) infective keratitis manifesting as peri-optic corneal melt (black arrow) and sloughed exudative material (red arrow) surrounding the intact optic (white arrow). On the one year follow-up (C), the retro-prosthetic membrane (red arrow) along with a hazy graft (green arrow) was noted.

Outcome:
- Postoperatively, the lamellar graft was found to be well integrated with the keratoprosthesis and hence no further surgical intervention was planned. On follow-up, the patient's visual acuity improved to 6/36 OD and the graft has remained stable up till his last six-month follow-up visit.

Supplementary Information and Additional Tips
- Patients with a keratoprosthesis implant are prone to develop inflammatory and infective retro-prosthetic membranes, vitreous exudates and eventually endophthalmitis (Figure 13.29), compromising visual outcomes in these cases.
- Suture-related problems and infections can lead to the formation of thick retro-prosthetic membranes with dense vascularisation (Figure 13.30) with keratoprosthesis implants.
- In patients with long-standing glaucoma associated with the keratoprosthesis surgery, implant extrusion and peri-optic corneal melting along with formation of ciliary staphyloma and choroidal detachment may be noted (Figure 13.31).

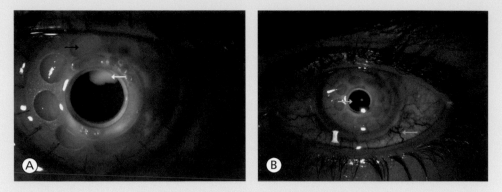

Figure 13.29 Slit lamp photograph of a patient with implanted Boston keratoprosthesis who developed endophthalmitis demonstrating (A) retro-prosthetic dense membrane (black arrow) with exudates (white arrow) with infective keratitis. The patient underwent vitrectomy with injection of intravitreal antibiotics, leading to (B) resolution of the endophthalmitis with a clear optic (yellow arrow). Note the dense vascularisation (green arrow) invading the host and donor cornea.

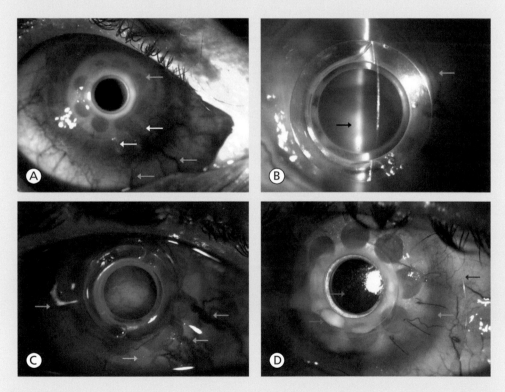

Figure 13.30 Slit lamp photograph of a patient with implanted Boston keratoprosthesis who developed endophthalmitis secondary to suture infection demonstrating (A) loose sutures (white arrows), dense vascularisation (green arrows) and hazy donor cornea (yellow arrow) due to corneal oedema. The patient developed (B) a thick retro-prosthetic membrane (black arrow) with surrounding vascularisation (green arrow), which became denser to form (C) giant tortuous episcleral vessels (green arrows) behind the prosthesis that invaded the donor cornea (yellow arrow). Endophthalmitis resolved following treatment to demonstrate (D) a clear optic (blue arrow), residual corneal infiltrates (grey arrow) and regressed vessels (green arrow). Note the bandage contact lens (red arrow) placed over the keratoprosthesis.

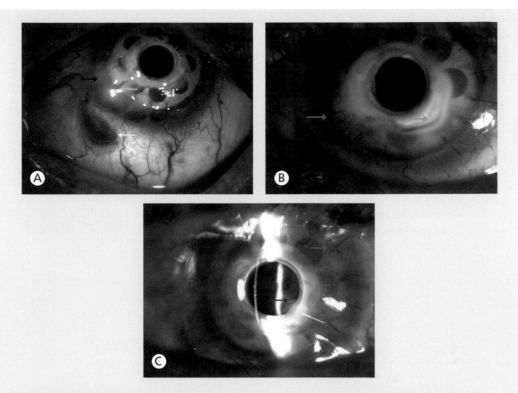

Figure 13.31 Slit lamp photograph of a patient with vascularised adherent leucoma with uncontrolled glaucoma who underwent keratoprosthesis implantation for visual rehabilitation demonstrating (A) impending extrusion (yellow arrow) of the keratoprosthesis with corneal melting (black arrow) ten months after surgery along with well-defined ciliary staphyloma (white arrow) and surrounding vascularisation (green arrow). On subsequent follow-up visits, the patient developed (B) peri-optic stromal melting (blue arrow) with loose sutures (grey arrow). Slit illumination (C) demonstrated early formation of retro-prosthetic membrane (red arrow) along with loose sutures (grey arrows).

REFERENCES

1. Hoskins EN, Oxford KW, Abbott RL, Jeng BH. Chapter 115. Infections after Penetrating Keratoplasty. In: Cornea; Volume 2 – Surgery of the Cornea and Conjunctiva. 4th ed. USA: Elsevier; 2017; 1324–37.

2. Özalp O, Atalay E, Köktaş Z, Yıldırım N. Distribution of microbial keratitis after penetrating keratoplasty according to early and late postoperative periods. Turk J Ophthalmol. 2020; 50(4):206–10.

3. Mathes KJ, Tran KD, Mayko ZM, Stoeger CG, Straiko MD, Terry MA. Reports of post-keratoplasty infections for eye bank-prepared and non-eye bank-prepared corneas: 12 years of data from a single eye bank. Cornea. 2019; 38(3):263–7.

4. Guilbert E, Bullet J, Sandali O, Basli E, Laroche L, Borderie VM. Long-term rejection incidence and reversibility after penetrating and lamellar keratoplasty. Am J Ophthalmol. 2013; 155(3): 560–9.e2.

14 Other Postsurgical Corneal Infections and Inflammation

Pooja Kumari, Amit K Das, Shikha Gupta, Noopur Gupta, Radhika Tandon

INTRODUCTION

Standard guidelines and preferred practice patterns have been developed to reduce the incidence of postoperative infections. Postsurgical infections are caused by organisms entering the eye during the surgical procedure or during the postoperative period. Infections depend on a multitude of factors including the technique and duration of surgery, inoculum load, host factors including systemic status and immune response of the body, postoperative therapy and hygiene, as well as the presence of any external risk factors like ocular trauma or contamination.

Infective keratitis and postoperative anterior segment inflammation can occur after cataract surgery, refractive surgery, pterygium excision and even trabeculectomy and vitreoretinal surgery.[1] Surgical infections in ophthalmic practice are most commonly associated with organisms from patient's local flora but can also involve more virulent hospital-acquired organisms.[2] Better instrumentation, surgical techniques, strict adherence to operating room sterilisation protocols, prophylactic antibiotics and optimum postoperative care play key roles in reducing the incidence of this complication.[3]

CASE 14.1

CLINICAL FEATURES

A 65-year-old female presented with sudden onset pain, redness and diminution of vision of the right eye following cataract surgery done in her hometown. On presentation, perception of light was present in the right eye with inaccurate projection of rays. The examination findings and slit lamp appearance are illustrated in Figure 14.1.

KEY POINTS

Diagnosis:
- The above clinical scenario describes a case of postsurgical infective keratitis.

Investigations:
- Microbiological investigations were performed from corneal scrapings: Gram stain, Giemsa stain, calcofluor white stain, KOH mount, bacterial culture on blood agar, fungal culture on Sabouraud dextrose agar and thioglycolate broth, and drug sensitivity testing. Bacterial culture demonstrated growth of *Staphylococcus epidermidis* that was sensitive to vancomycin and tobramycin.
- Ultrasound B-scan of the posterior segment demonstrated

mild-to-moderate amplitude spikes suggestive of vitreous exudates.

Treatment:
- The patient was treated with topical fortified vancomycin 5% and fortified tobramycin 1.3% every hour for 48 hours followed by tapering based on the clinical response, cycloplegic (homatropine hydrobromide 2% three times a day) and lubricants (preservative-free carboxymethylcellulose 0.5% six times a day), timolol maleate 0.5% twice a day.
- The patient was also prescribed systemic antibiotic (ciprofloxacin 500 mg twice a day) for a period of two weeks.

Outcome:
- The lesion responded to treatment and on subsequent follow-up visits, the size of the exudates in the anterior chamber (AC) reduced and the corneal lesion healed with healing and vascularisation noted at the corneal wound site.
- Eventually, a leucomatous corneal opacity was left behind with a final visual acuity of 6/60.

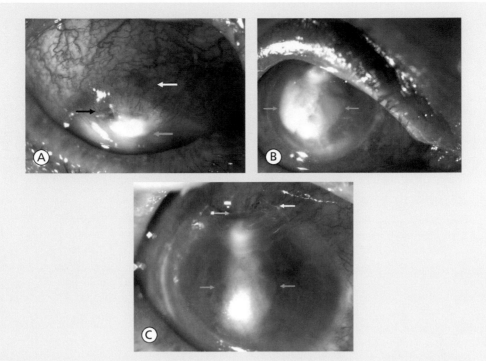

Figure 14.1 Slit lamp photograph of a patient with infective keratitis at the wound site following phacoemulsification demonstrating (A) corneal melt at the superior incision site (black arrow) along with anterior chamber exudate (green arrow) and circumcorneal congestion (white arrow). On diffuse illumination (B), dense anterior chamber exudates (green arrows) were noted. Response to medical therapy was noted with (C) reduction in size and density of anterior chamber exudates (grey arrows) and signs of healing in the form of increasing vascularisation at the wound site (white arrow) after two weeks; however, a small area of severe thinning (yellow arrow) remained at the wound site.

Supplementary Information and Additional Tips

- Elderly patients undergoing cataract surgery with a previous history of refractive surgery in adulthood are more prone to develop secondary infection at keratotomy sites due to compromised corneal morphology and function (Figure 14.2). In patients with operated radial keratotomy (RK), splaying of keratotomy incisions may occur leading to secondary infection during cataract surgery.
- Wound infection at the site of the phacoemulsification tunnel can lead to corneal melting and ulceration (Figure 14.3).
- Viral keratitis in the form of endotheliitis may also occur following phacoemulsification surgery (Figure 14.4) for cataract extraction.

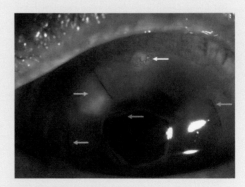

Figure 14.2 Slit lamp photograph of a patient with operated radial keratotomy (RK) for myopia who presented with corneal infiltrate (yellow arrow) at the wound site following phacoemulsification, with few infiltrates at 12 o'clock (white arrow). Note the central hexagonal keratotomy (grey arrow) and 10-0 monofilament nylon sutures at RK splayed incision sites (green arrows).

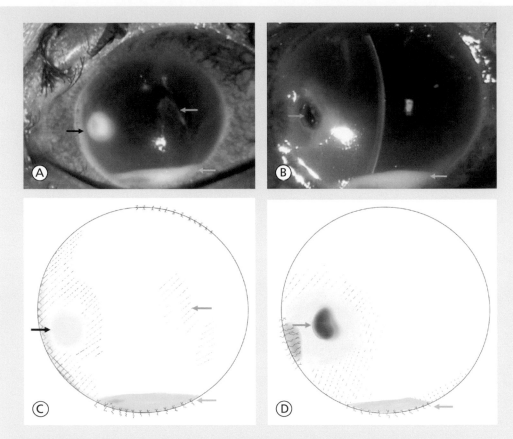

Figure 14.3 Slit lamp photograph of a patient who developed wound infection following phacoemulsification demonstrating (A) an area of localised corneal abscess (black arrow) at temporal wound site along with a hypopyon (yellow arrow) and an early inflammatory membrane in the anterior chamber (grey arrow). On follow-up (B), corneal melting (green arrow) at the site of infiltrate and hypopyon (yellow arrow) were noted. The corresponding schematic corneal diagrams at presentation (C) and at follow-up (D) depict the same clinical findings.

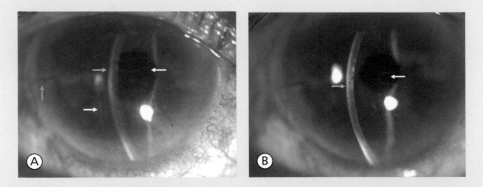

Figure 14.4 Slit lamp photograph of a patient who developed viral endotheliitis seven days after undergoing an uneventful phacoemulsification demonstrating (A) corneal oedema (yellow arrow) with Descemet's membrane folds (white arrows); note the single suture at the main wound site (grey arrow). One week after starting oral antiviral therapy (B), a reasonable reduction in corneal oedema (yellow arrow) and Descemet's folds (white arrow) was noted, which gradually resolved over another week.

CASE 14.2

CLINICAL FEATURES

A 65-year-old diabetic male presented with sudden onset redness, pain and diminution of vision of the left eye following cataract surgery in the village camp. He reported that he did not gain any useful vision after the surgery. His visual acuity was perception of light with inaccurate projection of rays in two quadrants. Examination findings and slit lamp appearance are illustrated in Figure 14.5.

KEY POINTS

Diagnosis:
- The above clinical scenario describes a case of infective keratitis with endophthalmitis following small incision cataract surgery (SICS).

Investigations:
- Microbiological investigations were performed from corneal scrapings: Gram stain, Giemsa stain, calcofluor white stain, KOH mount, bacterial culture on blood agar, fungal culture on Sabouraud dextrose agar and thioglycolate broth, and drug sensitivity testing.
- The bacterial culture demonstrated the growth of colonies of *Streptococcus pneumoniae* with negative fungal culture reports.
- Ultrasound B-scan of the posterior segment revealed vitreous exudates.

Treatment:
- The patient was managed with topical fortified antibiotics (cefazolin 5% and tobramycin 1.3%) due to the involvement of visual axis and presence of hypopyon. They were given hourly for the first 24 hours, then every two hours for 48 hours (round the clock), then given every four hours for one week, then every six hours for a week and then tapered as per the response. Antibiotic ointment and antiglaucoma medication were also prescribed.
- Intravitreal antibiotics (vancomycin 1 mg/0.1 ml and ceftazidime 2.25 mg/0.1 ml) were given and on follow-up patient responded to the treatment.

Outcome:
- The lesion responded to treatment and on follow-up, exudates in the AC reduced and the corneal lesion healed with explained poor visual prognosis.

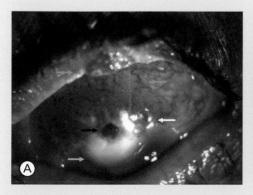 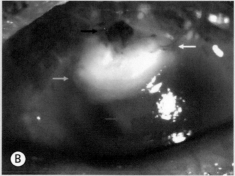

Figure 14.5 Slit lamp photograph of a patient who underwent small incision cataract surgery demonstrating (A) infective keratitis with a localised corneal abscess (yellow arrow), stromal melt and uveal tissue prolapse (black arrow) at the wound site, which also shows an infinity suture (white arrow); also note the surrounding circumcorneal and conjunctival congestion (green arrow) and severe blepharitis with upper eyelid crusting (blue arrow) in the affected eye. The magnified view reveal (B) the same findings in greater details; note the exudates in the anterior chamber along with the abscess (yellow arrow) and the relatively poor fundal glow (red arrow).

Supplementary Information and Additional Tips

- Occasionally, a filtering or non-filtering cystoid cicatrix may be observed following partial dehiscence or thinning at the site of the surgical incision created at the limbus during extracapsular cataract extraction (ECCE) or SICS (Figure 14.6).

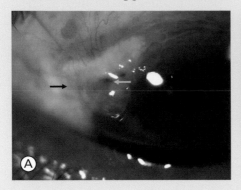
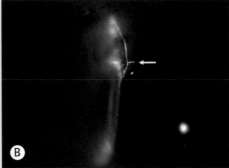

Figure 14.6 Slit lamp photograph of a patient with cystoid cicatrix demonstrating (A) cystic area at the site of previous extracapsular cataract extraction (ECCE) incision (black arrow) with surrounding superficial vascularisation and uveal show (yellow arrow) through the extremely thin wall of the cystoid cicatrix. Magnified slit illumination (B) demonstrated the elevated cystic spaces (white arrow) with corneal thinning.

CASE 14.3

CLINICAL FEATURES

A 22-year-old male underwent corneal collagen cross-linking to arrest progression of keratoconus. On the second postoperative day, he complained of sudden onset of painful diminution of vision in the right eye. He gave a history of rubbing his eyes after the procedure and splashing tap water into his eyes for excessive foreign body sensation. Examination findings and slit lamp appearance at presentation and follow-up are illustrated in Figure 14.7.

KEY POINTS

Diagnosis:
- The above clinical scenario describes a case of right eye infective keratitis following C_3R (corneal collagen cross linking) in a patient with keratoconus.

Investigations:
- Microbiological investigations were performed from corneal scrapings: Gram stain, Giemsa stain, calcofluor white stain, KOH mount, bacterial culture on blood agar, fungal culture on Sabouraud dextrose agar and thioglycolate broth, and drug sensitivity testing.
- Corneal scraping showed growth of *Staphylococcus aureus* that was sensitive to vancomycin, cefazolin, tobramycin, ciprofloxacin and chloramphenicol.

Treatment:
- The patient was managed with topical fortified antibiotics (cefazolin 5% and tobramycin 1.3%) due to the involvement of visual axis and presence of hypopyon. They were given hourly for the first 24 hours, then every two hours for 48 hours (round the clock), then given every four hours for one week, then every six hours for a week and then tapered as per the response. Antibiotic ointment and antiglaucoma medication were also prescribed.

Outcome:
- The lesion responded to treatment with decrease in the size of the infiltrate and hypopyon and initiation of corneal scarring.

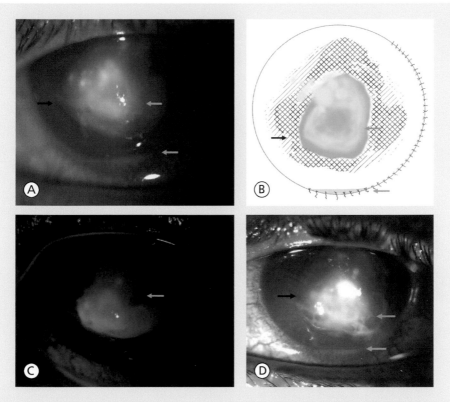

Figure 14.7 Slit lamp photograph of a patient who underwent corneal collagen cross linking to arrest progression of keratoconus showing (A) central necrotic ulcer (green arrow) confined to the debrided area (black arrow) along with hypopyon (grey arrow) and the same findings are shown in (B) the corresponding schematic diagram. The epithelial defect was well delineated (C) on slit lamp examination under cobalt blue filter (green arrow) after staining with sodium fluorescein dye. The patient responded to treatment (D) and within 72 hours there was reduction in the size of the ulcer (black arrow) with healing of the epithelial defect (green arrow) and decrease in height of the hypopyon (grey arrow).

CASE 14.4

CLINICAL FEATURES

A 37-year-old male presented with sudden-onset redness, pain and diminution of vision of the right eye. He had undergone RK for myopia at 25 years of age. He gave a history of dust falling in his eye while driving. There was no history of any steroid use or any systemic disease. His visual acuity at presentation was 3/60 in the involved eye. The examination findings and slit lamp appearance are illustrated in Figure 14.8.

KEY POINTS

Diagnosis:
- The above clinical scenario describes a case of infective keratitis in a myope with operated RK.

Investigations:
- Microbiological investigations were performed from corneal scrapings: Gram stain, Giemsa stain, calcofluor white stain, KOH mount, bacterial culture on blood agar, fungal culture on Sabouraud dextrose agar

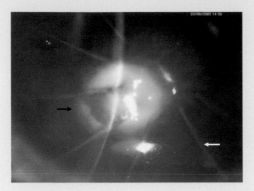

Figure 14.8 Slit lamp photograph of a patient demonstrating infective keratitis following radial keratotomy with central necrotic area and infiltrates (black arrow). Note the keratotomy incisions (white arrow) spanning the cornea.

due to the involvement of visual axis and presence of hypopyon. They were given hourly for the first 24 hours, then every two hours for 48 hours (round the clock), then given every four hours for one week, then every six hours for a week and then tapered as per the response. Antibiotic ointment and antiglaucoma medication were also prescribed.

Outcome:

- Poor visual outcome was explained to the patient as the ulcer healed with scarring that involved the visual axis.
- A scleral contact lens trial was attempted with good gain of best corrected visual acuity to 6/24.

and thioglycolate broth, and drug sensitivity testing.

- Corneal scraping showed growth of *S. epidermidis* that was sensitive to vancomycin, tobramycin, ciprofloxacin, cefazolin and chloramphenicol.

Treatment:

- The patient was managed with topical fortified antibiotics (cefazolin 5% and tobramycin 1.3%)

Supplementary Information and Additional Tips

- The altered structure of slowly healing keratotomy incisions coupled with redistribution of the tear film due to changes in corneal topography may result in intermittent epithelial irregularities. These changes in patients with RK scars make them prone to developing microbial keratitis, both bacterial and viral (Figure 14.9).

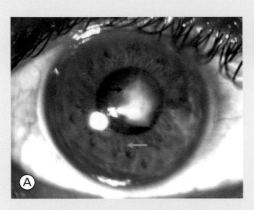
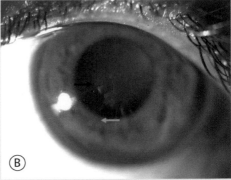

Figure 14.9 Slit lamp photograph of a patient with operated radial keratotomy showing (A) linear keratotomy scars (green arrow) and central leucomatous corneal opacity secondary to healed viral keratitis (black arrow) Examination of the other eye also revealed (B) scarred keratotomy incisions (green arrow) and central corneal haze (black arrow).

CASE 14.5

CLINICAL FEATURES

A 26-year-old female presented with foreign body sensation, intense photophobia and watering in the right eye. She had undergone small incision lenticule extraction (SMILE) refractive surgery for moderate myopia the day before. Postoperative visual acuity after the refractive surgery was 6/9 in the right eye and 6/6 in the left eye. The examination findings and slit lamp appearance in the right eye are illustrated in Figure 14.10.

KEY POINTS

Diagnosis:
- The above clinical scenario describes a case of post-SMILE corneal infiltrate.

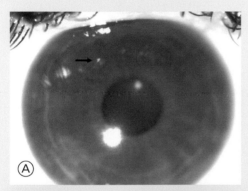

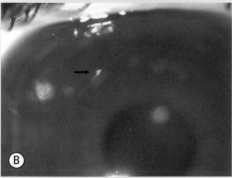

Figure 14.10 Slit lamp photograph of a young myope demonstrating (A) infiltrate at the supero-temporal tunnel incision site (black arrow) created by femtosecond laser during small incision lenticule extraction (SMILE) refractive surgery. The magnified view (B) demonstrates the corneal infiltrates in the interface (black arrow).

Investigations:
- Anterior segment optical coherence tomography of the right eye revealed haze below the SMILE flap and infiltrates at the supero-temporal entry site.

Treatment:
- She was started on topical antibiotics (moxifloxacin 0.5%) every hour and the frequency of lubricant eye drops was increased. Cycloplegic (homatropine 2%) was prescribed three times a day and steroid drops were withheld till the infection resolved.
- The frequency of the lubricant eye drop was increased gradually and topical antibiotic eye ointment was also added.

Outcome:
- The lesion completely healed in about two weeks along with the symptoms, as reported by the patient.
- Uncorrected visual acuity was 6/6 in both eyes.

Supplementary Information and Additional Tips

- Diffuse lamellar keratitis (DLK) is an uncommon complication after LASIK refractive surgery and usually manifests as sterile interface infiltrates (Figure 14.11), which, if untreated, may lead to stromal melting and secondary infection.

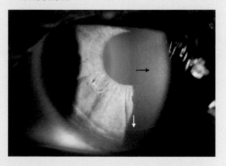

Figure 14.11 Slit lamp photograph of a young myope who underwent femtosecond-assisted laser in situ keratomileusis (LASIK) demonstrating sub-epithelial haze (black arrow) in the form of multiple, small sub-epithelial granular corneal precipitates resembling the characteristic 'sands of Sahara appearance' of diffuse lamellar keratitis. The edge of the LASIK flap is clearly visible (white arrow).

CASE 14.6

CLINICAL FEATURES

A 25-year-old female underwent insertion of implantable collamer lens (ICL) for correction of high myopia. On the first postoperative day, she complained of pain, photophobia and glare, and had a visual acuity of counting fingers. Intraocular pressure was noted to be 18 mm Hg. Examination findings and slit lamp appearance are illustrated in Figure 14.12.

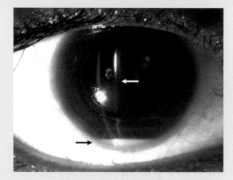

Figure 14.12 Slit lamp photograph of a young female demonstrating features of toxic anterior segment syndrome (TASS) following implantation of implantable collamer lens (ICL) for correction of myopia (white arrow). A mobile hypopyon measuring 3 mm (black arrow), minimal ciliary congestion and mild corneal oedema were evident on the first postoperative day.

KEY POINTS

Diagnosis:
- The above clinical scenario describes a case of toxic anterior segment syndrome and anterior segment inflammation following ICL implantation.

Investigations:
- Indirect ophthalmoscopy for posterior segment evaluation revealed no abnormalities. Posterior segment inflammation in the form of vitritis or vitreous exudates was characteristically absent.
- Anterior segment optical coherence tomography revealed corneal oedema with central corneal thickness measuring 692 microns.

Treatment:
- The patient was intensively treated with potent topical steroids, cycloplegic and antiglaucoma drugs. Oral prednisolone 50 mg in the morning was prescribed for a week along with oral omeprazole 20 mg once daily.

Outcome:
- Her vision improved drastically to 6/6 with the treatment after two weeks of surgery as the inflammation subsided completely.

CASE 14.7

CLINICAL FEATURES

A 50-year-old male presented with sudden pain, redness and discharge of the right eye. He had undergone pterygium excision in the same eye five days prior. On examination his visual acuity was 6/24. Examination findings and slit lamp appearance are illustrated in Figure 14.13.

KEY POINTS

Diagnosis:
- The above clinical scenario describes a case of surgically induced necrotising scleritis (SINS) that occurred following surgery for pterygium excision.

Investigations:
- Ultrasound B-scan revealed shallow peripheral retinal and choroidal detachments.

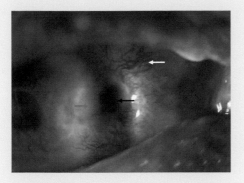

Figure 14.13 Slit lamp photograph of a patient showing corneoscleral melting and uveal show (black arrow) with surrounding congestion (white arrow) and corneal infiltrates (grey arrow). The patient had undergone pterygium excision three weeks prior.

- A scleral scraping revealed a moderate number of polymorphonuclear cells and occasional Gram-negative bacteria on microbiological study. No fungal elements were seen. Culture of scleral scraping showed no growth of organisms.
- Investigations were done to rule out collagen vascular diseases. The erythrocyte sedimentation rate (ESR) and chest X-ray were normal. Rheumatoid factor (RF), antinuclear antibodies (ANA) and antineutrophil cytoplasmic antibody (ANCA) were not detected.

- Postprandial blood sugar, serum immunoglobulin profile and uric acid estimation were within normal limits.

Treatment:
- The patient was started on topical antibiotic, cycloplegic and steroid combination eyedrops.
- The patient was given oral prednisolone 60 mg/day along with oral indomethacin 20 mg twice daily.

Outcome:
- The patient responded well to medical therapy and symptoms resolved over a period of four weeks with final best corrected acuity being 6/9.

Supplementary Information and Additional Tips

- The aetiology of SINS has not been established. It is also known to occur after cataract extraction, strabismus surgery, trabeculectomy, scleral buckling procedures and scleral perforation repair (Figure 14.14).
- SINS has also been associated with multiple surgical procedures, co-existent systemic collagen vascular disease, use of general anaesthesia, local ischaemia, the use of a higher concentration of mitomycin C, a chemotherapeutic agent, or use of excessive cautery on the scleral bed.

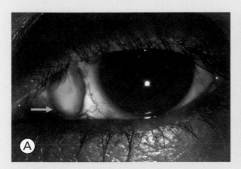
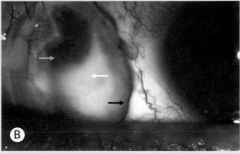

Figure 14.14 Slit lamp photograph of a patient with primary open-angle glaucoma with a surgical history of repaired post-traumatic scleral perforation in the left eye demonstrating (A) surgically induced necrotising scleritis on the medial aspect (yellow arrow) of the eye. The magnified view demonstrates (B) the underlying brown-coloured uveal tissue (yellow arrow), bare sclera (white arrow) and dilated vessel at the margin of necrotic area (black arrow).

CASE 14.8

CLINICAL FEATURES

A 41-year-old female with primary angle-closure glaucoma gave a history of loss of vision in the right eye following episodes of pain and redness over the past 3 years. The recorded visual acuity in the right eye was nil perception of light. Left eye trabeculectomy was performed for high intraocular pressure that was not controlled on maximal medical therapy. Visual acuity was recorded to be 6/9 at the time of first surgery. Bleb revision was planned in view of the thin cystic bleb, however, she was lost to follow-up and later presented with sudden diminution of vision, redness and pain in the left eye. Visual acuity in the left eye was hand movements close to face with accurate projection of rays. Examination findings and slit lamp appearance are illustrated in Figure 14.15.

KEY POINTS

Diagnosis:
- The above clinical scenario describes a case of post-trabeculectomy blebitis with bleb failure.

Investigations:
- Seidel test was noted to be positive, suggestive of a bleb leak.
- Ultrasound B-scan of the left eye was noted to be anechoic.

Treatment:
- The patient was initially treated with topical and systemic antibiotics after the diagnosis with bacterial and fungal culture sensitivity reports.
- Antiglaucoma medication was continued.

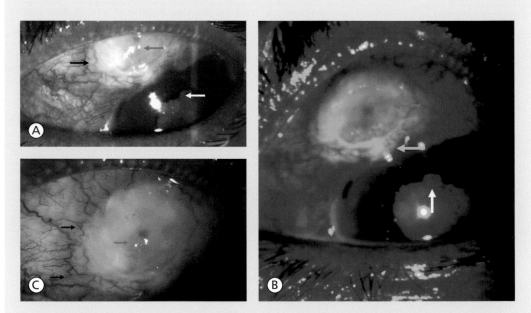

Figure 14.15 Slit lamp photograph of a patient with primary angle-closure glaucoma demonstrating features of post-phaco-trabeculectomy blebitis. The trabeculectomy bleb appears (A) cystic and avascular (grey arrow) associated with marked congestion (black arrow). Cataract, posterior synechiae and a shallow anterior chamber (white arrow) are also evident. Slit lamp examination under cobalt blue filter demonstrates (B) thin, cystic bleb (grey arrow) with leakage as shown by fluorescein dye (yellow arrow). Irregular pupil (white arrow) due to posterior synechiae can be seen. The magnified view (C) on slit lamp bio-microscopy reveals the same findings with greater detail.

Outcome:
- Patient was counselled regarding guarded outcomes in view of bleb failure and need for regular follow-up was reinforced.

Supplementary Information and Additional Tips
- Blebitis is characterised by conjunctival and ciliary injection, more around the bleb edges with periorbital chemosis, congestion with signs of bleb leak.
- Bleb-related endophthalmitis and keratitis can occur in children with primary congenital glaucoma due to bleb leak following trabeculectomy and glaucoma valve implantation for uncontrolled intraocular pressure (Figure 14.16).

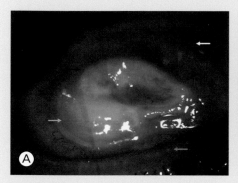 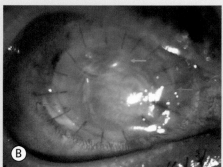

Figure 14.16 Slit lamp photograph of a child with operated glaucoma drainage device for primary congenital glaucoma who presented with a hypotonus globe and endophthalmitis showing (A) central corneal melt with sloughing (yellow arrow) and surrounding corneal oedema (black arrow). Diffuse conjunctival congestion, more pronounced at the area of the bleb (white arrow) and Meibomian gland dysfunction (grey arrow) of the lower lid can also be seen. The patient underwent therapeutic keratoplasty and the postoperative photograph shows (B) an oedematous donor cornea with well-apposed graft-host junction (blue arrows), multiple 10-0 monofilament nylon sutures and an air bubble in the anterior chamber (green arrow).

CASE 14.9

CLINICAL FEATURES

A 42-year-old female presented with sudden onset redness, pain and diminution of vision of the left eye due to the development of infective keratitis following surgery for retinal detachment. Her visual acuity in the left eye was 5/60 with accurate projection of rays. She underwent multiple surgeries in the left eye in view of glaucoma. Examination findings and slit lamp appearance on follow-up are illustrated in Figure 14.17.

KEY POINTS

Diagnosis:
- The above clinical scenario describes a case of healed keratitis following vitreoretinal surgery with secondary glaucoma.

Investigations:
- Intraocular pressure by applanation tonometry was recorded to be 20 mm Hg.

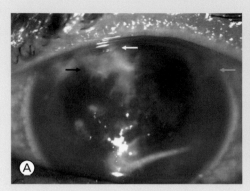 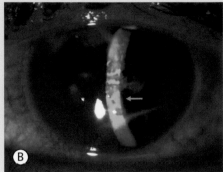

Figure 14.17 Slit lamp photograph of a patient with resolved keratitis following vitreoretinal surgery showing (A) maculo-leucomatous corneal opacity (black arrow) with surrounding conjunctival congestion (green arrow). 10-0 monofilament nylon suture (white arrow) can be seen in the superior part of the cornea. Slit lamp examination under cobalt blue filter (B) shows poor ocular surface with punctate staining (grey arrow) of the corneal surface.

- Ultrasound B-scan did not reveal any posterior segment exudates suggestive of endophthalmitis.

Treatment:
- The patient was initially managed with topical fortified antibiotics (cefazolin 5% and tobramycin 1.3%) every hour, homatropine 2% thrice a day and timolol 0.5% twice a day.

- Topical lubricants (carboxymethylcellulose 1%) were continued after the keratitis resolved.

Outcome:
- Poor visual outcome was explained to the patient due to poor ocular surface and failed vitreoretinal surgery.

REFERENCES

1. Trese MGJ, Sugar A, Mian SI. Chapter 95. Corneal Complications of Intraocular Surgery. In: Cornea; Volume 1 – Fundamentals, Diagnosis and Management. 4th ed. USA: Elsevier; 2017; 1120–34.

2. Ram J, Kaushik S, Brar GS, Taneja N, Gupta A. Prevention of postoperative infections in ophthalmic surgery. Indian J Ophthalmol. 2001 Mar; 49(1):59–69.

3. Anagol NC, Nisha D S, Ganesh S, Shree S. Post-operative infections at a tertiary eye hospital: a 5-year retrospective study. J Patient Saf Infect Control 2017; 5:24–9.

CORNEAL INFECTION AND INFLAMMATION IN SYSTEMIC DISORDERS

15 Corneal Involvement in Systemic Infections

Ritika Mukhija, Deeksha Rani, T Monikha, Nimmy Raj, Radhika Tandon

INTRODUCTION

Infectious diseases can affect all organs and tissues of the body, including the eye. While many symptoms and signs may be non-specific and subjective, ocular manifestations may provide valuable clinical insight. It is important for the ophthalmologist to identify these features, as they can aid in establishing the diagnosis and further management.[1] The cornea can be involved in a variety of systemic infections, such as tuberculosis, leprosy, acquired immunodeficiency syndrome, syphilis, Lyme disease and onchocerciasis.[2–4] This chapter gives a brief overview of corneal involvement in various systemic infections in relation to common clinical scenarios.

CASE 15.1

CLINICAL FEATURES

An 18-year-old female presented with gradually progressive redness, pain and watering in both her eyes for the past three weeks. There was no history of any such episodes previously, no associated diminution of vision or any other systemic disease. Examination findings and slit lamp appearance are illustrated in Figure 15.1.

KEY POINTS

Diagnosis:
- The above clinical scenario highlights a case of bilateral phlyctenular keratoconjunctivitis.

Investigations:
- The ocular diagnosis was based on clinical findings; systemic investigations, mainly complete blood count, erythrocyte sedimentation rate (ESR), C-reactive protein (CRP), Mantoux tuberculin skin test and a chest X-ray, were performed.
- All investigations were within normal limits, except for raised ESR.
- Patient was referred to the medicine department, where she was examined and investigated for tuberculosis (TB) and a diagnosis of TB lymphadenitis was made based on ultrasound and contrast-enhanced CT scan.

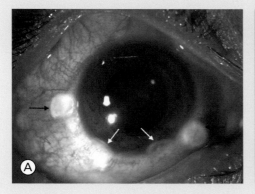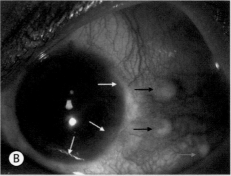

Figure 15.1 Slit lamp photograph showing a case of bilateral tubercular phlyctenulosis [right (A) and left (B)] in a 18-year-old patient with multiple limbal and scleral phlyctens (black arrows) and peripheral corneal involvement (white arrows) along with mucoid discharge (grey arrow).

Treatment:
- The patient was prescribed topical steroids (prednisolone acetate 1% six times a day), cycloplegic (homatropine hydrobromide 2% three times) and lubricants (carboxymethylcellulose 0.5% six times a day).
- A topical antibiotic (moxifloxacin hydrochloride 0.5% three times a day) cover was added for the first week in view of corneal involvement. After the first week, topical steroids were tapered.
- The patient was prescribed anti-tubercular treatment (ATT) [Isoniazid (INH, 100 mg/day), rifampicin (RIF, 300 mg/day), pyrazinamide (400 mg/day) for two months and INH (80 mg/day) and RIF (150 mg/day) for another four months] by the physician for tubercular lymphadenitis.

Outcome:
- A dramatic response in symptoms and signs was noted in the first week of therapy, and the phlyctens resolved completely in about four weeks.
- Patient completed six months of ATT and was confirmed as cured by the treating physician.

Supplementary Information and Additional Tips

- Phlyctenular keratoconjunctivitis, or phlyctenulosis, occurs as a result of an allergic response to a number of antigens, the most common being tubercular protein and staphylococcal antigen (Figure 15.2).
- Although the incidence of tubercular phlyctenulosis has diminished significantly over the decades, it should still be considered as one of the first differentials in endemic areas, especially in children, adolescents and young adults.
- Other anterior segment manifestations of TB can be subconjunctival nodular nonulcerative mass (tuberculoma), conjunctival granuloma (Figure 15.3), interstitial keratitis (Figure 15.4), peripheral ulcerative keratitis (PUK), scleritis (Figure 15.5) and granulomatous uveitis.

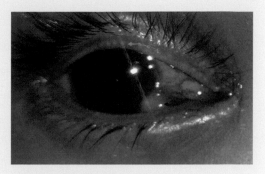

Figure 15.2 Slit lamp photograph showing a case of staphylococcal phlyctenulosis (black arrow) in a 10-year-old male with blepharitis (grey arrow).

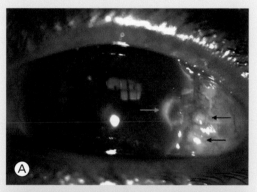

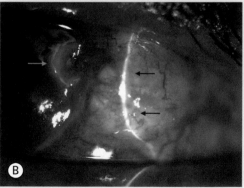

Figure 15.3 Slit lamp photograph showing left eye of a 31-year-old male with tubercular keratoconjunctivitis (A) showing bulbar conjunctival nodular mass (black arrows) in continuation with a localised peripheral corneal ulcer with stromal thinning (grey arrow); the magnified image (B) shows the findings more distinctly.

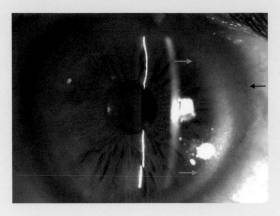

Figure 15.4   Slit lamp photograph showing a case of healed tubercular interstitial keratitis with peripheral corneal opacity (grey arrows) and vascularisation (black arrow).

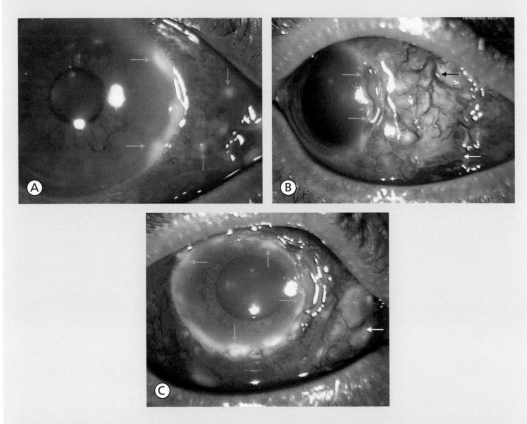

Figure 15.5   Slit lamp photograph (A) showing tubercular sclerokeratouveitis in a patient with Sweet syndrome; it started as peripheral corneal infiltrates (yellow arrows) and scleral infiltrates (grey arrows) in one quadrant, which progressed to (B) peripheral thinning (green arrows) and scleral melt (white arrow); note the dilated and tortuous vessels (black arrow). Eventually, (C) the patient developed 360° peripheral corneal infiltration (yellow arrows) with worsening of corneal thinning (green arrow) and uveal show (blue arrow) along with scleral necrosis (white arrow).

CASE 15.2

CLINICAL FEATURES

A 45-year-old male presented with pain, diminution of vision and redness in the right eye for the past two weeks. He also had an episode of similar complaints in the left eye three months ago. The patient had a known case of acquired immunodeficiency syndrome (AIDS) and was on highly active antiretroviral therapy (HAART). Examination findings and slit lamp appearance are illustrated in Figure 15.6.

KEY POINTS

Diagnosis:

- The above clinical scenario highlights a case of severe keratitis with diffuse corneal abscess in the right eye and healed keratitis in the left eye in a patient with human immunodeficiency virus infection.

Investigations:

- Corneal scraping was performed and specimens sent for Gram stain, KOH mount, bacterial and fungal culture and sensitivity testing. Growth of *Staphylococcus aureus* and *Aspergillus fumigatus* was noted.
- Posterior segment evaluation on B-scan ultrasonography was performed, which was within normal limits.

Treatment:

- He was empirically treated with frequent broad-spectrum fortified antibiotics (cefazolin 5% and tobramycin 1.3%), cycloplegic (homatropine hydrobromide 2% thrice a day), antiglaucoma medication (timolol 0.5% twice a day) and oral ciprofloxacin 500 mg twice a day.
- Cefazolin was replaced with topical vancomycin 5% after 72 hours in view of the culture sensitivity reports; topical natamycin 5% and oral ketoconazole 200 mg twice a day were additionally prescribed.

Outcome:

- The patient showed marked symptomatic improvement in the first ten days of treatment with reduction in size and density of infiltrates.
- However, due to progressive corneal thinning, therapeutic keratoplasty with a large graft had to be performed for an impending perforation.

Supplementary Information and Additional Tips

- AIDS is associated with an increased incidence of keratitis with viral, bacterial, filamentous and non-filamentous fungal and parasitic

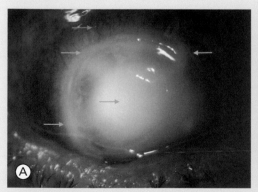
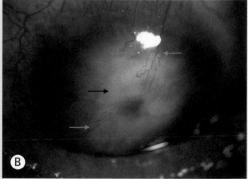

Figure 15.6 Slit lamp photograph showing a case of severe keratitis (A) with diffuse corneal abscess (green arrow) and scleral involvement (yellow arrows) in a patient with acquired immunodeficiency syndrome (AIDS). The other eye of the patient had features suggestive of healed keratitis (B) with dense corneal scarring (grey arrows) with vascularisation (black arrow).

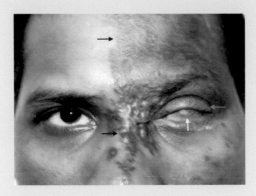

Figure 15.7 Clinical photograph showing a case of healing herpes zoster keratitis in a patient with acquired immunodeficiency syndrome (AIDS); note the healed skin lesions (black arrows), cicatricial lid changes (grey arrow) and healing keratitis with diffuse corneal opacity (white arrow) in a shrunken globe.

pathogens like varicella zoster virus, herpes simplex virus, herpes zoster virus (Figure 15.7), cytomegalovirus, *Candida* (Figure 15.8), *Fusarium* (Figure 15.9), *Aspergillus* and microsporidial keratitis.

- Keratitis is often severe and needs a combination of topical and systemic antibiotics along with continuation of systemic treatment (HAART).
- Drug interactions of oral anti-microbials with those of HAART should be kept in mind and appropriate dose adjustment may be needed in consultation with the physician.

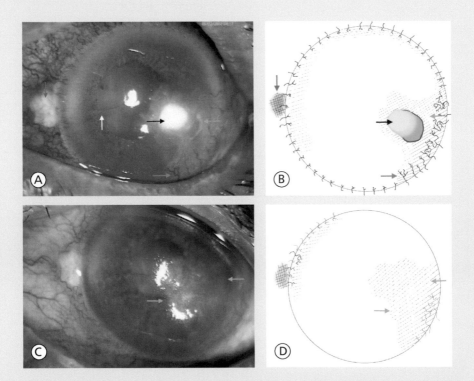

Figure 15.8 Slit lamp photograph (A) and corresponding corneal diagram (B) showing *Candida* keratitis (A) in a patient with acquired immunodeficiency syndrome (AIDS); note the localised corneal abscess (black arrow) with surrounding scarring (green arrow) and vascularisation (grey arrow) along with a focal area of scleral involvement (blue arrow) and posterior synechiae (white arrow). Patient showed a good response to medical management (C) and the ulcer healed with nebular corneal scarring (green arrows) after six weeks of treatment; corresponding corneal diagram (D) is also shown.

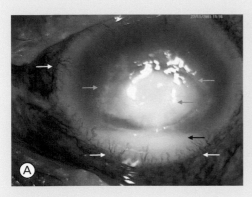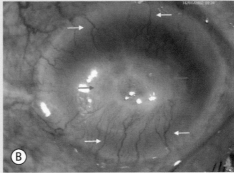

Figure 15.9 Slit lamp photograph showing *Fusarium* keratitis (A) in a patient with AIDS showing a central corneal ulcer (green arrow) and hypopyon (black arrow); note the dense infiltrates (grey arrow) with feathery margins (yellow arrow) and diffuse superficial vascularisation (white arrows). Patient showed good response to medical management (B) and the ulcer healed with macular corneal scarring (blue arrows) and dense superficial vascularisation (white arrows) after about eight weeks of treatment.

CASE 15.3

CLINICAL FEATURES

A 70-year-old male presented with complaints of diminution of vision, pain, redness and eyelid swelling in the left eye over the past four days. The patient was a known case of diabetes mellitus with chronic kidney disease and was on regular haemodialysis. He also gave history of high-grade fever, malaise and headache for previous ten days. The examination findings and slit lamp appearance are illustrated in Figure 15.10.

KEY FEATURES

Diagnosis:
- The above clinical scenario highlights a case of metastatic endophthalmitis with severe necrotising keratitis in a patient with septicaemia.

Investigations:
- Gentle debridement and scraping were performed and specimens sent for Gram stain, KOH mount along with bacterial and fungal culture and sensitivity testing; the latter revealed growth of *S. aureus* and *Aspergillus flavus*, respectively.

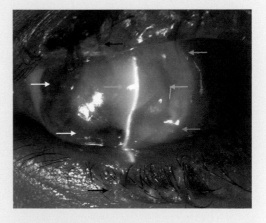

Figure 15.10 Slit lamp photograph showing a case of metastatic endophthalmitis with keratitis in a patient with septicaemia with diffuse corneal infiltrates (yellow arrow), stromal melting (green arrow) and large areas of total corneal melt with uveal tissue prolapse (white arrows) along with limbal involvement (grey arrows). Note the matting and muco-purulent discharge in the upper and lower lid lashes (black arrows).

- In addition, posterior segment B-scan ultrasonography revealed mild-to-moderate amplitude spikes in the vitreous cavity suggestive of vitreous exudation.
- A complete blood count showed severe leucocytosis (total leucocyte count = 28,000/mm^3) and blood culture also revealed growth of *S. aureus*.

Treatment:
- He was empirically treated with frequent broad-spectrum fortified antibiotics (topical vancomycin 5% and tobramycin 1.3%), topical natamycin 5% and oral ketoconazole 200 mg twice a day, cycloplegic (homatropine hydrobromide 2% thrice a day), antiglaucoma medication (timolol 0.5% twice a day) and oral ciprofloxacin 500 mg twice a day.
- Parenteral antibiotics (intravenous vancomycin and intravenous ceftriaxone) were started after five days as there was minimal improvement and the patient started developing a mild restriction of extraocular movements.

Outcome:
- The patient showed significant improvement after starting intravenous antibiotics, which were continued for two weeks; thereafter the patient was shifted to oral antibiotics.
- The infection was controlled in about six weeks; however, the eye eventually shrunk in size and resulted in phthisis bulbi.

Supplementary Information and Additional Tips

- Diabetes mellites and chronic kidney disease can both lead to a state of chronic immunosuppression and predispose the patient to septicaemia; regular haemodialysis is another risk factor for septicaemia.
- Such patients may have multiple foci of infection including the eye. Ophthalmic presentation may manifest as keratitis, endophthalmitis or panophthalmitis.

CASE 15.4

CLINICAL FEATURES

A 3-year-old female (informant: mother) presented with complaints of diminution of vision, pain and redness in both eyes for the past month. There was also an associated history of whitish discoloration, which started superiorly and gradually progressed to the current clinical picture. The mother gave a history of a mild skin rash on the child's abdomen in infancy which resolved on its own. Examination findings under anaesthesia and clinical appearance are illustrated in Figure 15.11.

KEY FEATURES

Diagnosis:
- The above clinical scenario highlights a case of bilateral stromal syphilitic (interstitial) keratitis presenting as a sign of late congenital syphilis.

Investigations:
- For diagnosis a treponemal test (indirect immunofluorescence; fluorescent treponemal antibody absorption (FTA-ABS) test) was performed, which tested positive for immunoglobulins to *Treponema pallidum* polypeptides.
- In addition, bilateral posterior segment B-scan ultrasonography was performed which was within normal limits.
- Serological testing of the mother was also positive, indicating prior exposure to the pathogen.

Treatment:
- The child was treated with aqueous penicillin G (50,000 units/kg intravenously every 8–12 hours) for

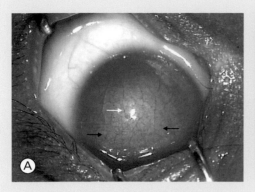
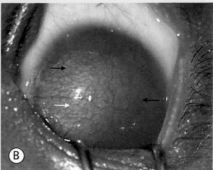

Figure 15.11 Clinical photographs showing congenital syphilitic infection with bilateral stromal keratitis (right eye A; left eye B) with ground-glass appearance of the cornea, diffuse stromal haze and oedema (black arrows) and diffuse superficial and deep vascularisation in an arborescent and intertwining pattern (white arrows).

two weeks in consultation with the paediatrician.

■ In addition, topical steroids (prednisolone acetate 1% six times a day) were given to reduce inflammation and consequent scarring.

Outcome:

■ The child showed significant improvement after starting treatment with a decrease in stromal oedema and inflammation.

■ The keratitis healed in about three months leaving behind bilateral nebulo-macular scarring with vascularisation.

Supplementary Information and Additional Tips

■ Stromal keratitis is the most common, and at times, the only sign of late congenital syphilis. Stromal neovascularisation occurs frequently and with varying severity; the classically described 'salmon patch' is nothing but a pannus of intertwining vessels on a pale stromal backdrop.

■ Stromal keratitis can also occur in acquired syphilis (Figure 15.12), although it is relatively uncommon; many patients may not recall a primary chancre or previous symptoms of secondary syphilis.

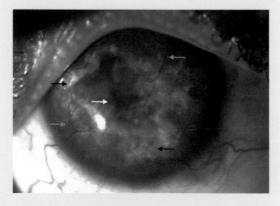

Figure 15.12 Slit lamp photograph showing a case of healed keratitis in a patient with acquired syphilis; note the diffuse corneal haze with dense vascularisation (grey arrows), lipid keratopathy (black arrows) and overlying pigmentation (white arrow).

- PUK and associated scleritis are rare manifestations of syphilis (Figure 15.13) and may also present as infective ulceration with

hypopyon (Figure 15.14). Treatment includes parenteral penicillin or oral erythromycin and doxycycline.

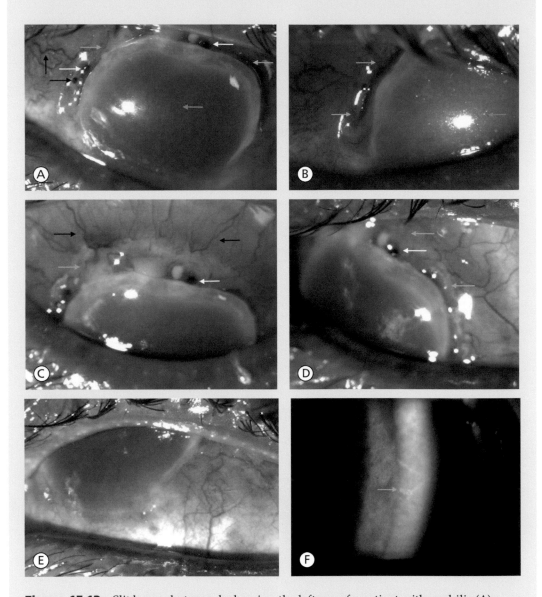

Figure 15.13 Slit lamp photograph showing the left eye of a patient with syphilis (A) with findings suggestive of sclerokeratouveitis; note the diffuse corneal haze (grey arrow) and severe peripheral thinning (yellow arrows) with areas of early melt and uveal show (white arrows) along with peripheral neovascularisation (black arrows); magnified views of the superonasal (B), superior (C) and superotemporal cornea (D) reveal the findings more distinctly. The presence of vascularised corneal and scleral scarring (blue arrow) in the inferotemporal quadrant (E) may be suggestive of a previous episode of sclerokeratouveitis. On slit illumination (F), pigments and keratic precipitates on the endothelium (green arrow) can be seen clearly.

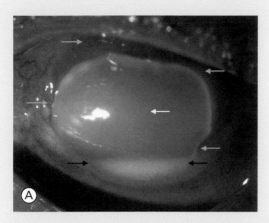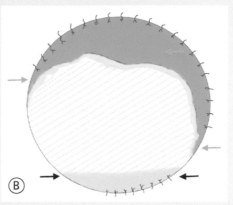

Figure 15.14 Slit lamp photograph (A) and corresponding corneal diagram (B) showing the right eye of the same patient with diffuse corneal haze (white arrow), severe peripheral thinning spanning almost nine clock hours (yellow arrows) and severe anterior uveitis resulting in a hypopyon (black arrows).

CASE 15.5

CLINICAL FEATURES

A 3-month-old infant was referred from the paediatrics department for signs suggestive of corneal ulceration. The mother gave a history of fever and difficulty in feeding the infant around three weeks before, following which there was the development of rash and skin lesions on the right forehead and around the eye. The infant started developing redness and discharge in the right eye around ten days ago, which was eventually followed by whitish discoloration. Examination findings and clinical appearance are illustrated in Figure 15.15.

KEY FEATURES

Diagnosis:
- The above clinical scenario highlights a case of neonatal varicella infection with severe necrotising stromal keratitis and corneal melt.

Investigations:
- The diagnosis was made primarily on the clinical presentation; however, gentle corneal scraping was performed to rule out secondary infection. No organisms were identified on Gram stain or KOH mount and bacterial and fungal cultures did not reveal any growth.

- In addition, posterior segment B-scan ultrasonography was performed which was within normal limits.

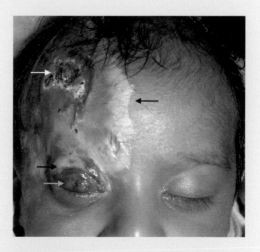

Figure 15.15 Clinical photograph showing severe keratitis in an infant with congenital varicella infection showing with diffuse corneal infiltrates and central melt (yellow arrow) along with ipsilateral skin lesion involving the scalp, forehead and lids. Note the active lesion (white arrow) along with scarring (black arrows).

■ A Tzanck smear of the material scraped from the base of a skin vesicle was performed by the dermatologist in consultation with the paediatrics team at the time of active skin lesions, which showed multinucleated giant cells and characteristic acidophilic intranuclear inclusions, thereby confirming the diagnosis of varicella zoster virus infection.

Treatment:

■ The infant had received intravenous acyclovir (30 mg/kg/day) for ten days.

■ A broad-spectrum topical antibiotic (moxifloxacin 0.5%), topical antiviral ointment (acyclovir 3%), atropine ointment (1%) and preservative-free lubricants (carboxymethylcellulose) were prescribed. In addition, topical antiglaucoma medication (betaxolol 0.25%) twice a day was also added.

Outcome:

■ Keratitis healed with the formation of a total adherent leucoma in about three months. In addition, a mild cicatricial ectropion developed in the upper eyelid. The surrounding skin lesions also healed with scarring.

Supplementary Information and Additional Tips

■ Although varicella is generally a mild disease, it is more severe in neonates, young adults and immunocompromised individuals.

■ Ocular manifestations of varicella generally involve the periocular skin, eyelids, cornea, conjunctiva and rarely the intraocular structures.

CASE 15.6

CLINICAL FEATURES

A 44-year-old female presented with chief complaints of sudden diminution of vision, redness and discharge in her right eye for the past three weeks. The patient was receiving treatment for bacterial keratitis elsewhere; however, the condition rapidly worsened. She noticed extrusion of some material from her eye, following which she presented to the ophthalmic casualty department. The patient's husband was diagnosed with leprosy around five months prior and was being treated for the same. Examination findings and slit lamp appearance are illustrated in Figure 15.16.

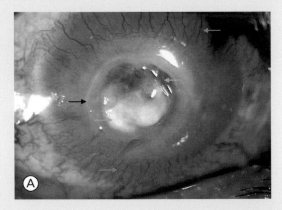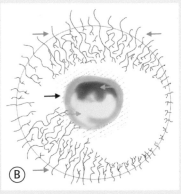

Figure 15.16 Slit lamp photograph (A) and corresponding corneal diagram (B) showing severe infective keratitis and corneal melt in a patient with leprosy-related corneal hypoesthesia; note the central ulcer (black arrow) with corneal melt (green arrow) and stromal infiltrates (yellow arrow) and diffuse superficial vascularisation (grey arrows).

KEY FEATURES

Diagnosis:
- The above clinical scenario highlights a case of severe infective keratitis and corneal melt in a patient with leprosy.

Investigations:
- The diagnosis was provisionally made on the clinical presentation and the patient was taken for an emergency tectonic keratoplasty. The host cornea specimen was sent for histopathological and microbiological diagnosis, which revealed growth of *S. aureus*.
- After restoring globe integrity, the patient was referred to the dermatology department, wherein a detailed workup and examination revealed skin lesions that tested positive for acid-fast bacilli on Ziehl-Neelsen staining.

Treatment:
- The patient was treated with dapsone, rifampicin and clofazimine as per the recommendations of the infectious disease department.
- For the ocular involvement, she was prescribed topical antibiotics, cycloplegics and lubricants; topical steroid drops were started after two weeks of keratoplasty after ruling out fungal infection in the host corneal button specimen.

Outcome:
- The patient maintained a clear graft for about one year after the surgery, following which the graft decompensated.

Supplementary Information and Additional Tips

- Corneal nerve involvement in terms of opacification and enlargement and corneal hypoesthesia are common ocular manifestations of leprosy. These can predispose the eye to secondary infections as in the above case.
- Exposure keratopathy, secondary to lagophthalmos and lower lid ectropion because of facial nerve involvement, is also common (Figure 15.17).
- Other corneal manifestations are chronic ocular surface disease and inferior vascularised corneal opacity (Figure 15.18), avascular keratitis, chalk-dust opacities, diffuse stromal haze and vascular pannus.

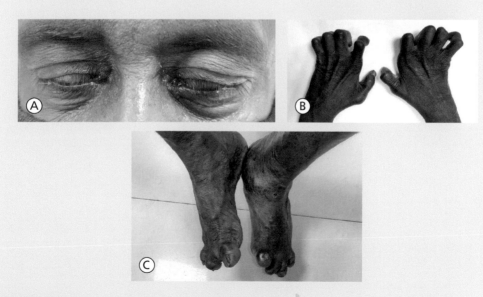

Figure 15.17 Clinical photograph showing bilateral lagophthalmos (A) in a patient with prior leprosy; note the inability to completely close the eyes (yellow arrows). External photographs of the hands (B) and feet (C) of the same patient showing characteristic deformities of leprosy sequelae.

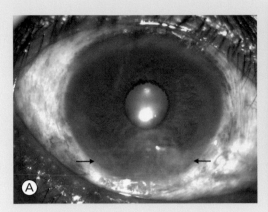 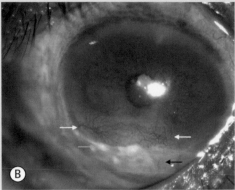

Figure 15.18 Slit lamp photograph showing bilateral healed exposure keratitis (right eye: A; left eye: B) in the same patient with leprosy-related lagophthalmos; note the characteristic inferior corneal involvement (black arrows) in both eyes and vascularisation (white arrows) and lipid keratopathy (green arrow) in the left eye.

REFERENCES

1. Lee SH, Schwab IR. Chapter 64. Infectious Disease: Ocular Manifestations. In: Cornea; Volume 1 – Fundamentals, Diagnosis and Management. 4th ed. USA: Elsevier; 2017; 719–31.
2. Cutrufello NJ, Karakousis PC, Fishler J, Albini TA. Intraocular tuberculosis. Ocul Immunol Inflamm. 2010; 18(4):281–91.
3. Gharai S, Venkatesh P, Garg S, Sharma SK, Vohra R. Ophthalmic manifestations of HIV infections in India in the era of HAART: analysis of 100 consecutive patients evaluated at a tertiary eye care center in India. Ophthalmic Epidemiol. 2008; 15(4):264–71.
4. Wilhelmus KR. CHAPTER 83. Syphilitic Keratitis. In: Cornea; Volume 1 – Fundamentals, Diagnosis and Management. 4th ed. USA: Elsevier; 2017; 996–1012.

16 Corneal Involvement in Non-Infective Systemic Disorders

Ritika Mukhija, Rachna Meel, Vipul Singh, Noopur Gupta

INTRODUCTION

The eye is sometimes called the gateway to the human body. Various systemic diseases have different ocular presentations, which sometimes may even herald the onset of the systemic disease.[1,2] The cornea can be involved in a variety of autoimmune, skeletal and connective tissue disorders and endocrine and metabolic diseases.[3–6] It is important to identify these features as the management in most of these cases relies on adequate treatment of the underlying systemic pathology. This chapter gives a brief overview of corneal infective and inflammatory pathologies in various non-infective and auto-immune systemic disorders.

CASE 16.1

CLINICAL FEATURES

A 45-year-old female presented with painful diminution of vision in her left eye for the last two weeks, along with the appearance of a brown patch in the eye two days ago. She had a history of undergoing tectonic keratoplasty in the same eye five months ago, which was performed for a sterile corneal melt. The patient was a known case of rheumatoid arthritis (RA) and was on treatment for the same. Examination findings and slit lamp appearance are illustrated in Figure 16.1.

KEY POINTS

Diagnosis:
- The above clinical scenario highlights a case of recurrent sterile corneal melt in a patient with RA.

Investigations:
- The ocular diagnosis was primarily clinical; however, a referral was made to the treating rheumatologist to review the patient's systemic status and investigations revealed a high non-steroidal rheumatoid factor (RF) titre.

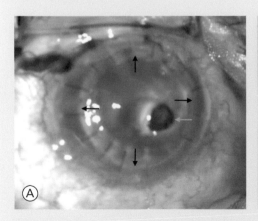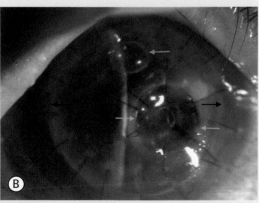

Figure 16.1 Clinical photograph of a 45-year-old female with rheumatoid arthritis showing (A) sterile corneal graft melt with iris prolapse (yellow arrow) in a previously operated tectonic penetrating keratoplasty; note that the graft is otherwise well-apposed (black arrows) with all sutures in situ. Slit lamp photograph of the same patient showing (B) the eye four days after a full-thickness patch graft (green arrows) was performed. Note the well-apposed graft host junction (black arrows) of the previous keratoplasty and the air bubble (grey arrow) in the anterior chamber.

Treatment:
- The patient was treated with topical and oral broad-spectrum antibiotics and artificial tear drops and was taken for an emergency tectonic patch graft.
- After the surgery, topical steroids (prednisolone acetate 1% four times a day) were also added.
- She was also simultaneously prescribed a course of oral steroids by the rheumatologist along with some modifications in her treatment regimen, consisting of disease-modifying antirheumatic drugs (DMARDs) and non-steroidal anti-inflammatory drugs (NSAIDs).

Outcome:
- The graft uptake was good in the early postoperative period; however, three weeks later the patient developed a recurrent melt involving the graft-host junction (Figure 16.2), following which a lamellar overlay corneal graft was performed.

- After the third surgery and after achieving good systemic control, the patient has remained stable with no recurrence of ocular inflammation; however, the graft opacified in about six months.

Supplementary Information and Additional Tips

- Extra-articular disease in RA is relatively less common than before; this is due to better understanding of the pathophysiology and aggressive treatment early in the course of the disease. However, patients presenting with ophthalmic disease often have severe, long-standing course and/or high RF titres (Figure 16.3).
- Keratoconjunctivitis sicca is the most common ocular manifestation in RA and may present as punctate keratopathy, mucus stranding and filamentary keratitis (Figure 16.4).

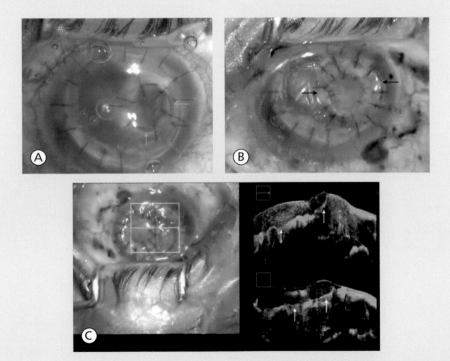

Figure 16.2 Clinical intraoperative photograph of the same patient who developed recurrent graft melt showing (A) areas of early graft melt apparent as gaps in the graft-host junction (yellow arrows). Clinical photograph at the end of the surgery showing (B) a larger overlay lamellar patch graft (black arrows) and an intraoperative OCT image (C) clearly demonstrating the graft-host interface (white arrows).

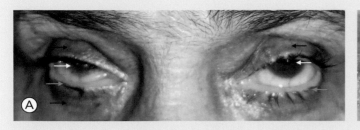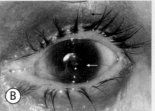

Figure 16.3 Clinical photograph of a 55-year-old female with rheumatoid arthritis showing (A) bilateral sterile corneal melt (white arrows) along with inflamed lid margins (grey arrows) and mild periocular skin erythema and excoriation (black arrows). Magnified view of the left eye distinctly showing (B) the area of corneal melt with uveal prolapse.

- Scleritis, including diffuse anterior, nodular and necrotising types, and episcleritis are also common anterior segment manifestations of RA (Figure 16.5). Keratitis occurring as marginal infiltrates, peripheral ulcerative keratitis (PUK) and sterile corneal stromal melts may also occur (Figure 16.6).

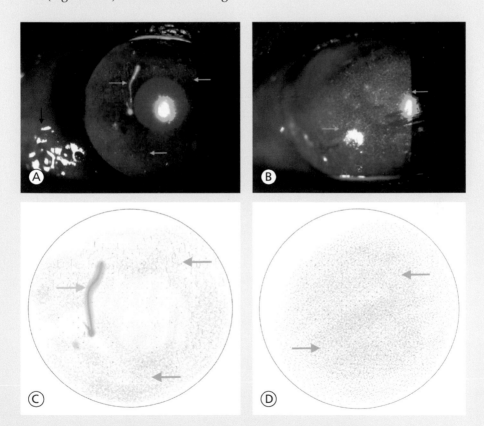

Figure 16.4 Slit lamp photographs of a patient with rheumatoid arthritis and secondary Sjögren's syndrome showing bilateral keratoconjunctivitis sicca (right eye: A; left eye: B) with diffuse punctate staining (green arrows); also note the filamentary keratitis (yellow arrow) and conjunctival xerosis (black arrow) present in the right eye. The corresponding corneal diagrams (right eye: C; left eye: D) illustrate the same findings.

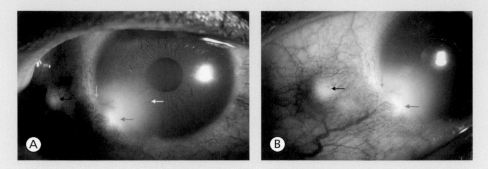

Figure 16.5 Slit lamp photographs of a patient with rheumatoid arthritis showing (A) nodular scleritis (black arrow) and peripheral corneal infiltrates (grey arrow); note the localised conjunctival congestion, superficial vascularisation (yellow arrow) and peripheral corneal opacity (white arrow) possibly due to a prior episode of keratitis or sclerokeratitis. Magnified view (B) shows the same findings more distinctly.

- Small corneal perforations can be managed well with tissue adhesives and bandage contact lens (Figure 16.7); larger ones may require tectonic patch grafts, which may be sutured, as in this case, or sutureless (Figure 16.8) or even penetrating keratoplasty.

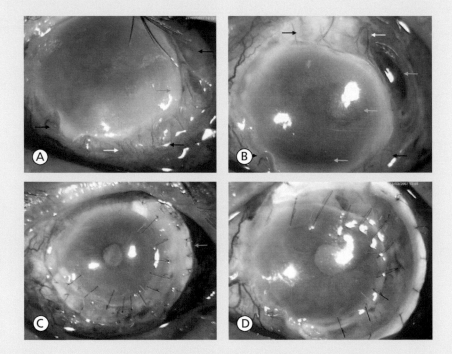

Figure 16.6 Slit lamp photographs of a patient with rheumatoid arthritis showing bilateral severe peripheral ulcerative keratitis (right eye: A; left eye: B) with severe peripheral thinning (black arrows) spanning in up to three quadrants and corneal neovascularisation (white arrows); note the few stromal infiltrates (grey arrow) in the right eye and uveal tissue prolapse (yellow arrow) and hyphaema with endothelial staining (green arrows) in the left eye. Tectonic crescentic patch grafts (blue arrows) tailored to the extent of involvement were performed for both eyes (right eye: C; left eye: D); note the pupillary peaking (red arrow) in the left eye.

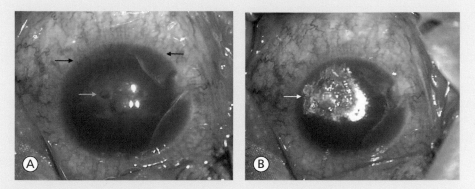

Figure 16.7 Clinical intraoperative photographs of a patient with rheumatoid arthritis showing (A) a small area of sterile corneal melt with uveal show (yellow arrow) and severe ciliary congestion (black arrows) at the start of the procedure and (B) showing the eye after application of cyanoacrylate glue (white arrow); a bandage contact lens is placed after adequate glue application.

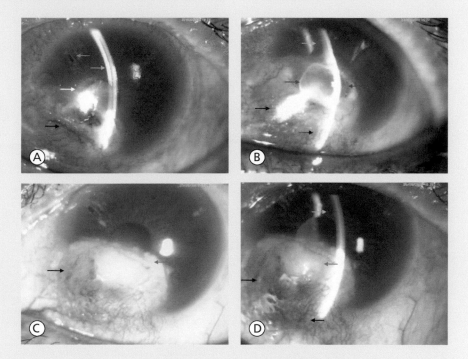

Figure 16.8 Slit lamp photographs of a patient with rheumatoid arthritis showing (A) recurrent sclerokeratitis with spontaneous corneal perforation (yellow arrow); note the peripheral dense scarring and vascularisation (black arrow) and mild nebular haze in the surrounding cornea (white arrow) along with a flat anterior chamber (green arrow) as seen on slit illumination. As the patient also had primary-angle closure glaucoma, a peripheral laser iridotomy (grey arrow) was previously performed. Slit lamp photograph in the immediate postoperative period showing (B) a circular sutureless patch graft (red arrows) at the site of perforation performed using fibrin-glue; note that the anterior chamber is now formed (green arrow). Late postoperative photographs at three months follow-up showing (C) a well-healed scar (blue arrow) and an increase in the peripheral vascularised corneal opacification (black arrow); the parallelepiped illumination (D) shows that the anterior chamber (AC) depth is adequate (green arrow).

CASE 16.2

CLINICAL FEATURES

A 45-year-old male presented with complaints of pain, redness and watering in his right eye for the last three weeks. He was taking over-the-counter medications (antibiotic-steroid combination eye/ear drops) and reported some relief in the initial days; however, he started to notice a brown mass for the last three days, following which he presented to our ophthalmic emergency. Patient gave a history of a similar episode of redness and pain two months back, which resolved in about two weeks. He also gave a history of recurrent sinusitis for which he took on/off treatment from a local physician. Examination findings and slit lamp appearance are illustrated in Figure 16.9.

KEY POINTS

Diagnosis:

- The above clinical scenario highlights a case of necrotising scleritis with peripheral corneal infiltrates in a patient with Wegener's granulomatosis (WG).

Investigations:

- A gentle scraping was performed at the site of corneal infiltrates and some specimen was also collected from the area of sclera necrosis using a cotton-tipped applicator. These were sent for microbiological analysis to rule out any infective organisms, and no microbe was identified or cultured.
- A basic panel of systemic investigations, vis-à-vis complete blood count, erythrocyte sedimentation rate (ESR), RF and chest X-ray was ordered. ESR was found to be elevated along with a positive RF and an abnormal X-ray, following which the patient was referred to the rheumatology department.
- A thorough systemic workup and investigations led to the diagnosis of WG with high levels of antineutrophil cytoplasmic antibody (c-ANCA).

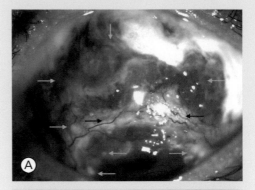
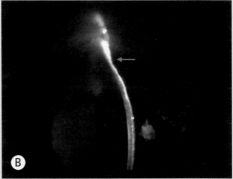
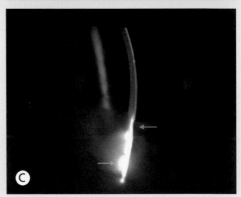

Figure 16.9 Slit lamp photographs of a patient with Wegener's granulomatosis showing (A) severe sclerokeratitis with diffuse areas of scleral melt and uveal show (green arrows), sterile corneal and scleral infiltrates (yellow arrows) and vascularisation (black arrows); magnified parallelepiped views of the superior (B) and inferior (C) cornea show peripheral corneal thinning (grey arrows).

Treatment:
- The patient was treated with topical and oral broad-spectrum antibiotics; artificial tear drops and oral ascorbate.
- He was also prescribed oral prednisone (1 mg/kg) and cyclophosphamide (2 mg/kg) by the rheumatology team; steroids were tapered and cyclophosphamide continued.
- After one week of therapy, an amniotic membrane transplant was performed to cover the large area of scleral necrosis.

Outcome:
- Acceptable response to therapy was noted in the initial week; the margins of scleral necrosis displayed signs of healing and the peripheral corneal infiltrates started regressing.

- The amniotic membrane melted in about two weeks after transplantation; however, the defect eventually healed with scarring, scleral thinning and mild uveal show.

Supplementary Information and Additional Tips
- Scleritis and keratitis may often present as the first sign of WG, hence it is important for the ophthalmologist and/or cornea specialist to be aware and alert about the same. Other anterior segment manifestations are conjunctivitis, episcleritis and uveitis.
- Secondary Sjögren's syndrome and dry eye also occurs frequently (Figure 16.10); in severe cases, peripheral corneal guttering, necrosis and perforation may be seen (Figure 16.11).

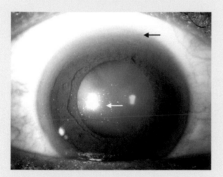

Figure 16.10 Slit lamp photograph of a patient with Wegener's granulomatosis showing mild dry eye; note areas of tear-film breakup (white arrow) visible without cobalt blue filter and fluorescein staining and diffuse limbal pigmentation (black arrow).

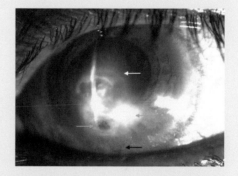

Figure 16.11 Slit lamp photograph of a patient with Wegener's granulomatosis with secondary Sjögren's syndrome showing peripheral corneal ulceration (green arrow), infiltrates (yellow arrow), vascularisation (black arrow), and surrounding corneal haze (white arrow).

CASE 16.3

CLINICAL FEATURES

A 50-year-old male presented with complaints of diminution of vision, pain, redness and photophobia in his left eye for the last ten days. Patient was a known case of polyarteritis nodosa (PAN) with chronic renal disease and was on treatment for the same. Examination findings and slit lamp appearance are illustrated in Figure 16.12.

KEY POINTS

Diagnosis:
- The above clinical scenario highlights a case of PUK in a patient with PAN.

Investigations:
- As there were no clinical signs suggestive of infective aetiology, corneal scarping was not performed.

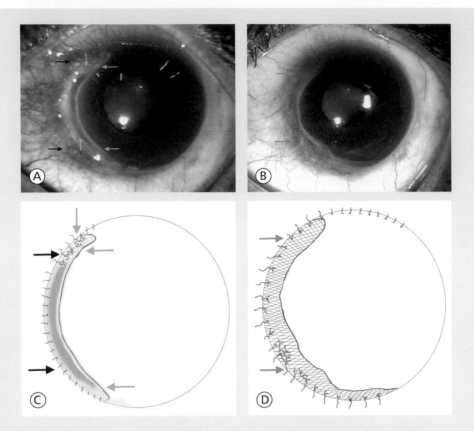

Figure 16.12 Slit lamp photograph of a patient with polyarteritis nodosa (PAN) showing (A) peripheral ulcerative keratitis (PUK) with peripheral thinning and gutter formation (green arrows), few infiltrates (yellow arrows) and associated ciliary and conjunctival congestion (black arrows); follow-up picture after two months (B) showing healed PUK with peripheral vascularised corneal scarring (grey arrows). Corresponding corneal diagrams (C, D) illustrate the same findings.

■ There is no specific diagnostic test for the disease; however, Hepatitis B surface antigens (HbSAg) have been found in around 50% of the patients; antineutrophil perinuclear antibody (P-ANCA) testing may also be positive.

Treatment:
■ Apart from the ongoing systemic immunosuppression, a short course of oral steroids was prescribed after consultation with the treating physician.
■ He was also treated with topical broad-spectrum antibiotic (moxifloxacin 0.5% QID), steroid (loteprednol 0.5% QID), cycloplegic (homatropine 2% BD), antiglaucoma

(timolol 0.5% BD) and lubricants. In addition, oral doxycycline was also prescribed for four weeks.

Outcome:
■ The patient showed significant improvement with treatment, and the ulcer healed with scarring and peripheral conjunctivalisation in about four weeks.

Supplementary Information and Additional Tips
■ Anterior segment findings are not very common in PAN; however, scleritis, sclerokeratitis and PUK can occur; cases with bilateral recurrent severe PUK have also been reported (Figures 16.13 and 16.14).

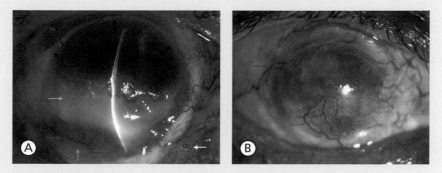

Figure 16.13 Slit lamp photograph of the right eye of a patient with polyarteritis nodosa (PAN) and bilateral recurrent severe PUK (A) showing areas of inferior graft melt (grey arrow) four weeks after a crescentic patch graft (black arrows pointing towards the edge of the graft superiorly) was performed; note the inferior host corneal melt and infiltration (yellow arrow), vascularisation (red arrows) and remnant of vicryl sutures (white arrow). The photograph on the right (B) shows the same eye after two sittings of multilayered amniotic membrane transplantation were performed; note the diffuse corneal opacity (blue arrow) and vascularisation (red arrows).

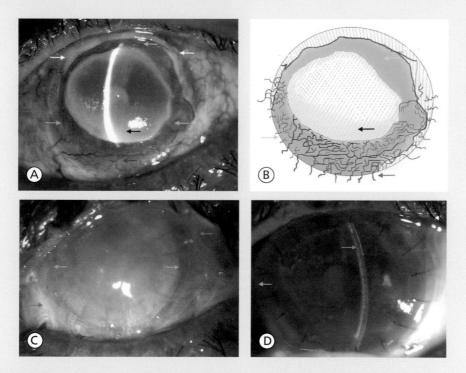

Figure 16.14 Slit lamp photograph of the left eye of the above patient with polyarteritis nodosa (PAN) and bilateral recurrent severe PUK (A) circumferential 360 degree corneal melt (yellow arrows) six weeks after being operated for an annular patch graft (white arrows pointing towards the edge of the remnant graft tissue superiorly); note the inferior host corneal haze and infiltration (black arrow) and diffuse vascularisation (red arrow). The corresponding clinical diagram (B) illustrates the same findings. Slit lamp photograph at follow-up after a large diameter lamellar keratoplasty and amniotic membrane transplantation was performed (C) showing a limbus-to-limbus graft (green arrows pointing towards graft-host junction) with overlying amniotic membrane graft (blue arrows); parallelepiped view (D) also shows the graft-host interface (grey arrow).

CASE 16.4

CLINICAL FEATURES

A 32-year-old female presented with a history of gradually progressive painful diminution of vision in her right eye for the last six weeks. She gave a history of undergoing laser in the same eye around two weeks back. She also had a history of recurrent oral ulcers, multiple pustular lesions on her leg and joint pain for the past year, for which she was taking treatment from the local dermatologist. Examination findings and slit lamp appearance are illustrated in Figure 16.15.

KEY POINTS

Diagnosis:

- The above clinical scenario highlights a case of keratouveitis associated with suspected Behcet's disease.
- The patient had undergone multiple laser peripheral iridotomies to relieve the pupillary block as a result of severe anterior chamber inflammation.

Investigations:

- The ocular diagnosis was based on clinical findings; systemic workup under the rheumatology department

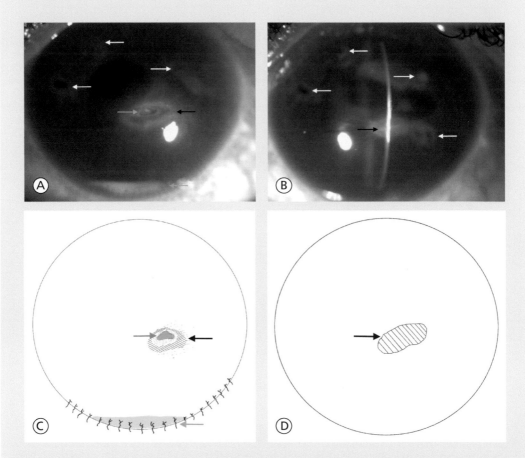

Figure 16.15 Slit lamp photograph of a patient with Behcet's disease showing (A) healing keratitis with a small epithelial defect (green arrow) and surrounding scarring (black arrow) along with severe uveitis and hypopyon (yellow arrow). Photograph (B) shows the same eye two weeks later with healed keratitis with scarring (black arrow). Note the multiple mid-peripheral iridotomies (white arrows) performed to release pupillary block. The corresponding corneal diagrams (C, D) illustrate the same findings.

revealed that the patient was HLA-B51 positive and had a positive pathergy test.

Treatment:

- She was treated with topical steroids (prednisolone acetate 1%) every two hours for the first 48 hours followed by tapering, cycloplegic (homatropine hydrobromide 2% thrice a day) and antiglaucoma (timolol 0.5% twice a day).
- For the keratitis, that had already started resolving, a broad-spectrum topical antibiotic (moxifloxacin hydrochloride 0.5% four times a day) cover and lubricating eye drops (carboxymethylcellulose 0.5% four times a day) were added.
- After consultation with the treating rheumatologist, the patient was also prescribed oral azathioprine (2.5 mg/kg/day).

Outcome:

- The patient showed improvement with resolution of inflammatory hypopyon

in a week and healing of corneal ulcer leaving a macular corneal opacity in about two weeks.

Supplementary Information and Additional Tips

- Behcet's disease may present with severe keratouveitis with hypopyon in a relatively white eye; this is sometimes referred to as the 'cold hypopyon.' However, limited anterior segment involvement is uncommon, and a thorough posterior segment evaluation is warranted in all cases.
- Intense anterior chamber reaction may lead to the formation of fibrinous membrane and even pupillary block in some cases; the latter may be relieved by performing multiple peripheral iridotomies as in this case.
- Isolated corneal involvement is rare; however, a few cases of PUK have been reported (Figure 16.16).

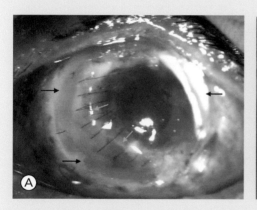 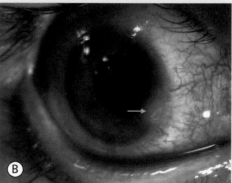

Figure 16.16   Slit lamp photograph of a patient with Behcet's disease with bilateral peripheral keratitis; the left eye (A) shows an operated crescentic patch graft (black arrows) for severe PUK (green arrows pointing towards corneal graft-host junction); the right eye (B) shows a small peripheral corneal ulcer (yellow arrow) along with localised ciliary and conjunctival congestion (grey arrows).

CASE 16.5

CLINICAL FEATURES

A 60-year-old male presented with complaints of pain, redness and watering

in his left eye for three weeks, which was followed two weeks later by the appearance of a brown mass. There were

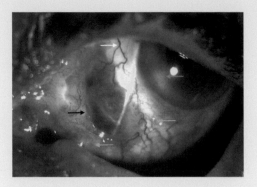

Figure 16.17 Slit lamp photograph of a patient with inflammatory bowel disease showing necrotising scleritis with an area of diffuse scleral necrosis and melt in the nasal quadrant (black arrow), vascularisation (white arrow) and peripheral corneal opacity (grey arrow). Amniotic membrane transplantation was performed, but the AMG melted in a few days owing to inflammation; note the residual vicryl sutures (green arrows).

no prior similar episodes or any history of preceding trauma. He was a known case of inflammatory bowel disease and was on treatment for the same. Examination findings and slit lamp appearance are illustrated in Figure 16.17.

KEY POINTS

Diagnosis:
- The above clinical scenario highlights a case of necrotising scleritis in a patient with inflammatory bowel disease.

Investigations:
- Gentle debridement around the area of scleral necrosis was performed and specimens sent for microbiological testing; no organism was identified or cultured.
- In addition, posterior segment B-scan ultrasonography (USG) was performed, which was within normal limits.

Treatment:
- Patient was prescribed systemic NSAIDs, topical broad-spectrum antibiotic (moxifloxacin 0.5% QID), cycloplegic (homatropine 2% TDS) and lubricants.
- A referral was sought from the treating gastroenterologist; the patient was subsequently taken for an amniotic membrane transplantation (AMT).

Outcome:
- The initial outcome to the AMT was not very encouraging as the graft melted in a few days owing to the inflammation; thereafter, a tectonic scleral patch graft had to be performed.

CASE 16.6

CLINICAL FEATURES

A 46-year-old female presented with complains of diminution of vision, severe pain, redness and mild discharge in her right eye for the last ten days. She also gave history of hearing loss for the last six months, following which she was diagnosed as a case of relapsing polychondritis; since then she has been on oral NSAIDs. There was no history of any prior ocular complaints. Examination findings and slit lamp appearance are illustrated in Figure 16.18.

KEY POINTS

Diagnosis:
- The above clinical scenario highlights a case of sclerokeratouveitis in a patient with relapsing polychondritis.

Investigations:
- The necrotic debris was carefully removed and sent for microbiological testing; no organism was identified or cultured.
- There is no specific investigation of choice for relapsing polychondritis; conjunctival and scleral biopsies may be performed if needed.

Treatment:
- The patient was prescribed a short course of oral steroids in addition to topical broad-spectrum antibiotic, cycloplegic and lubricants. Topical steroids were not given, as they are usually not helpful and there was no active uveitis.
- She was also referred to the treating physician to assess and modify

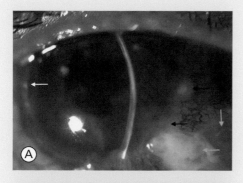

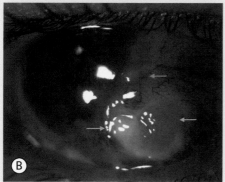

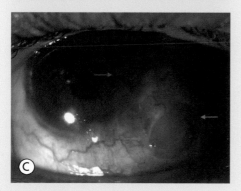

the systemic therapy and to add immunomodulators as necessary.

Outcome:

- There was a good response to treatment and an improvement in both symptoms and signs was noted; the lesions healed with a corneoscleral scarring in about four weeks.

Supplementary Information and Additional Tips

- Scleritis and episcleritis are the most frequent findings; scleritis can be either diffuse, nodular or necrotising (Figures 16.19 and 16.20). It is believed to be a marker of the severity of the underlying disease, and

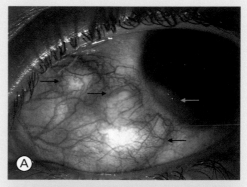

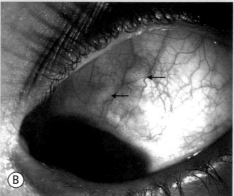

Figure 16.18 Slit lamp photographs of a patient with relapsing polychondritis and sclerokeratouveitis (A, B) showing localised scleritis (green arrows), necrotic debris (yellow arrows), diffuse conjunctival congestion (grey arrow) along with a few adjacent peripheral corneal infiltrates (black arrows) and a few infiltrates (white arrow) away from the main site of involvement. Slit lamp photograph at two weeks follow-up (C) showing healing scleritis with distinct margins of involvement (blue arrows) and a decrease in necrotic debris; also note the posterior synechiae (red arrow).

Figure 16.19 Slit lamp photographs of a patient with relapsing polychondritis with bilateral nodular scleritis; note the multiple nodules (black arrows) in the inferotemporal quadrant in the right eye (A) and superotemporal quadrant in the left eye (B), along with peripheral corneal scarring in the right eye (grey arrow), which could be suggestive of a healed peripheral ulcer.

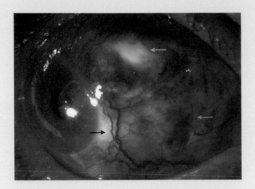

Figure 16.20 Slit lamp photograph of a patient with relapsing polychondritis with necrotising scleritis showing an area of diffuse scleral necrosis and melt (grey arrow), scleral infiltrates (yellow arrow) and dilated tortuous vessels (black arrow).

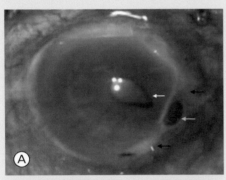

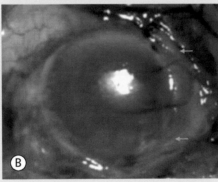

Figure 16.21 Clinical intraoperative photographs of a patient with relapsing polychondritis and peripheral ulcerative keratitis showing (A) perforated corneal ulcer (black arrows) with iris tissue prolapse (yellow arrow) and pupillary peaking (white arrow) at the beginning of the surgery; and (B) a well-apposed crescentic sutured patch graft (green arrows) at the end of the surgery.

often suggests a need for aggressive immunomodulatory treatment.

■ Corneal manifestations can occur in the form of PUK, infiltrates, crystalline deposits and spontaneous perforations (Figures 16.21 and 16.22).

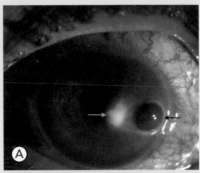

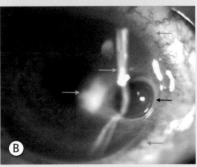

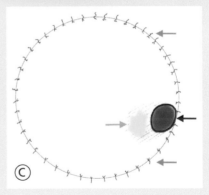

Figure 16.22 Slit lamp photographs of a patient with relapsing polychondritis (A) showing a peripheral perforated corneal ulcer with iris tissue prolapse (black arrow), adjacent stromal infiltrates (yellow arrow), likely due to secondary infection, and ciliary and conjunctival congestion (grey arrows). Photograph with parallelepiped illumination (B) shows the flat anterior chamber (green arrow) and the corresponding corneal diagram (C) illustrates the same findings.

CASE 16.7

CLINICAL FEATURES

A 40-year-old female presented with complaints of pain, redness and photophobia in her left eye for the last four days. She was a known case of psoriasis and typical scaly lesions were evident on her scalp. She was on regular treatment from her dermatologist. Examination findings and slit lamp appearance are illustrated in Figure 16.23.

KEY POINTS

Diagnosis:
- The above clinical scenario highlights a case of peripheral corneal infiltrates in a patient with psoriasis.

Investigations:
- The diagnosis was primarily clinical; no specific investigations were performed.

Treatment:
- She was prescribed a course of topical broad-spectrum antibiotic, cycloplegic, artificial tears and lubricating eye ointment.
- Lid hygiene and warm compresses were additionally advised for the blepharitis.

Outcome:
- There was significant improvement with the treatment and the infiltrates regressed in about two weeks; treatment for blepharitis was continued.

Supplementary Information and Additional Tips

- Corneal disease is uncommon in psoriasis; peripheral keratitis and vascularisation, punctate epithelial keratopathy, corneal opacities, ulceration and melting can occur (Figure 16.24).

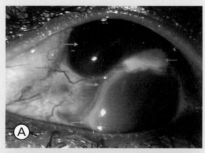

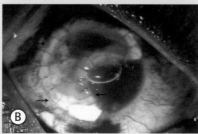

Figure 16.24 Slit lamp photograph of a patient with psoriasis and severe PUK (A) showing peripheral corneal melt and thinning (green arrows), large area of superior uveal tissue prolapse (yellow arrow), vascularisation (grey arrow) and necrotic debris (blue arrow). Slit lamp photograph at first-operative day (B) showing a large crescentic patch graft (black arrows) sutured using 10-0 monofilament nylon sutures along with some areas of subconjunctival haemorrhage and a small air bubble in the anterior chamber.

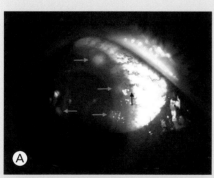

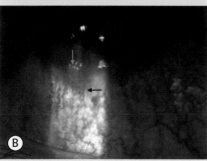

Figure 16.23 Slit lamp photographs of a patient with psoriasis (A) showing peripheral corneal infiltrates (grey arrows) and ciliary congestion (black arrow) and (B) showing similar findings in the inferior cornea.

CASE 16.8

CLINICAL FEATURES

A 65-year-old male presented with complaints of diminution of vision, pain and redness in both his eyes for the last three months. He gave a history of taking medications for myalgia around six months back, following which he developed high-grade fever, vomiting and diarrhoea, which was followed by the development of multiple rashes over the face, trunk, arms and feet and redness and discharge from both the eyes. The patient was diagnosed as a case of toxic epidermal necrolysis (TEN) by the treating physician and dermatologist and was receiving treatment for the same. Subsequently, the patient consulted a local ophthalmologist after

he developed ocular symptoms, where he initially received treatment in the form of topical antibiotics and lubricants, and later underwent bilateral AMT. Following the surgery, there was marked improvement for three weeks; however, the complaints recurred, with no improvement with further conservative management for a month. He was then referred to a tertiary-care centre. On presentation, the visual acuity was 6/12 in the right eye and finger counting at two metres in the left eye; bilateral intraocular pressure was within normal limits. Examination findings and slit lamp appearance at presentation are illustrated in Figure 16.25 and the healed skin lesions are shown in Figure 16.26.

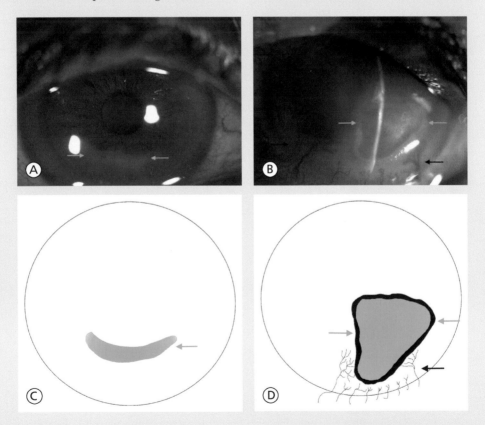

Figure 16.25 Slit lamp photographs of a patient with toxic epidermal necrolysis (TEN) sequelae with bilateral neurotrophic keratitis; the right eye (A) showing a small linear epithelial defect (green arrows) and the left eye (B) showing a large epithelial defect with punched out margins (green arrows) along with unhealthy epithelium at the edges and active vascularisation (black arrows). The corresponding schematic corneal diagram of the right (C) and left eye (D) depict the same findings.

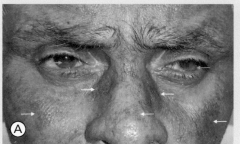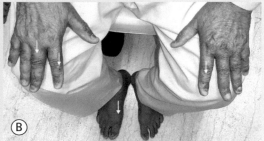

Figure 16.26 Clinical photographs of a patient with toxic epidermal necrolysis (TEN) sequelae showing (A) multiple healed scars (white arrows) on the face along with grossly visible fluorescein stained epithelial defects (green arrows); photographs of the hands and feet of the patient (B) also show similar scars.

KEY POINTS

Diagnosis:
- The above clinical scenario highlights a case of bilateral TEN sequalae with ocular surface disorder, partial limbal stem-cell deficiency (LSCD) and neurotrophic keratitis, with a worse disease in the left eye.

Investigations:
- Diagnosis was made on clinical findings; no specific investigations were performed.
- Impression cytology may be performed in chronic cases to determine the extent of LSCD.

Treatment:
- The patient was treated with broad-spectrum topical antibiotics (chloramphenicol 0.5% TDS) and a combination of preservative-free lubricating eye drops (carboxymethyl cellulose 1% every two hours; polyethylene and propylene glycol QID) and ointment (hydroxypropylmethylcellulose 0.3% TDS).
- In addition, topical autologous serum (20%) was prescribed four times a day in both eyes.

Outcome:
- The patient showed significant improvement with the above treatment. After ten days, the epithelial defect healed completely in the right eye and partially in the

left eye; the latter showed unhealthy heaped-up epithelium, owing to severe ocular surface disease (OSD) and LSCD (Figure 16.27).
- Autologous serum was continued for three weeks in the left eye and was stopped after complete healing of epithelial defect was noted. Thereafter, the patient was asked to continue lubricating eye drops and ointment.
- Snellen chart visual acuity improved to 6/9 in the right eye and 6/36 in the left eye; the latter owing to a nebulo-macular corneal opacity.

Supplementary Information and Additional Tips

- TEN is a disease at the extreme end of the severity spectrum in erythema multiforme and is characterised by involvement of over 30% of the epidermis in the body.
- Ocular sequelae of TEN can be severe and involve eyelids, conjunctiva and cornea. They can be either acute, in the form of nonspecific conjunctivitis, ulceration and uveitis, or chronic. The latter includes conjunctival or corneal scarring; corneal neovascularisation; symblepharon formation; cicatricial changes in the conjunctiva, lids and lacrimal ducts; keratinisation of lid margins, conjunctiva and cornea; and LSCD and persistent epithelial defects (PEDs) (Figure 16.28).

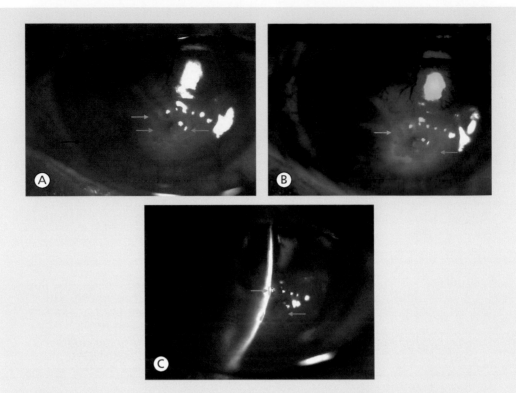

Figure 16.27 Slit lamp photographs of the left eye of the above two weeks after treatment (A) showing healing neurotrophic ulcer with dense vascularisation (black arrows); note the heaped-up unhealthy epithelium (grey arrows) with bullae (yellow arrow). The photograph under cobalt flue filter with fluorescein staining (B) shows that there is no epithelial defect (grey arrow) and delineates the bullae (yellow arrow) better, which can also be seen as on parallelepiped illumination (C).

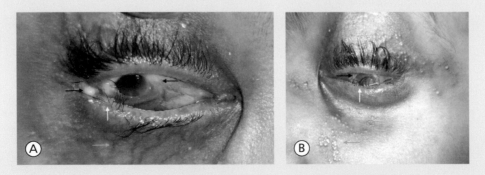

Figure 16.28 Clinical photographs of a 7-year-old female with toxic epidermal necrolysis (TEN) (right eye: A; left eye: B) showing severe entropion and lash-globe contact (white arrows) and inflamed conjunctiva (grey arrow) with mucoid discharge (black arrows); note the skin erythema with dilated vessels (green arrow) in the right eye and multiple small lesions (yellow arrows) in the left eye.

CASE 16.9

CLINICAL FEATURES

An 18-year-old male presented with diminution of vision, redness and discoloration in both his eyes for the last two months. He gave a history of recurrent ocular redness and photophobia in the past. Patient was a known case of xeroderma pigmentosum (XP) and had multiple melanotic lesions and scarring on his face. Examination findings and slit lamp appearance are illustrated in Figures 16.29 and 16.30.

KEY POINTS

Diagnosis:
- The above clinical scenario describes a case of bilateral healed keratitis and conjunctival melanosis in a patient with XP.

Investigations:
- Diagnosis was primarily clinical; anterior segment optical coherence tomography was performed to assess the extent and depth of corneal opacity.
- Frequent examinations and early detection of cutaneous and ocular malignancies are essential; impression cytology from any doubtful lesion on ocular surface may be helpful.

Treatment:
- Treatment of XP primarily revolves around avoidance of sun exposure and protection from UV light with liberal use of sunscreen and symptomatic treatment for ocular complaints.
- This patient was prescribed lubricating eye drops and ointment, advised to wear protective eye-wear and to follow up regularly.

Outcome:
- The patient had some improvement in redness and photophobia with treatment. Surgical intervention in the form of keratoplasty was not performed in view of poor prognosis for graft survival.

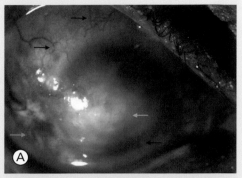

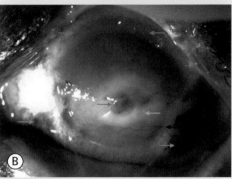

Figure 16.29 Slit lamp photographs of a patient with xeroderma pigmentosum showing (right eye: A; left eye: B) bilateral healed keratitis with corneal opacity (yellow arrows) and conjunctival melanosis (grey arrows); note the vascularisation (black arrows) and pigmentation over the cornea and limbus (blue arrows).

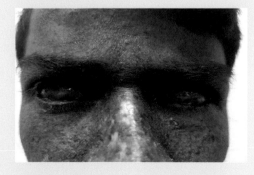

Figure 16.30 Clinical photograph of a patient showing the multiple facial scars and freckling in sun-exposed areas that is diagnostic of xeroderma pigmentosum with corneal opacification due to resolved keratitis and resultant loss of vision.

Supplementary Information and Additional Tips

- Ophthalmic manifestations of XP are mainly restricted to sun-exposed areas, i.e. eyelids, interpalpebral zone of the bulbar conjunctiva, cornea and iris. Common ocular features are progressive atrophy of the lower eyelid leading to exposure of ocular surface, inflammation and ulceration; conjunctival hyperaemia, keratinisation and melanosis and pannus formation, LSCD, corneal neovascularisation and opacity are also seen (Figure 16.31).

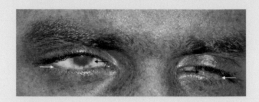

Figure 16.31 Clinical photograph of a 14-year-old male with xeroderma pigmentosa showing bilateral lid margin inflammation (white arrows) and corneal opacity (black arrows).

CASE 16.10

CLINICAL FEATURES

An 8-year-old female (informer: father) presented with a history of diminution of vision in both her eyes for the last six months. There was no history of associated pain or photophobia and the child was comfortably opening her eyes. She was diagnosed as a case of type 1 diabetes mellitus (DM) one year prior; however, she had uncontrolled blood glucose levels in view of poor compliance to treatment. Examination findings and slit lamp appearance are illustrated in Figure 16.32.

KEY POINTS

Diagnosis:
- The above clinical scenario highlights a case of bilateral diabetic keratopathy in a child with type 1 DM.

Investigations:
- The ocular diagnosis was based on clinical findings; systemic investigations revealed a random blood sugar of 420 mg/dl.

Treatment:
- The patient was immediately referred to the paediatric department, where she was admitted for management of diabetes.
- She was simultaneously treated with topical antibiotic (moxifloxacin hydrochloride 0.5% four times a day), cycloplegic (homatropine hydrobromide 2% twice a day) and plenty of lubricants (preservative-free carboxymethylcellulose 0.5% every hour).
- The patient was planned for bilateral AMT for non-healing epithelial defects; however, the same could not be performed in view of the lack of systemic clearance for general anaesthesia.

Outcome:
- There were signs of healing of the ulcer with control of blood sugar levels and ocular treatment. The patient was lost to follow up after one month of treatment and presented six months later with bilateral macular corneal opacity.

Supplementary Information and Additional Tips

- Diabetic keratopathy encompasses a clinical spectrum which includes superficial punctuate epitheliopathy, persistent epithelial erosions, corneal hypoesthesia, non-healing PEDs and corneal oedema.
- Infective keratitis may occur more commonly in patients with diabetes owing to the compromised ocular surface and the high risk of infection with opportunistic organisms in cases with uncontrolled blood sugars (Figure 16.33); PUK, albeit rare, may also be seen in association with DM (Figure 16.34).

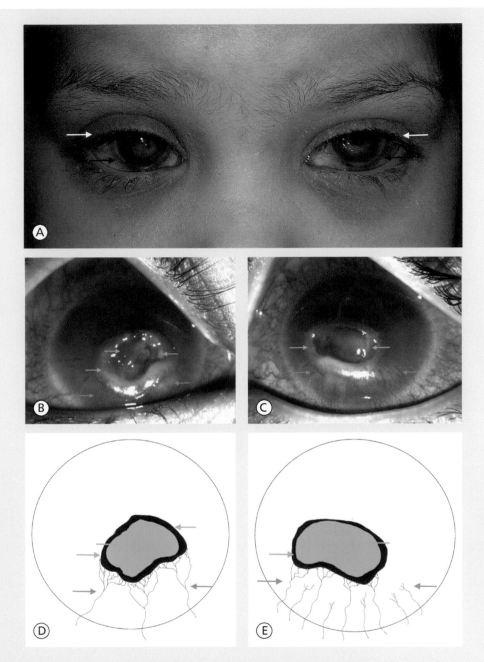

Figure 16.32 Clinical photograph of an 8-year-old female with type 1 diabetes mellitus (A) showing bilateral severe neurotrophic keratitis (black arrows); note how the child is comfortably opening her eyes (white arrows). Slit lamp photographs (right eye: B; left eye: C) showing bilateral central punched out epithelial defect with stromal tissue loss (green arrows), heaped-up unhealthy epithelium at the edges (yellow arrows) and extensive corneal neovascularisation (grey arrows). The corresponding corneal diagrams (right eye: D; left eye: E) depict the same findings.

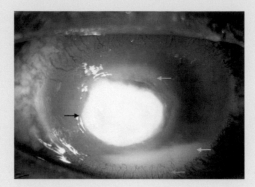

Figure 16.33 Slit lamp photograph showing a case of fungal hypopyon ulcer in a patient with uncontrolled diabetes mellitus; note the dense infiltrates (black arrow) with fuzzy margins (green arrow), hypopyon (yellow arrow) and intense ciliary congestion (grey arrows).

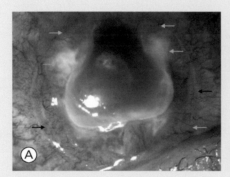
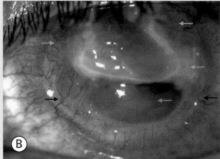

Figure 16.34 Slit lamp photographs of a 12-year-old male child with type 1 diabetes mellitus and bilateral severe PUK (right eye: A; left eye: B) showing severe circumferential thinning and stromal melt (green arrows) with intense corneal neovascularisation (black arrows); also note the necrotic slough (yellow arrows) and haze in the rest of the cornea, and large area of uveal prolapse (grey arrow) in the left eye.

CASE 16.11

CLINICAL FEATURES

A 62-year-old female presented with complaints of bilateral protrusion of both eyeballs, which was progressively worsening for the past few months. She also gave history of diminution of vision, grittiness, redness, pain and watering in both her eyes, more in the left eye over the past 15 days. Patient was a known case of thyroid disorder and was on treatment for the same. At presentation to us, the Snellen visual acuity was 6/12 in the right eye and finger counting at 3 m in the left eye; intraocular pressure was 18 and 22 mm Hg in right and left eye, respectively. Examination findings and clinical appearance are shown in Figure 16.35.

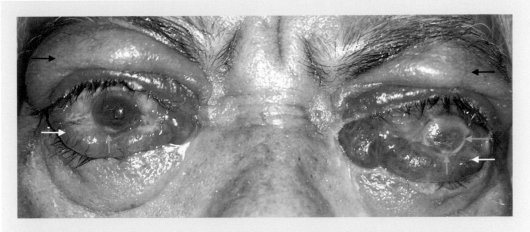

Figure 16.35   Clinical photograph of a patient with bilateral severe thyroid eye disease showing proptosis and lid oedema and fullness (black arrows) and diffuse conjunctival chemosis (white arrows). Corneal involvement can be seen in the form of inferior exposure keratitis (yellow arrows) in both eyes and corneal xerosis and haze (green arrow) in the left eye.

KEY POINTS

Diagnosis:
- The above clinical scenario highlights a case of bilateral severe thyroid eye disease (TED) with proptosis, eyelid oedema, conjunctival congestion and chemosis and left-eye exposure keratopathy.

Investigations:
- Bilateral B-scan USG revealed a normal posterior segment and tendon sparing extraocular muscle thickening; contrast-enhanced computed tomography (CECT) of the orbits and paranasal sinuses was performed to look for the extent of the pathology in consultation with the oculoplastics department.
- A referral was made to the treating endocrinologist and the thyroid function tests were found be abnormally deranged.

Treatment:
- The patient was advised to frequently instil lubricating eye drops as well as nighttime instillation of antibiotic ointment followed by lid taping in both eyes; additional prophylactic antibiotics (moxifloxacin 0.5%) were prescribed for the left eye.
- A 12-week course of intravenous steroids was prescribed for active TED.

Outcome:
- The patient showed significant improvement with a decrease in proptosis and improvement on ocular surface.
- Orbital decompression may be needed in severe cases not responding to conservative management or those with signs of optic nerve compression.

Supplementary Information and Additional Tips

- Anterior segment manifestations in TED are mainly as a result of ocular surface exposure due to proptosis and/or lid retraction; inadequate treatment may lead to sight-threatening complications such as corneal ulceration and melting (Chapter 12, Figure 12.1).
- Conjunctival chemosis, hyperaemia and punctate keratopathy are some other features of TED.

UNUSUAL/ATYPICAL CASE SCENARIOS

- A 28-year-old male presented with swelling in the left upper eyelid, redness and diminution of vision for the last month. On examination, a port-wine stain was noted involving the left forehead and eyelid, along with proptosis, upper lid fullness, conjunctival and episcleral vascular tortuosity and telangiectasia and inferior band-shaped keratopathy (BSK) in the left eye. A diagnosis of Sturge-Weber syndrome (SWS) with proptosis, secondary glaucoma and BSK was made (Figures 16.36 and 16.37).

- A 2-year-old female child presented with history of bilateral redness and watering in both eyes for one month. An examination under anaesthesia was performed; findings revealed bilateral conjunctival vascular tortuosity and sterile keratitis (Figure 16.38). A small central ulcer was noted in the right eye and a peripheral ulcer with circumferential thinning and uveal show was noted in the left eye. There were no signs to suggest an infective aetiology, and the corneal scraping did not reveal any micro-organism. On detailed paediatric evaluation, the child was also found to have lesions suggestive of ichthyosis and dermatitis. It is unclear whether the findings were incidental, or if this presentation was a variant of keratitis-ichthyosis-deafness (KID) syndrome.

- A 26-year-old female presented with gradually progressive whitish opacity and diminution of vision in both her eyes for the last three years. She also gave a history of intermittent dull pain and redness. Ocular examination demonstrated bilateral disc oedema with scleral thinning with hypotony and the best corrected visual acuity was 2/60 in the right eye and 3/60 in the left eye. A physician referral was sought in view of the atypical presentation and a thorough evaluation revealed the presence of hypophysitis on magnetic resonance imaging (MRI) of the brain. A diagnosis of bilateral non-ulcerative perilimbal kerato-scleromalacia (idiopathic non-necrotising scleritis) with hypotonic maculopathy was made and bilateral overlay corneoscleral patch grafts were performed (Figure 16.39).

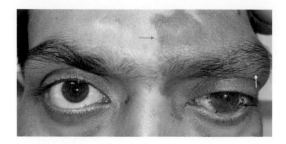

Figure 16.36 Clinical photograph of a patient with Sturge-Weber syndrome (SWS) showing port-wine stain (grey arrow), proptosis in the left eye along with upper lid fullness (white arrow); also note the conjunctival and episcleral vascular tortuosity and telangiectasia (black arrow) and inferior BSK (green arrow).

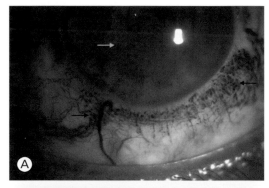

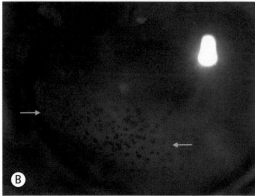

Figure 16.37 Slit lamp photograph of the left eye of the same patient with Sturge-Weber syndrome (SWS) showing (A) conjunctival and episcleral vascular tortuosity and telangiectasia (black arrows) and band-shaped keratopathy (green arrow). Under higher magnification(B), the keratopathy (green arrows) is better appreciated.

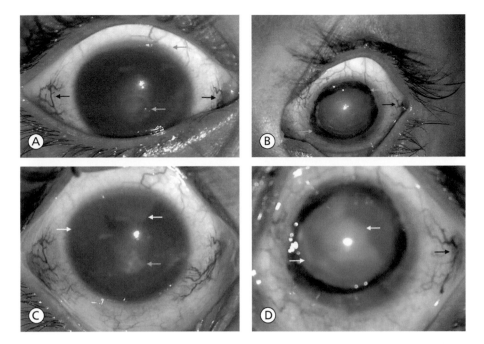

Figure 16.38 Clinical photographs of a 2-year-old female child with ichthyosis and dermatitis and bilateral keratitis; the right eye shows (A) a small central ulcer (yellow arrow) and the left eye shows (B) peripheral ulcer with circumferential thinning and uveal show (green arrows); also note the peripheral corneal vascularisation (grey arrow) and the dilated and tortuous episcleral vessels (black arrows) present nasally and temporally in both the eyes. Corresponding pictures (right eye: C; left eye: D) taken after fluorescein staining delineate the area of epithelial defects (white arrows).

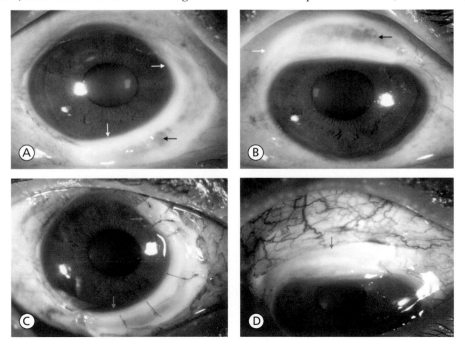

Figure 16.39 Slit lamp photographs of a patient with bilateral non-ulcerative perilimbal kerato-scleromalacia (right eye: A; left eye: B) showing scleral thinning and corneal opacification (white arrows) with cystic areas and mild uveal show (black arrows). Corresponding postoperative photographs (right eye: C; left eye: D) showing bilateral overlay sutured corneoscleral patch grafts (blue arrows).

REFERENCES

1. Freissler KA, Lang GE. The cornea and systemic diseases. Current Opinion in Ophthalmology. 1996 Aug; 7(4):22–7.
2. Ladas JG, Mondino BJ. Systemic disorders associated with peripheral corneal ulceration. Current Opinion in Ophthalmology. 2000 Dec; 11(6):468–71.
3. Taylor S, Li JY. CHAPTER 89. Corneal Disease in Rheumatoid Arthritis. In: Cornea; Volume 1 – Fundamentals, Diagnosis and Management. 4th ed. USA: Elsevier; 2017; 1050–65.
4. Cortina MS, Sugar CJ. CHAPTER 90. Corneal Disease Associated with Nonrheumatoid Collagen-Vascular Disease. In: Cornea; Volume 1 – Fundamentals, Diagnosis and Management. 4th ed. USA: Elsevier; 2017; 1066–75.
5. Gregory DG, Holland EJ. CHAPTER 50. Erythema Multiforme, Stevens–Johnson Syndrome, and Toxic Epidermal Necrolysis. In: Cornea; Volume 1 – Fundamentals, Diagnosis and Management. 4th ed. USA: Elsevier; 2017; 558–72.
6. Zargar MD, Bartow RM. CHAPTER 62. Endocrine Disease and the Cornea. In: Cornea; Volume 1 – Fundamentals, Diagnosis and Management. 4th ed. USA: Elsevier; 2017; 696–704.

SECTION F

PAEDIATRIC CORNEAL DISORDERS

17 Approach to Paediatric Patients with Corneal Disease

Nimmy Raj, Akash D Saha, Yogita Gupta, Nikita Sharma, Noopur Gupta

INTRODUCTION

Paediatric patients present unique challenges in terms of examination and diagnosis as well as management of corneal diseases. The medical history comes primarily from the parents/caregivers and needs to be correlated with clinical findings. Socioeconomic history, especially in developing countries, assumes importance in children as compliance to therapy and regular follow-up guide response to therapy and outcomes in these cases. Different examination strategies are needed depending upon the age of the patient ranging from feeding and swaddling an infant to using colourful toys and movies to distract toddlers. An initial torch-light examination should be done to evaluate the overall status of the ocular surface and the quality of the light reflex. A slit lamp biomicroscopy should be performed in a child wherever possible. The child can be made to sit on the parent's lap to ensure compliance and correct positioning. Since many corneal conditions have a hereditary component, it is advisable to perform a quick slit lamp examination of the parents and cooperative siblings, too.[1] Use of a topical anaesthetic and lubricant can help in slit lamp examination of uncooperative and photophobic children. An examination under anaesthesia (EUA) often becomes necessary and should be undertaken to ensure a thorough ocular examination and to establish correct diagnosis. Ophthalmic images, obtained using simple smartphone cameras with relatively low light settings, can also aid the examination.[2]

COMMON CORNEAL DISEASES AND CORNEAL EMERGENCIES IN CHILDREN

Children can present with similar signs and symptoms for a myriad of disorders; hence examination and accurate diagnosis pose a great challenge. The common complaints with which a child presents in the emergency services include acute red eye, white reflex, excessive watering, sensitivity to light, sudden increase in size of eyeball, eye discharge, history of trauma or child not following lights or objects. The common corneal diseases in children are summarised in Table 17.1.

CLINICAL EXAMINATION IN A PAEDIATRIC PATIENT

Visual acuity can be assessed through appropriate preverbal methods or specific vision charts based on the age of the child and their cooperation. The assessment for functional outcome is imperative to provide a realistic picture to the anxious parents expecting a good visual outcome in these cases. Examination for fixation, ocular axis deviation helps to obtain a fair assessment of visual prognosis in children. Visual evoked potential should be done wherever indicated and is paramount in cases where surgical intervention is planned for visual rehabilitation.

Table 17.1: Common Corneal Disorders in Children

Underlying etiology	Corneal diseases
Infection	Corneal ulcers/keratitis, Keratoconjunctivitis, TORCH infections, sclerokeratitis, peripheral ulcerative keratitis (these may be viral, bacterial, fungal or miscellaneous infections)
Immune mediated	Phlyctenular keratoconjunctivitis, Allergic Keratoconjunctivitis, Vernal Keratoconjunctivitis, Stevens-Johnson Syndrome (SJS), Toxic epidermal necrolysis (TEN)
Nutritional and Metabolic	Keratomalacia, xerophthalmia, mucopolysaccharidosis
Trauma/Injury	Corneal lacerations, birth trauma, corneal foreign bodies, chemical injury (lime related injuries, household chemicals), thermal injuries (firecracker injuries)
Malignancy	Corneal involvement in a case of retinoblastoma and other tumours
Congenital	Sclerocornea, anterior segment mesodermal dysgenesis, buphthalmos and congenital glaucoma, other miscellaneous lesions like dermoid, keloid
Hereditary	Corneal dystrophy including CHED, CHSD

*TORCH=Toxoplasma, Rubella, Cytomegalovirus, Herpes virus; CHED=Congenital Hereditary Endothelial Dystrophy; CHSD=Congenital Hereditary Stromal Dystrophy

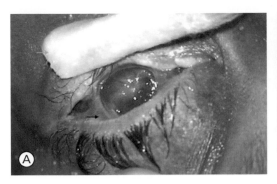
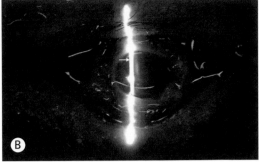

Figure 17.1 Examination under anaesthesia performed in a child with bilateral chemical injury sequelae to plan management strategies for visual rehabilitation showing (A) symblepharon formation (black arrow) and corneal opacification with vascularisation (blue arrow) upon retracting the eyelids using cotton tipped applicator (yellow arrow). Examination of the other eye (B) under thin slit illumination (white arrow) under microscope reveals conjunctival chemosis with congestion (grey arrow).

Various tools needed for paediatric ocular examination include a torch with a bright light, a direct ophthalmoscope, fluorescein strips, a blue light source and magnifying loupes when examining a child in the ophthalmic emergency room.

EXAMINATION UNDER ANAESTHESIA FOR CORNEAL DISORDERS

EUA for all infants and children with corneal inflammation or infection is important for detailed evaluation and deciding on appropriate management (Figure 17.1). Though older children may permit a slit lamp biomicroscopic evaluation, assessment for intraocular pressure and axial length measurement needs to be performed under EUA. In neonates and infants, a preoperative EUA can be scheduled for a complete evaluation with handheld slit lamp and other diagnostic imaging to ascertain the indication and prognosticate the surgical intervention. Alternatively, the EUA for evaluation can be performed prior to scheduled surgery, whenever indicated. General anaesthesia should be used judiciously in infants and young children, as they respond differently to anaesthesia medications in comparison to adults due to many factors, including body composition, protein binding, body temperature, distribution of cardiac output and functional maturity of the liver and kidneys.

With an EUA, a comprehensive examination of both eyes, including details of the limbus, corneal diameter, anterior chamber, angle evaluation (when possible), anterior and posterior synechia, iris and pupil abnormalities, lens status and fundus (when possible), is performed under the

operating microscope or handheld slit lamp. In cases of corneal ulceration and opacification, intraocular pressure (IOP), keratometry measurement with handheld keratometer (for fellow eye when possible), ultrasound examination for axial length and posterior segment evaluation also need to be done (Video 17.1).

Videos for Chapter 17 can be accessed at: www.routledge.com/9780367761561

Video 17.1: Paediatric examination under anaesthesia (EUA).

Video 17.2: Corneal scraping in a child with corneal ulcer.

Preoperative anterior segment optical coherence tomography (OCT) or high frequency ultrasound biomicroscopy (UBM) during an EUA can help to delineate the depth of involvement favouring an anterior lamellar therapeutic keratoplasty instead of full-thickness keratoplasty. Operating microscopes with integrated OCT facilities now enable both preoperative evaluations in determining the depth of stromal involvement as well as intraoperative assessments on depth and corneal thickness in cases with keratitis and other inflammatory corneal disorders.

During an EUA of a child with corneal infection or inflammation, diagnostic scraping and noting the size and depth of the infiltration and epithelial defect are paramount (Video 17.2). The parameters to be noted during evaluation of corneal opacification (Table 17.2) resulting from infective and inflammatory diseases broadly include:

a. Corneal diameters: Limbal to limbal horizontal and vertical corneal diameters measured by Vernier callipers

Table 17.2: Scheme for Examination under Anaesthesia for Corneal Disorders

S. No.	Detail	OD	OS
1.	Corneal clarity, any opacity		
2.	Corneal surface, fluorescein staining pattern		
3.	Peripheral corneal examination		
4.	Central corneal examination		
5.	Any limbal lesion		
6.	Any associated conjunctival (bulbar/palpebral/forniceal) lesion Perform double eversion of lids, if required		
7.	Any associated lid or adnexal lesion		
8.	Any limbal stem cell deficiency		
9.	Any foreign body on the ocular surface		
10.	Corneal diameters		
11.	Corneal keratometry		
12.	Corneal pachymetry (central, 9 point)		
13.	Digital ocular tension		
14.	Fundus details (if visible)		
15.	Investigations done in EUA		

- Ultrasonography
- Ultrasonic biomicroscopy

b. Central corneal thickness measured from the centre inner surface of the corneal endothelium to the outer epithelial surface by handheld ultrasound pachymeter SP-3000 or integrated i-OCT microscopy

c. Clinical photographs for documentation and follow-up

d. AS-OCT to assess corneal thinning in cases with full-thickness corneal opacity

e. Corneal contour, especially in ectatic disorders

f. Presence/absence of iris adhesions

g. IOP assessed digitally or through a Perkins tonometer (Haag Streit Perkins Mk3 handheld applanation tonometer)

h. B-Scan USG and axial length (Sonomed EZ Scan AB5500+ Ophthalmic Ultrasound Scanner)

i. AC depth: Axial distance between corneal endothelium to anterior lens surface

j. Anterior chamber angle: Anterior chamber angle measured by constructing a line along the inner surface of the cornea into the anterior chamber recess and joining it with a line on the anterior iris surface

k. Ultrasound biomicroscopic examination: (Sonomed VuMax UBM 35 MHz transducer) performed using the specially designed scleral cup fixed to the patients' eyes with 5% freshly prepared methyl cellulose being used as a coupling medium

In cases of paediatric keratoplasty, sequential and regular EUAs are indicated, and parameters related to graft status (Table 17.3) and functional and morphological outcomes of the corneal graft need to be documented at each follow-up visit to ensure successful outcomes in paediatric grafts.

CONCLUSION

Successful patient outcome in paediatric ocular emergencies related to corneal infection and inflammation depend on proper recognition and evaluation as well as appropriate management and referral. A comprehensive evaluation involving a concise history, general observation, pupil examination and basic ocular tests can lead to a probable diagnosis and thereby appropriate management and timely referral that will go a long way to achieving successful outcomes in these children.

Table 17.3: Pediatric Keratoplasty: Proforma for Postoperative "Examination under Anaesthesia" in Children

Date of EUA: __/____/_____   EUA performed by Dr._____

Name/Age/Sex of patient: Unique Identification Number:

Diagnosis:

Surgery type: Surgery date: Surgeon:

OCULAR FINDINGS	DIAGRAMATIC REPRESENTATION
Graft Clarity, Graft-Host Junction	
Sutures	
Anterior Chamber details:	
Keratometry:	
K1	
K2	
Refraction:	
Fundus	
WTW	
AL	
USG B Scan	
UBM	
IOP	

EUA=Examination under anaesthesia; WTW=White-to-white diameter; AL=Axial length; USG=Ultrasonography; UBM=Ultrasound Biomicroscopy; IOP=Intraocular pressure

REFERENCES

1. Colby K. Corneal Diseases in Children: Challenges and Controversies. Cham, Switzerland: Springer; 2017.
2. Myung D, Jais A, He L, Chang R. Simple, low-cost smartphone adapter for rapid, high quality ocular anterior segment imaging: a photo diary. J Mob Technol Med. 2014 Mar; 1;3:2–8.

18 Paediatric Corneal Infection and Inflammation

Yogita Gupta, T Monikha, Neiwete Lomi, Radhika Tandon

INTRODUCTION

Paediatric corneal infective and inflammatory disorders, albeit rare, are important due to their potentially serious effects on the visual development with long-term consequences.[1] Unlike adults, paediatric corneal abnormalities pose great challenges to clinicians for both diagnosis and management due to poor cooperation for slit lamp examination, review and follow-up. Any delay in management may lead to complications and eventually visual impairment and amblyopia. Common conditions affecting the cornea in childhood include infections (local or systemic), metabolic conditions, malnutrition and systemic inflammatory and autoimmune conditions.[2,3] This chapter illustrates the paediatric infective and inflammatory disorders affecting the cornea and ocular surface.

CASE 18.1

CLINICAL FEATURES

An 8-year-old male presented to our outpatient department with symptoms of pain, diminution of vision, redness and discharge over the last five days. The parents gave history of matting of eyelashes. There was no history of ocular trauma or fever. Visual acuity at presentation was hand motions close to face (HMCF) with accurate projection of rays and 6/6 in the right and left eye, respectively. Careful examination revealed healed folliculitis lesions on the skin of the nose and scalp. Clinical findings and schematic diagram of the cornea are illustrated in Figure 18.1.

KEY POINTS

Diagnosis:
- The clinical picture describes a case of paediatric bacterial keratitis presenting as a stromal abscess with hypopyon secondary to folliculitis of the face and the scalp, seen as healed lesions on the skin.

Investigations:
- Corneal scrapings were collected and sent for microscopy (Gram stain and KOH mount), bacterial culture on blood agar, fungal culture on Sabouraud dextrose agar and thioglycolate broth, and drug sensitivity testing.

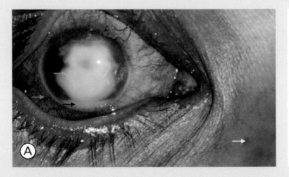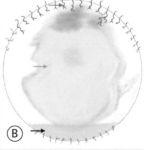

Figure 18.1 External photograph of an 8-year-old male showing (A) large corneal ulcer with hypopyon (black arrow) approximately 2 mm in height, dense corneal stromal infiltrates (yellow arrow) and conjunctival congestion (grey arrow). Superficial vascularisation was noted (green arrow) at superior three clock hours of cornea at the site of the infiltration. Careful facial examination revealed healed folliculitis lesions (white arrow) on the skin of the nose as a possible source of infection. (B) Corresponding schematic diagram shows the same findings.

- The bacterial culture was positive for growth of *Staphylococcus aureus*, that was sensitive to fluoroquinolones, tobramycin and cefazolin.

Treatment:
- The patient was managed with systemic and topical antibiotics. Amoxicillin clavulanate 30 mg/kg/day was administered orally. Fortified cefazolin 5% and tobramycin 1.3% were administered every hour for 48 hours, then every two hours for 48 hours and then six times per day for the next 48 hours. Antibiotics were slowly tapered as per clinical response. Ointment gatifloxacin 0.3% was applied at night.

Outcome:
- The patient did not show significant improvement with medical management. Therapeutic keratoplasty was performed for the case in view of impending corneal perforation and non-resolution of stromal abscess. A good outcome was achieved with best corrected visual acuity (BCVA) (6/12) six weeks after keratoplasty with a clear graft and no infiltrates or recurrence in the postoperative period.

Supplementary Information and Additional Tips
- Often, bacterial keratitis can develop following any local folliculitis on the face in the paediatric population. Deep stromal abscess with hypopyon may be a presentation of bacterial keratitis.
- Organisms such as *Staphylococcus epidermidis* and *Staphylococcus albus* usually cause a small localised suppurative reaction in the cornea (Figure 18.2) and are usually self-limiting but occasionally may respond differently in children.

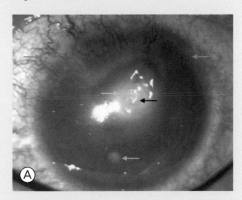 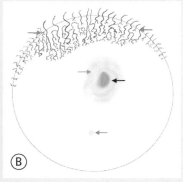

Figure 18.2 Clinical photograph of a child with (A) a small, well-defined, round central corneal ulcer (black arrow), caused by *Staphylococcus epidermidis*, with oedema limited to the surrounding cornea (yellow arrow). Also note the superficial corneal vascularisation (grey arrows) involving three clock hours, a sign of healing, and a satellite lesion (green arrow). The corresponding schematic image (B) illustrates the findings.

CASE 18.2

CLINICAL FEATURES

A 10-year-old male presented to our outpatient department with symptoms of mild pain, diminution of vision and redness over the past 14 days. There was a history of finger nail trauma for which he was prescribed topical eyedrops that were a combination of mild steroid and antibiotic. On experiencing worsening of symptoms after an initial relief, the parents brought the child to our tertiary eye care hospital. Visual acuity at presentation was HMCF and 6/6 in the right and left eye, respectively. The clinical findings captured under the operating microscope during the examination under anaesthesia (EUA) are illustrated in Figure 18.3.

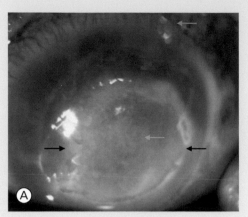
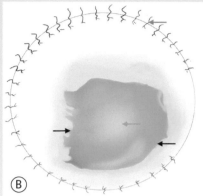

Figure 18.3 Clinical photograph of a child with (A) a large central corneal ulcer with well-defined margins (black arrows), minimal corneal stromal infiltrates (yellow arrow) and diffuse conjunctival congestion (grey arrow). Note that the surrounding cornea is relatively clear. The corresponding schematic diagram (B) depicts the same findings.

KEY POINTS

Diagnosis:

- The clinical picture describes a case of fungal keratitis with a large corneal ulcer involving the visual axis. The ulcer exhibited the classic dry texture and feathery margins of a fungal corneal ulcer.

Investigations:

- Corneal scrapings were collected and sent for microscopy (Gram stain and KOH mount), bacterial culture on blood agar, fungal culture on Sabouraud dextrose agar and thioglycolate broth, and drug sensitivity testing.
- The corneal scraping specimen from the ulcer base and margins obtained during EUA revealed septate hyphae with V-shaped branching on KOH mount. The diagnosis was confirmed by a culture that demonstrated growth of *Aspergillus flavus*.

Treatment:

- The patient was managed with systemic and topical antifungals. Oral ketoconazole 50 mg twice a day was given for ten days along with topical natamycin ophthalmic suspension (5%) every hour for 48 hours followed by tapering the frequency based on the clinical response, prophylactic topical antibiotic (moxifloxacin hydrochloride 0.5% four times a day), cycloplegic (homatropine hydrobromide 2% three times a day) and copious lubricants (preservative-free carboxymethylcellulose 1% every two hours).

Outcome:

- The child responded well to medical management. Corneal opacity was noted at the third month follow-up. An optical keratoplasty was later performed after six months of resolution of keratitis. Good outcomes were achieved with best corrected visual acuity (BCVA) (6/18) after all sutures were removed one year after keratoplasty with a clear graft.

CASE 18.3

CLINICAL FEATURES

A 6-year-old female presented to the cornea clinic of our tertiary eye care hospital with symptoms of pain, diminution of vision, redness and discharge over the past five days. The parents gave history of trauma with a

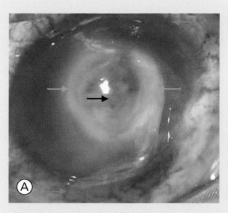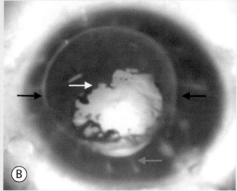

Figure 18.4 Clinical photograph of a child with post-traumatic infective keratitis caused by *Aspergillus niger* demonstrating (A) a sloughing corneal ulcer (yellow arrows), conjunctival congestion (grey arrows), a central perforation (black arrow) with iris tissue and corneal infiltrates organising to form a pseudocorneal membrane in the region of perforation. Therapeutic keratoplasty with pupilloplasty was performed for this case and the postoperative picture (B) reveals a clear corneal graft with a healthy graft-host junction (black arrows), visible suture tracks (grey arrow) and a surgically enlarged pupil (white arrow) with few irido-capsular adhesions.

pencil while attending school. Visual acuity at presentation was hand movements close to face with accurate projection of rays in the affected eye. The examination findings under anaesthesia are illustrated in Figure 18.4.

KEY POINTS

Diagnosis:
- The clinical picture describes a case of post-traumatic perforated fungal corneal ulcer involving the visual axis.

Investigations:
- Corneal scrapings were collected and sent for microscopy (Gram stain and KOH mount), bacterial culture on blood agar, fungal culture on Sabouraud dextrose agar and thioglycolate broth, and drug sensitivity testing.
- The host corneal button was sent for microbiological and histopathological evaluation.

Treatment:
- The patient was administered systemic and topical antifungals (Oral ketoconazole 50 mg twice a day for ten days along with topical natamycin 5% drops every two hours and tapered as per response).
- Emergency therapeutic penetrating keratoplasty (TPK) was performed

along with pupilloplasty to clear the dense infiltrates.

Outcome:
- The patient had good postoperative outcomes with BCVA being 6/18 six months after the keratoplasty with a clear graft seen 12 months after surgery.

Supplementary Information and Additional Tips

- Penetrating injuries are also a fairly common cause of corneal infections in the paediatric age group.
- Simple injuries may present as self-sealing corneal wounds and may often present as keratitis at a later date (Figure 18.5).
- TPK may also be needed for cases not responding to maximal medical therapy alone.
- At times, TPK may require an eccentrically placed graft to achieve control of infection with good morphological and functional outcome (Figure 18.6).
- In cases of paracentral perforations secondary to trauma and infective keratitis, corneal patch grafts secured with sutures (Figure 18.7) prove to be successful in providing tectonic support and optical rehabilitation.

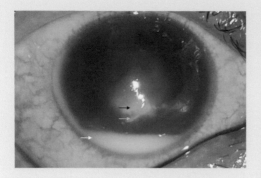

Figure 18.5 Clinical photograph of a case of infective keratitis occurring after penetrating ocular injury in a child showing a self-sealed corneal perforation wound (yellow arrow) with a small, well-demarcated corneal ulcer along with surrounding localised infiltrates (black arrow) and hypopyon of 1.5-mm height (white arrow). Note that the surrounding cornea is relatively clear.

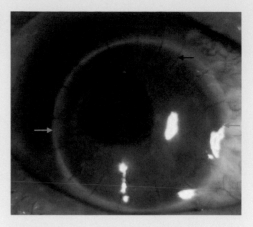

Figure 18.6 Clinical photograph of a child who underwent therapeutic keratoplasty for a large perforated corneal ulcer and presented with a clear eccentric graft three months after surgery, with well-apposed graft-host junction (grey arrows) and intact sutures (black arrow). TPK may require an eccentrically placed graft as this picture depicts to ensure complete removal of infective tissue.

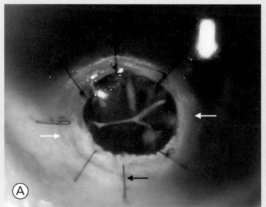

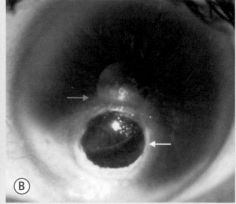

Figure 18.7 Clinical photograph of a child presenting with viral keratouveitis with descemetocele and spontaneous corneal perforation with iris plugging the wound that was managed by performing (A) tectonic patch graft secured with sutures (black arrow). Note the surrounding stromal oedema near the limbal area and the well-apposed graft-host junction (white arrows). Sutures were removed (B) after nine months and a clear, paracentral patch graft with healthy graft-host junction (white arrow) and adjacent corneal opacification (grey arrow) can be observed.

CASE 18.4

CLINICAL FEATURES

A 2-week-old female neonate was brought by her parents to the ophthalmic emergency with a history of purulent discharge from both eyes (left eye more than right eye) over the previous ten hours. There was a history of full-term normal vaginal delivery with uneventful perinatal period. There was no history of ocular prophylaxis soon after delivery to the baby. Clinical findings are illustrated in Figure 18.8.

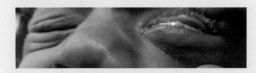

Figure 18.8 External photograph of a 2-week-old neonate presenting with purulent discharge (white arrow), swollen eyelids and conjunctival chemosis with high suspicion of ophthalmia neonatorum due to gonococcal infection.

KEY POINTS

Diagnosis:
- The clinical picture with swollen eyelids and conjunctival chemosis describes a case of ophthalmia neonatorum with purulent conjunctival discharge with a high clinical suspicion of gonococcal infection.

Investigations:
- Conjunctival swab sample was obtained from the baby's eyes that tested positive for *Neisseria gonorrhoeae*.

Treatment:
- The child was administered oral ceftriaxone 50 mg/kg intramuscularly along with topical tobramycin drops and moxifloxacin ointment.

Outcome:
- The patient had good outcomes with healing and resolution of discharge within five days after initiation of antibiotic therapy. There was no recurrence on further follow-ups.

CASE 18.5

CLINICAL FEATURES

A 2-year-old female presented with parents noticing the child having pain, swelling, redness and purulent discharge in the left eye over the past 17 days. Similar episodes were noted in the last four months and were treated with traditional eye medications. At the age of six months, she had been diagnosed with unilateral retinoblastoma for which enucleation was advised. However, the parents were reluctant to give consent for enucleation a year ago. There was no history of fever. Examination findings are illustrated in Figure 18.9.

KEY POINTS

Diagnosis:
- The above clinical scenario describes a case of unilateral infective keratitis in a child with retinoblastoma.

Investigations:
- Corneal scrapings were sent for microbiological investigations. Ultrasonography B-scan was done for posterior segment examination (Figure 18.9C) that revealed intraocular calcified mass, consistent with the diagnosis of retinoblastoma. Magnetic resonance imaging (MRI) was performed to look for any extraocular spread of the tumour.

Treatment:
- The case was initially managed conservatively with oral antibiotics and topical fortified antibiotics: 5% cefazolin and 1.3% tobramycin administered every hour, then slowly tapered down as per clinical response, to achieve local infection control. After three weeks of therapy, enucleation was performed after obtaining written informed consent from the parents.

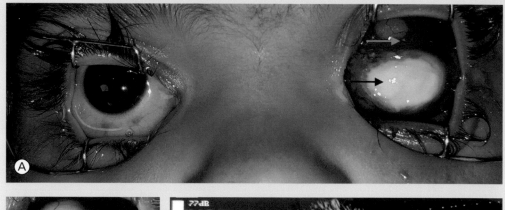

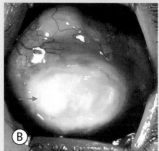

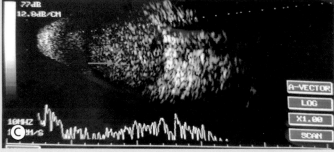

Figure 18.9 External photograph of a 2-year-old with (A) unilateral retinoblastoma and infective keratitis (black arrow) with diffuse conjunctival congestion (grey arrow) in the left eye. On magnified view (B), limbus-to-limbus involvement with dense corneal infiltrates (green arrow) with calcification was observed. The diagnosis was confirmed on B-scan ultrasonography (C) that revealed an intraocular mass with dense, hyperreflective foci of calcification (yellow arrow).

Outcome:

- A good outcome from surgical resection was achieved with no tumour residue on MRI on one-year follow-up.

Supplementary Information and Additional Tips

- Retinoblastoma or other orbital tumours may present with infective keratitis in cases with proptosis and enlargement of the tumour. In extraocular retinoblastoma (EORB), the tumour may present as a case of orbital cellulitis (Figure 18.10) with purulent discharge, chemosis and prolapsed conjunctival tissue. Infective keratitis results in these cases due to inadequate closure of the eyelids due to the tumour mass and resulting exposure keratopathy with secondary infection due to xerosis and absence of blinking.

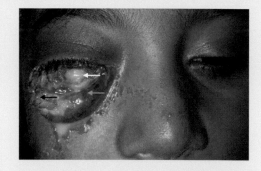

Figure 18.10 External photograph of a child with unilateral extraocular retinoblastoma (EORB) presenting as right orbital cellulitis. Corneal ulceration (white arrow) with conjunctival chemosis (yellow arrow) and congestion were seen along with mucopurulent discharge and crusting (black arrow) in the right eye of this child.

CASE 18.6

CLINICAL FEATURES

An 8-year-old male presented to an ophthalmic emergency room with parents complaining of yellowish discharge in both the eyes over the past two weeks. As per the history from the parents, the redness lasted for five days and then 'whites of both the eyes were noted to turn yellow-white since last 1 week.' There was no history of similar episodes in past. The four elder siblings had normal findings on ocular examination. The child was malnourished and had muscle wasting with delayed milestones. Examination findings are illustrated in Figure 18.11.

KEY POINTS

Diagnosis:

- The above clinical scenario describes a case of severe malnutrition with bilateral keratomalacia due to vitamin A deficiency.

Investigations:

- The case was thoroughly examined by the paediatrician for muscle wasting and growth stunting. Measurement of head circumference, mid-upper arm circumference, height-for-age and weight-for-height were all below third centile for age for this case. Immunisation and nutritional status were assessed.

Treatment:

- The patient was managed for severe malnutrition by the paediatrician. The mother was counselled regarding 'nutritious diet' to treat malnutrition. Proper immunisation (including vitamin A doses) was ensured through referral to the paediatrics department. Ocular management comprised topical antibiotic (drops and ointment) and topical lubricants.

Outcome:

- There was poor outcome in this case with healing of corneal ulcer and formation of corneal scar in both the eyes. The BCVA was perception of light in both eyes, six weeks after initiation of therapy. Optical keratoplasty was required sequentially in both the eyes. Five months after corneal transplantation in the right eye, there was a graft infection, which resolved with therapy, leading eventually to graft opacification.

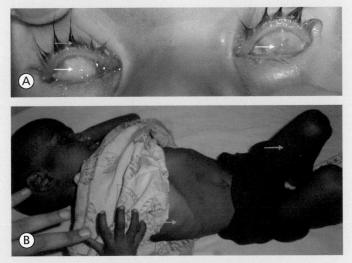

Figure 18.11 External photograph of child with (A) bilateral keratomalacia suffering from grade 4 malnutrition presenting bilateral total corneal ulceration (white arrows) along with matted eyelashes (yellow arrows) and (B) stunting and wasting: pigeon chest (yellow arrow), dry and scaly skin, reduced muscle mass at the thigh region (grey arrow) with poor, stunted growth was observed.

CASE 18.7

CLINICAL FEATURES

A 2-month-old male infant weighing 2.6 kg presented to the ophthalmology emergency department with excessive crying, redness and watering of eyes over the past 15 days. He was not breastfed as the mother had stopped breastfeeding when the child was hospitalised with pneumonia at 15 days of life. The child was now bottle-fed with diluted cow's milk with water (1:2) after discharge from the hospital. He was immunised in accordance to his age. Examination findings under anaesthesia are illustrated in Figure 18.12.

KEY POINTS

Diagnosis:
- The above clinical presentation describes a case of bilateral keratomalacia with diffuse stromal melting in an infant.

Investigations:
- EUA was performed and corneal scraping specimens were retrieved and cultures yielded growth of *S. aureus*.
- Paediatric consultation was sought for systemic illness, immunisation and nutritional advice and vitamin A supplementation.

Treatment:
- Systemic workup and treatment were provided in consultation with the paediatrician.
- The patient was started on topical fortified cefazoline (5%) and tobramycin (1.4%) every hour with a cycloplegic. As part of his treatment for vitamin A deficiency, the patient was given 100,000 IU of vitamin A, by intramuscular injection, on each of three days (days 1, 2 and 14 post-presentation).
- TPK was performed in right eye for impending corneal perforation.

Outcome:
- With this treatment, the patient showed improvement and the corneal ulcer healed in the left eye, albeit with residual corneal opacity.
- The right eye underwent therapeutic keratoplasty for tectonic support but eventually resulted in corneal opacification and formation of anterior staphyloma due to the occurrence of secondary glaucoma.

Supplementary Information and Additional Tips

- Keratomalacia, the most severe manifestation of vitamin A deficiency, may present with bilateral (Figures 18.13

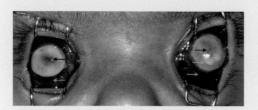

Figure 18.12 External photograph captured while performing examination under anaesthesia for an infant with bilateral corneal ulceration and melting (black arrows) in a case of severe keratomalacia. Diffuse conjunctival congestion (grey arrow), corneal sloughing and dense exudates (yellow arrow) suggesting infective keratitis due to vitamin A deficiency were observed.

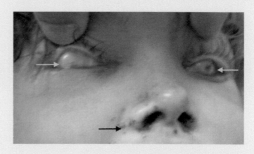

Figure 18.13 External photograph of a 6-year-old child with bilateral corneal ulceration (yellow arrows) in a case of bilateral keratomalacia secondary to malnutrition. Small petechiae-like lesions were visible on the face near the ala of the nose suggesting poor wound healing due to malnutrition (black arrow).

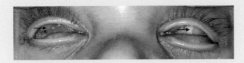

Figure 18.14 External photograph of a child with bilateral corneal melting due to keratomalacia (black arrows). Note the conjunctival congestion, diffuse corneal haze and impending corneal perforation in the right eye.

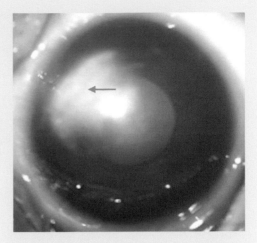

Figure 18.16 Clinical photograph taken under the operating microscope while performing examination under anaesthesia demonstrating paracentral corneal opacity (grey arrow) in a child with a history of keratomalacia and resolved keratitis.

and 18.14) or unilateral (Figure 18.15) involvement of the cornea.

- The visual prognosis in children with keratomalacia is guarded due to delayed presentation and poor response to corneal grafting due to concomitant systemic co-morbidities. Eventual outcomes include paracentral corneal opacity (Figure 18.16) or a central corneal opacity obscuring the visual axis (Figure 18.17) that are amenable to visual rehabilitation through refractive correction, pupilloplasty or corneal grafting.
- Irreversible blindness may result in some cases wherein the eventual outcome includes vascularised corneal opacities with or without corneal thinning (Figure 18.18) or anterior staphyloma with secondary glaucoma (Figure 18.19).

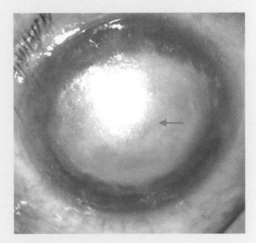

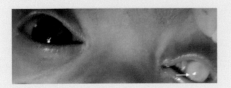

Figure 18.15 Clinical photograph of an infant with unilateral keratomalacia presenting as severe infective keratitis and total corneal involvement (white arrow) in the left eye while the right eye was normal.

Figure 18.17 Clinical photograph of a child with a previous history of keratomalacia that demonstrates total leucomatous corneal opacity with xerosis (green arrow) with perilimbal superficial vascularisation.

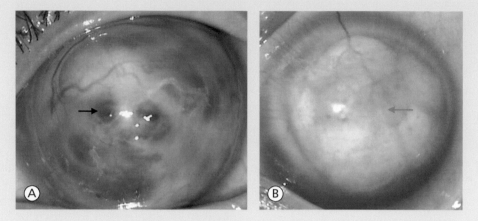

Figure 18.18 Clinical photograph of a child with bilateral keratomalacia suffering from grade 4 malnutrition presenting with (A) staphylomatous corneal scar with vascularisation and areas of corneal thinning (black arrow). Examination of the other eye revealed (B) dense corneal scar with vascularisation (green arrow) occurring secondary to resolution of graft infection following optical keratoplasty performed for visual rehabilitation in the right eye. Note the bulging of the eye due to an increase in axial length of the eye because of raised intraocular pressure.

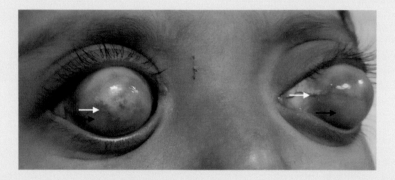

Figure 18.19 External photograph of a child showing chronic sequelae of bilateral keratomalacia in the form of total corneal opacity with secondary glaucoma manifesting as bilateral anterior staphyloma (black arrows) with superficial vascularisation (white arrows).

CASE 18.8

CLINICAL FEATURES

An 8-year-old female presented with complaints of pain, redness and purulent discharge from the left eye over the past seven days, as noted by the parents. The redness started a week following a low-grade fever (temperature ~99.5°F). Visual acuity at presentation was 6/6 in both eyes. There was no history of any ocular injury. Examination findings and slit lamp appearance are illustrated in Figure 18.20.

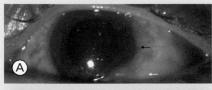

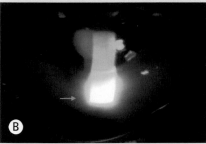

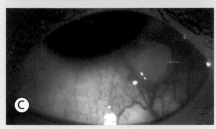

Figure 18.20 Slit lamp photograph of 8-year-old female presenting with (A) purulent keratoconjunctivitis in the left eye. Note the conjunctival congestion (black arrow), few infiltrates in peripheral cornea (grey arrow), mucopurulent discharge (white arrow) and (B) corneal epithelial defect with conjunctival staining (yellow arrow) as evidenced under cobalt blue filter after instillation of fluorescein dye. Note the presence of (C) a cystic lesion (green arrow) in the inferotemporal conjunctiva that resolved with a course of oral and topical antibiotics.

KEY POINTS

Diagnosis:
- The above clinical scenario describes a case of unilateral purulent conjunctivitis.

Investigations:
- A conjunctival swab was sent for microbiological investigations, namely, Gram stain, Giemsa stain, calcofluor white stain, KOH mount, bacterial culture on blood agar, fungal culture on Sabouraud dextrose agar and thioglycolate broth, and drug sensitivity testing. Blood haemogram was also tested.
- Ultrasonography B-scan was done for posterior segment examination.
- X-ray paranasal sinuses was performed to rule out any sinusitis which revealed a fluid level in the left maxillary sinus.

Treatment:
- The case responded well to topical fortified antibiotics: 5% cefazolin and 1.3% tobramycin initially instilled every two hours and then slowly tapered down as per clinical response.
- After one week of therapy, a small cystic lesion was noted, which finally disappeared after starting oral amoxicillin with clavulanic acid in consultation with an otorhinolaryngologist.

Outcome:
- There was good clinical response to treatment three weeks after initiation of therapy.

CASE 18.9

CLINICAL FEATURES

A 5-year-old male presented to the outpatient department with parents noticing severe redness, photophobia and watering in both the eyes for the past three days. The parents further disclosed that the child was diagnosed with Down syndrome. There was no history of any ocular injury. Examination findings and slit lamp appearance are illustrated in Figure 18.21.

KEY POINTS

Diagnosis:
- The above clinical scenario describes a case of Down syndrome with bilateral acute conjunctivitis with cystic lesions.

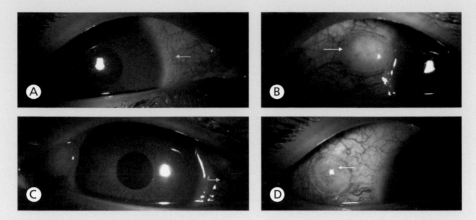

Figure 18.21 Slit lamp photograph of 5-year-old child with Down syndrome presenting with (A) purulent keratoconjunctivitis and diffuse conjunctival congestion (yellow arrow) On examination of the left eye (C), conjunctival congestion (yellow arrow) with nasal and temporal cystic lesions were seen. On left gaze (D), the nasal cyst (white arrow) could be seen clearly.

Investigations:
- A conjunctival swab was sent for microbiological investigations. Gram stain, Giemsa stain, calcofluor white stain, KOH mount, bacterial culture on blood agar, fungal culture on Sabouraud dextrose agar and thioglycolate broth, and drug sensitivity testing were conducted.

Treatment:
- This case was managed conservatively with topical antibiotics (gatifloxacin 0.5%), started hourly and tapered slowly as per response. Ciprofloxacin ointment 0.3% was applied at night.

Outcome:
- The redness and swelling subsided over two weeks after the initiation of therapy, with good outcome on follow-up.

CASE 18.10

CLINICAL FEATURES

A 12-year-old male, suffering from insulin-dependent diabetes mellitus (IDDM), presented to the ophthalmic emergency room with complaints of redness, watery discharge, eyelid oedema, photophobia and foreign body sensation in both the eyes over the last two weeks. The parents reported taking treatment from a local ophthalmologist but there was no relief. He was on insulin for type 1 diabetes mellitus for the past four years. the clinical picture is illustrated in Figure 18.22.

KEY POINTS

Diagnosis:
- The above clinical scenario describes a case of bilateral peripheral ulcerative keratitis (PUK) with scleritis in a case of IDDM.

Investigations:
- Corneal scrapings from the ulcer bed were collected and sent for microbiological investigations (the same as mentioned in Case 3). Ultrasonography B-scan was done

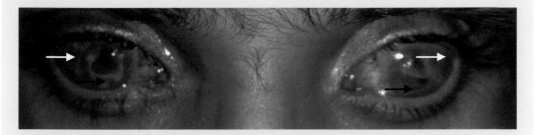

Figure 18.22 External photograph of a 12-year-old male with insulin-dependent diabetes mellitus showing bilateral severe peripheral ulcerative keratitis (black arrows). Note the diffuse conjunctival congestion (white arrows) and corneal oedema with peripheral guttering.

for posterior segment examination and was found to be anechoic. Rheumatological and other autoimmune diseases were ruled out with tailored history and examination.

- Blood plasma glucose was noted to be 323 mg/dl at presentation. HbA1c (glycosylated haemoglobin) of 9.5 was detected.
- A meticulous systemic workup in consultation with a paediatrician was performed, including laboratory investigations like complete haemogram with erythrocyte sedimentation rate (ESR), viral serology (tests for HIV, Hepatitis B and C), VDRL (for syphilis), Mantoux test, chest X-ray, baseline kidney and liver function tests, peripheral blood smear, blood culture and urine routine and microscopic evaluation. All of these tests were negative and all other differential diagnoses for PUK were ruled out.

Treatment:

- Insulin therapy was titrated with fluctuating blood sugar levels in consultation with the endocrinologist. Strict diabetic control helped in healing the peripheral keratitis.
- The patient was managed on topical steroids: prednisolone actetate (1%) drops (started at two-hourly frequency for the first week then every six hours for two weeks then tapered slowly according to clinical response), topical cyclosporine 0.05% twice a day, topical antibiotics (moxifloxacin 0.5% QID for two weeks) and topical lubricants (carboxymethylcellulose 0.5% every two hours). An ointment combination of carbomer 3.5 mg with vitamin A 1000 IU was applied at night.

- Oral doxycycline 100 mg twice a day and oral vitamin C 500 mg thrice a day were added to promote epithelial healing.
- Oral steroids were contraindicated due to high blood glucose levels.

Outcome:

- A close follow-up was kept and the ulcer healed with medical therapy along with strict control of the diabetic status.
- A fair outcome was achieved in this case with healing of the peripheral ulcer in both the eyes. The BCVA was OD 6/12 and OS 6/60 six weeks after initiation of therapy.

Supplementary Information and Additional Tips

- Diabetes is associated with corneal changes which include increased epithelial fragility; defects and recurrent erosions; non-healing ulcers and corneal oedema due to altered epithelial barrier function. The disease affects the corneal epithelium, corneal nerves, tear film and, to a lesser extent, endothelium.
- Common manifestations in the cornea include non-healing ulcers and neurotrophic keratopathy with abnormally slow and often incomplete epithelial healing (Figure 18.23), especially in paediatric patients with IDDM. Neuropathy/loss of corneal sensitivity and tear film changes in uncontrolled diabetes contribute to the condition.
- These abnormalities may appear or become exacerbated following trauma, including any ocular surgery or stressor.
- A dramatic improvement is usually seen with control of blood sugar levels.

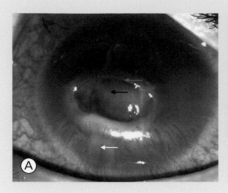
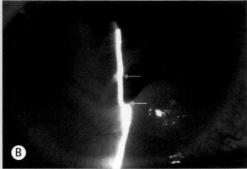

Figure 18.23 Slit lamp photograph of a 9-year-old female suffering from uncontrolled blood glucose levels due to type 1 diabetes mellitus demonstrating (A) neurotrophic corneal ulcer (black arrow) with sharp, heaped-up margins (green arrow) and peripheral nearly 3 o'clock hours of corneal vascularisation (white arrow). Examination of ulcer in thin slit illumination revealed (B) the excavated epithelial defect (grey arrow) and raised, steep margins (yellow arrow).

CASE 18.11

CLINICAL FEATURES

A 6-year-old female presented to the ophthalmic emergency department with profuse redness in both eyes accompanied by photophobia and sticky discharge, running nose, cough and fever of ~102°F. Parents gave a history of a prescription of trimethoprim-sulfamethoxazole by a paediatrician for fever and sore throat three days back, following which fever and rash developed with sore eyes. Examination findings under anaesthesia are illustrated in Figure 18.24. There were tender macular skin lesions (Figure 18.25), all over the trunk, back, face and limbs (>30% of body surface area was involved).

KEY POINTS

Diagnosis:
- The above clinical scenario describes an acute presentation of toxic epidermal necrolysis (TEN) with widespread macular skin rash and bilateral ocular involvement.

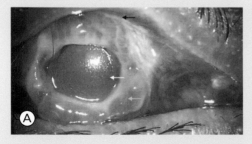
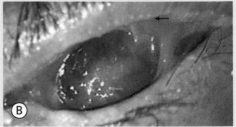

Figure 18.24 Clinical photograph of a child with an acute episode of toxic epidermal necrolysis presenting with (A) intense mucosal proliferative response with conjunctival chemosis (yellow arrow), upper lid symblepharon (black arrow) with dry ocular surface and hazy cornea (white arrow) in the right eye and left eye showing (B) upper lid symblepharon (black arrow) and cojunctivalisation of corneal surface along with xerosis (green arrow).

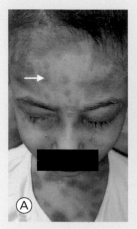 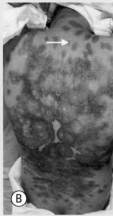 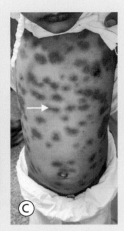 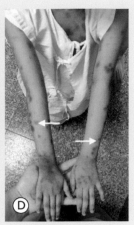

Figure 18.25 External photographs of the child with toxic epidermal necrolysis demonstrating multiple healed erythematous macules and targetoid lesions and involvement of more than 30% of the cutaneous surface. The targetoid lesions (white arrows) were widespread and can be seen on (A) face, (B) back, (C) chest and abdomen and (D) extensor surfaces of both upper limbs.

Investigations:
- EUA revealed severe ocular surface inflammation and extensive symblepharon formation.
- Conjunctival swab sent for microbiological investigations did not grow any microorganism.
- Ultrasonography B-scan revealed that the posterior segment examination was within normal limits.
- Complete haemogram and kidney and liver function tests were also checked.

Treatment:
- The case was initially managed conservatively with topical lubricants (carboxymethylcellulose 1%), sodium ascorbate 10% drops and sodium citrate 10% drops to ensure healing of conjunctival and corneal epithelial defects. Topical steroid (prednisolone acetate 1% QID) drops were started after the epithelial defect healed to reduce surface inflammation. Topical antibiotic drops and ointment application were administered to prevent superinfections. Oral vitamin C 250 mg thrice a day was prescribed to promote healing.
- Sweeping the fornices with a glass rod was advised to prevent formation of adhesions between the eyelid and conjunctiva.

Outcome:
- The acute inflammatory phase settled with healing of the epithelial defects. However, there were bilateral upper lid symblepharon, keratinisation and limbal stem cell deficiency which responded well to ocular surface reconstruction and mucous membrane grafting.

Supplementary Information and Additional Tips
- TEN involves extensive sloughing of skin and mucosal surfaces with oral and ocular involvement. It is a hypersensitive reaction to certain classes of drugs (e.g. anticonvulsants, non-steroidal anti-inflammatory drugs and antibiotics) in some individuals.
- Severe ocular surface disease with limbal stem cell deficiency occurs secondary to Stevens-Johnson syndrome (SJS), which affects the mucosal lining of the eye resulting in lid abnormalities, cicatrisation, loss of cilia, keratinisation with severe dry eye and loss of corneal transparency (Figure 18.26).

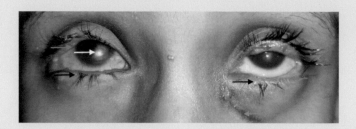

Figure 18.26 External photograph of a 13-year-old female with severe bilateral keratoconjunctivitis sicca due to chronic sequelae of Stevens-Johnson syndrome (SJS). Conjunctival congestion, corneal xerosis and opacification (white arrow) secondary to limbal stem cell deficiency can be clearly seen in the right eye. Upper lid cicatricial ectropion (green arrow) and lower lid skin scar (yellow arrow) due to healing of skin lesions of SJS were seen on examination of the left eye. Bilateral lid keratinisation (grey arrow) and swelling with loss of cilia (black arrow) due to cicatrisation of hair follicles are observed.

- SJS and TEN are now believed to be variants of the same condition. These are potentially fatal conditions involving the loss of sheets of mucosal and skin surfaces. They are medical emergencies and present with painful rash with blisters.

CASE 18.12

CLINICAL FEATURES

A 2-year-old male presented with pain, redness and swelling in the left eye of two weeks' duration, noted by the parents. There was no history of any ocular injury. Bilateral blue sclera was noted on ocular examination with peripheral corneal thinning (nearly four clock hours) in the left eye. BCVA was 6/15 and 6/60 (at 50 cm) in the right and left eye, respectively, as assessed through Cardiff paediatric visual acuity charts. Examination findings and clinical appearance are illustrated in Figure 18.27.

KEY POINTS

Diagnosis:
- The above clinical scenario describes a case of connective tissue disease with bilateral blue sclera and left eye peripheral corneal thinning.
- Clinically, Brittle cornea syndrome (BCS) was suspected, which is a rare autosomal recessive connective tissue disease, characterised by blue sclera, corneal thinning, and often with red hair, with normal skin and ligament elasticity.

Investigations:
- A thorough musculoskeletal examination was performed by the paediatrician for evaluating skin and ligament hyper elasticity.
- To rule out collagen vascular disease, a geneticist referral was sought.
- 2D-echocardiography was advised to look for any cardiac defects. Osteogenesis imperfecta was ruled out after looking for bone fractures and deafness.

Treatment:
- The left eye was treated with topical steroid drops (prednisolone acetate 1% six times a day and then tapered down gradually as per response) to control inflammation. Topical antibiotic (moxifloxacin hydrochloride 0.5% four times a day) was added to prevent superinfections. Oral ascorbic acid (250 mg twice a day) was added to promote healing. Parental counselling was done regarding the diagnosis of

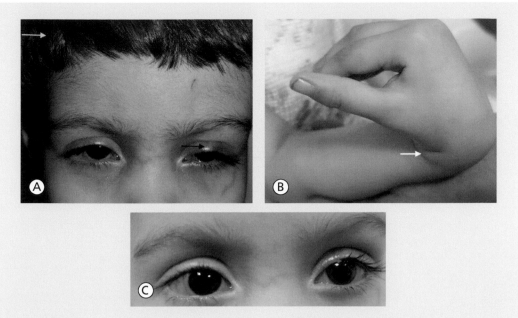

Figure 18.27 External photograph of a child with blue sclera and peripheral corneal melt showing (A) characteristic facial features with red colour of the hair (yellow arrow), bilateral blue sclera and mild lid oedema (black arrow), mechanical ptosis, watery discharge and redness in the left eye. Musculoskeletal examination showed (B) normal elasticity of skin and ligaments and normal extensibility of wrist joint (white arrow) and ocular examination revealed (C) resolution of peripheral corneal ulceration in the left eye with evidence of signs of healing in the form of corneal opacification of peripheral cornea (green arrow), after management with topical steroids and antibiotics.

BCS, explaining the treatment and further follow-up schedule with the paediatrician.

Outcome:
- Pain and redness subsided two weeks after initiation of treatment. BCVA of 6/24 (Cardiff acuity test at 1 m) in the left eye was achieved after medical management with adequate healing of the peripheral cornea.

Supplementary Information and Additional Tips
- A few important systemic causes of congenital blue sclera and peripheral corneal thinning are osteogenesis imperfecta (brittle bone disease), Ehlers-Danlos syndrome, pseudoxanthoma elasticum and Marfan syndrome.

CASE 18.13

CLINICAL FEATURES

A 15-year-old female presented with complaints of pain, redness and foreign body sensation in the left eye over the last seven days. Visual acuity at presentation was 6/6 in both eyes. There was no history of any ocular injury. The mother reported that the child had loss of weight, evening rise of temperature and anorexia for the last two months. A history of tuberculosis was positive in the paternal uncle who resided with them. Examination findings and clinical appearance are illustrated in Figure 18.28.

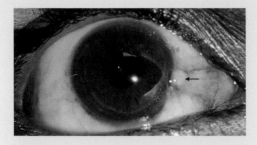

Figure 18.28 Clinical photograph of a child with phlyctenular conjunctivitis showing a raised, gelatinous limbal nodule (phlyctenule), of 2 mm diameter (black arrow) along with conjunctival injection (grey arrow). The rest of the conjunctiva and cornea is clear and uninvolved.

KEY POINTS

Diagnosis:
- The above clinical scenario describes a case of phlyctenular conjunctivitis in a case with systemic tuberculosis.

Investigations:
- Chest X-ray and computed tomography of the abdomen were performed to look for tubercular focus of infection and to rule out any sinusitis which revealed a fluid level in the left maxillary sinus.
- A Mantoux test and complete haemogram help in the diagnosis of tuberculosis.

Treatment:
- Systemic antitubercular treatment in consultation with a physician is important.
- Phlyctenular conjunctivitis, a hypersensitivity reaction to tubercular antigens, responded to low potency topical steroid, fluorometholone ophthalmic suspension 0.1% administered thrice a day, and then tapered as per clinical response.
- Carboxymethylcellulose 1% four times a day was also prescribed.

Outcome:
- There was good clinical response to treatment three weeks after initiation of therapy.

CASE 18.14

CLINICAL FEATURES

A 10-year-old male presented with parents complaining of a whitish mass growing in the left eye of the child since birth. The right eye had on-and-off symptoms of redness and had peripheral corneal opacification. The BCVA was 6/24 and 6/12 in the right eye and left eye, respectively. On facial examination, pre-tragal skin appendages were noted. Examination findings and slit lamp appearance are illustrated in Figure 18.29.

KEY POINTS

Diagnosis:
- The above clinical scenario describes a case of limbal dermoid with lipodermoid and lid coloboma in a case of Goldenhar syndrome (oculo-auriculo-vertebral syndrome). Peripheral corneal opacification with limbal stem cell deficiency and upper lid coloboma was seen in the other eye of the child.

Investigations:
- A dilated fundus examination was performed to rule out any associated posterior segment abnormality. To evaluate the depth of the lesion, an anterior segment optical coherence tomography (AS-OCT) can often be performed. However, paediatric patients may not cooperate for the same. An intraoperative optical coherence tomography (iOCT) and ultrasonic biomicroscopy (UBM) were performed during EUA, that ruled out any intraocular extension.

Treatment:
- Dermoid excision with corneal patch graft secured with fibrin glue was performed under general anaesthesia for the child.

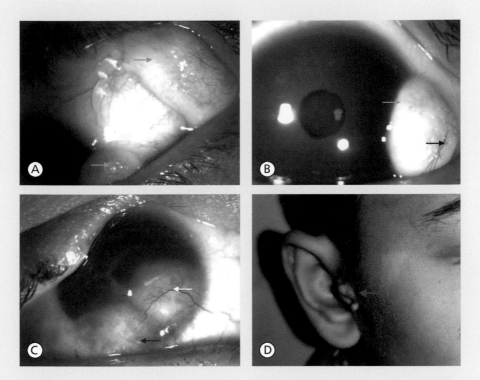

Figure 18.29 Clinical photograph of a child with Goldenhar syndrome and limbal dermoid showing (A) lipodermoid (grey arrow) in superotemporal location with inferotemporal limbal dermoid (yellow arrow) seen in the left eye and (B) growth of ectodermal tissue remnants e.g. cilia (black arrow) on the surface of a dermoid (yellow arrow). The right eye of the same patient revealed (C) the presence of lid coloboma (green arrow) and inferonasal three clock hours of limbal stem cell deficiency (LSCD) (blue arrow) seen with superficial vascularisation and corneal opacification (white arrow). External photograph of the same patient (D) showing a pre-tragal skin tag anterior to the right ear (red arrow).

Outcome:

- The anatomical outcomes were excellent with adequate wound healing, achieving good cosmesis. BCVA achieved after surgery in this case was 6/9 (one month postoperatively), owing to amblyopia resulting due to corneal astigmatism caused by the limbal dermoid. Patching and orthoptic treatment were advised.

Supplementary Information and Additional Tips

- Goldenhar syndrome classically presents as a triad of (a) midfacial hypoplasia causing facial asymmetry (b) auricular and ocular manifestations and (c) vertebral anomalies.
- Limbal dermoid may be associated with eyelid colobomas, loss of cilia

(Figure 18.30) and corneal exposure with secondary inflammation and infection.

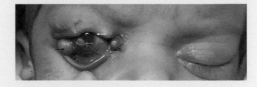

Figure 18.30 External photograph of an infant with Goldenhar syndrome with limbal dermoid (black arrow), corneal opacification and exposure with conjunctival congestion, upper lid coloboma (white arrow), lower lid coloboma (yellow arrow), loss of upper eyelid cilia and pre-tragal skin tag (green arrow). Corneal ulceration (grey arrow) was noted due to corneal exposure occurring to the upper lid defect.

CASE 18.15

CLINICAL FEATURES

A 4-year-old female was brought to the ophthalmic emergency by the parents with complaints of sudden onset pain, redness, watering and diminution of vision in the left eye for the last ten days. There was a history of fever followed by the appearance of vesicular skin eruptions on the left side of the face four days before the appearance of the ocular symptoms. Clinical appearance and examination findings under anaesthesia are illustrated in Figure 18.31.

KEY POINTS

Diagnosis:
- The above clinical scenario describes a case of herpes zoster ophthalmicus in a child presenting with necrotising stromal keratitis and corneal melting with surrounding stromal opacification.

Investigations:
- Posterior segment was within normal limits on B-scan ultrasonography.

- Blood investigations to rule out immunocompromised status were done which came out to be normal.
- Paediatric evaluation did not reveal any systemic abnormality.

Treatment:
- The patient was started on oral acyclovir 100 mg five times a day and topical antibiotics.
- Tectonic penetrating tectonic keratoplasty was performed to maintain corneal integrity.

Outcome:
- On first postoperative day following penetrating keratoplasty, the child was following light with accurate projection of rays.
- The graft was clear and the graft-host junction was well apposed with all the sutures intact and buried. Globe integrity was restored.
- The child was kept on topical antibiotics, steroids and cycloplegic and oral acyclovir.

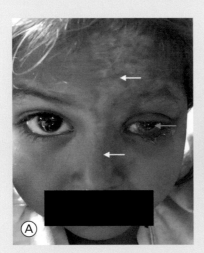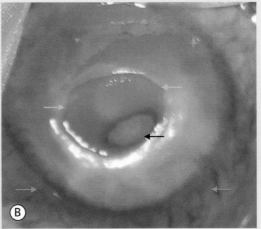

Figure 18.31 Clinical photograph of a young female child demonstrating (A) unilateral facial lesions of herpes zoster ophthalmicus involving a dermatome supplied by the trigeminal nerve (white arrows), including the tip of the nose and involvement of the ipsilateral eye (grey arrow) showing congestion and corneal opacification. Examination under anaesthesia revealed (B) a punched-out ulcer with a well-delineated epithelial defect (yellow arrows) with stromal lysis, surrounding conjunctival congestion (green arrows) and central perforation (black arrow).

CASE 18.16

CLINICAL FEATURES

An 11-month-old female child presented to the outpatient department when the parents noticed watering, frequent rubbing of eyes and redness in the right eye over the previous two weeks. The child had undergone optical keratoplasty in the same eye for congenital hereditary endothelial dystrophy (CHED) six months ago. The examination findings are illustrated in Figure 18.32.

KEY POINTS

Diagnosis:
- The above clinical scenario describes a case of suture infiltrates and graft infection in a case of operated optical keratoplasty performed for visual rehabilitation in a child with CHED.

Investigations:
- An emergency EUA was performed.
- The removed suture was sent for microbiological investigations to rule out any microbial infection.

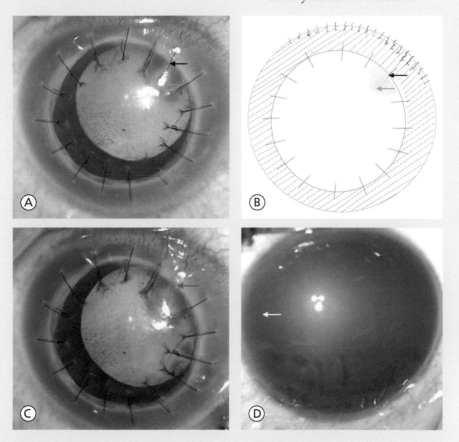

Figure 18.32 Clinical photograph (A) and corresponding corneal diagram (B) of a child with operated right-eye optical keratoplasty for congenital hereditary endothelial dystrophy (CHED) showing a clear graft with well-apposed graft-host junction in the right eye. Superonasally, the 2 o'clock suture was loose (black arrow) and there were demonstrable corneal infiltrates (yellow arrow) at the site of the loose suture. The loose suture in the right eye was removed under general anaesthesia and minimal corneal opacification was seen (C) with a well-apposed graft-host junction (green arrow) after loose suture removal. Clinical photograph of the left eye (D) with cloudy ground-glass appearance (white arrow) of left eye cornea consistent with the diagnosis of CHED.

Treatment:

- Following removal of the loose suture, the child was started on fortified topical antibiotics (cefazolin 5% and tobramycin 1.3%) along with cycloplegic (homatropine hydrobromide 2%). The antibiotic was tapered as per clinical response.
- Topical steroid drops were stopped for a week and then restated after the infection resolved.

Outcome:

- There was a good outcome in this case with resolution of the corneal infiltrates at the site of the loose suture.
- Peripheral corneal opacity was observed on follow-up at the site of the suture infection.

Supplementary Information and Additional Tips

- Keratoplasty in the paediatric age group has a higher incidence of early healing and occurrence of loose sutures, allogenic graft rejection, post-keratoplasty glaucoma, poor graft survival and poor outcomes in general when compared to that in adults.
- Frequent scheduling of EUAs decreases the occurrence of severe complications and helps in early management of any adverse events, if they occur.

- Secondary glaucoma may lead to localised ectasia and anterior staphyloma formation in a post-penetrating keratoplasty follow-up in paediatric age group (Figure 18.33).

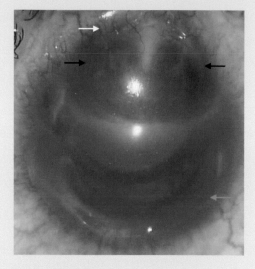

Figure 18.33 Clinical photograph of a child with operated optical penetrating keratoplasty showing a localised superior ectasia (black arrows) with superficial corneal vascularisation (white arrow). Note the clear graft and healthy graft-host junction (yellow arrow) in the inferior cornea.

REFERENCES

1. Wagner RS. Ocular allergy: pediatric concerns of ocular inflammation. Immunol Allergy Clin North Am. 1997; 17:161–77.
2. Singh M, Gour A, Gandhi A, Mathur U, Farooqui JH. Demographic details, risk factors, microbiological profile, and clinical outcomes of pediatric infectious keratitis cases in North India. Indian J Ophthalmol. 2020; 68(3):434–40.
3. Gupta N, Tandon R. Sociodemographic features and risk factor profile of keratomalacia in early infancy. Cornea. 2012; 31(8):864–6.

MISCELLANEOUS CORNEAL INFECTIONS AND INFLAMMATION

19 Contact Lens-Related Corneal Infection and Inflammation

Sneha Agarwal, Nimmy Raj, Noopur Gupta, Radhika Tandon

INTRODUCTION

Contact lens (CL) wear is becoming more and more prevalent according to a number of reasons, including cosmetic, refractive, myopia control, and therapeutic uses. It has been estimated that over 140 million people around the world use CLs.[1] The resurgence of scleral lenses, with their ability to vault the cornea by creating a tear reservoir between the cornea and lens, not only aids visual rehabilitation with enhanced comfort but also leads to a myriad of complications as some patients may experience poor tolerance and diminished comfort over time due to impaired CL surface wettability and poor CL hygiene.[2–4]

CL-related eye disease can have many different manifestations which can be both non-infectious and infectious. The non-infectious manifestations include inflammatory conditions like CL-induced acute red eye (CLARE) response and CL-associated peripheral ulcers (CLPU), CL-induced papillary conjunctivitis (CLPC), CL-related discomfort, dryness, meibomian gland dysfunction and allergic and toxic reactions to the lens material. The most important and dreadful consequence of CL wear among infectious causes is CL-related microbial keratitis (CLMK). The infection is most frequently caused by bacteria, mainly *Pseudomonas aeruginosa* and *Staphylococcus* species.[5] Fungi and Acanthamoeba species are now being commonly implicated in corneal infections related to CL wear.

CASE 19.1

CLINICAL FEATURES

A 29-year-old female patient using monthly disposable CLs for the past four years presented with redness, pain, watering and discharge for the last five days. The clinical examination findings and slit lamp features are shown in Figure 19.1.

KEY POINTS

Diagnosis:
- The above scenario describes a case of CLMK.

Investigations:
- Microbiological investigations were performed from corneal scrapings: Gram stain, Giemsa stain, calcofluor

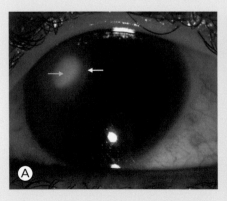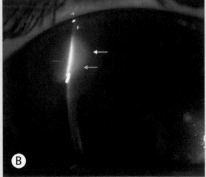

Figure 19.1 Slit lamp photograph of a 29-year-old female patient with contact lens-related microbial keratitis showing (A) corneal epithelial defect measuring approximately 4.4×5 mm (white arrow) with central 3.5×3 mm dense corneal infiltrate with abscess formation (green arrow). On slit illumination (B), appreciable corneal thinning with tissue loss (blue arrow) and corneal abscess (green arrow) with surrounding epithelial defect (white arrow) are noted.

white stain, KOH mount, bacterial culture on blood agar, fungal culture on Sabouraud dextrose agar and thioglycolate broth, and drug sensitivity testing.

- In addition, the CL with its case and the solution were sent for microbiological examination.
- The corneal scrapings came out as sterile with no growth after seven days. However, the CL and the solution showed growth of *P. aeruginosa* after three days that was sensitive to amikacin, moxifloxacin and polymyxin.

Treatment:
- The patient was started on moxifloxacin 0.5% empirically every two hours along with homatropine hydrobromide 2% four times a day. The patient was shifted to amikacin 1% and polymyxin B every two hours after receiving the culture and sensitivity report.

Outcome:
- The patient responded well to the treatment with the vessels regressing in three weeks leaving behind a residual macular corneal opacity measuring approximately three mm with a best corrected visual acuity of 6/6.

Supplementary Information and Additional Tips

- CL-related infections should be treated aggressively.
- The patient needs to be counselled about the need to handle the lens with the utmost care and to follow strict hygiene practices.
- The use of CL and the splashing of dirty water are important risk factors in development of *Acanthamoeba* keratitis (Figure 19.2) that can also occur secondary to swimming with CL on. A history of splashing of water into the eye or any kind of exposure to water should be carefully investigated in all cases of CL-associated keratitis.

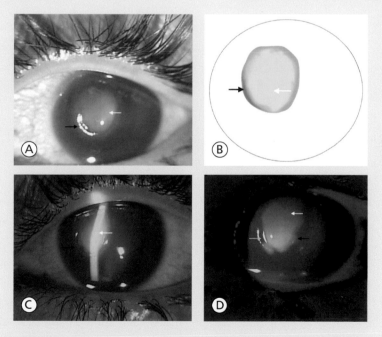

Figure 19.2 Slit lamp photograph of a patient with contact lens-related *Acanthamoeba* keratitis showing (A) ring-shaped central corneal ulcer with 5×4.5 mm epithelial defect (black arrow) with dense corneal infiltrates (white arrow); the same findings are illustrated (B) in a schematic corneal diagram. On slit examination (C), dense corneal infiltrates involving the full-thickness of the cornea (white arrow) with the associated epithelial defect (black arrow) can be seen. Examination under cobalt blue filter after fluorescein staining of the lesion (D) highlights the clinical findings of the central epithelial defect (black arrow) with infiltrate (white arrow) and surrounding corneal melt (yellow arrow).

CASE 19.2

CLINICAL FEATURES

A 26-year-old female patient presented with complaints of the sudden development of redness, pain, profuse watering and photophobia in her left eye over the last six hours. She gave a history of daily disposable CL use for the past month which she forgot to remove the previous night and had difficulty removing in the morning. Her clinical examination findings and slit lamp appearance on presentation and follow-up are shown in Figure 19.3.

KEY POINTS

Diagnosis:
- The above scenario describes a case of CL-induced keratitis.

Investigations:
- Corneal scraping of the lesion showed the presence of Gram-positive cocci in groups and clusters on Gram stain and bacterial culture showed growth of *Staphylococcus epidermidis* after three days.

Treatment:
- The patient was started on fortified antibiotics cefazolin 5% with tobramycin 1.3% every two hours for the first three days and then decreased to six times a day along with homatropine 2% four times a day.

Outcome:
- The ulcer completely healed in 21 days leaving behind a nebulo-macular corneal opacity.

Supplementary Information and Additional Tips

- Overnight use or extended wear of disposable CL is an important risk factor for keratitis. Removal of the CL by the patient themselves should not be attempted so as to prevent unwanted injuries to the corneal epithelium.
- CLs are a suitable surface for bacterial adhesion and biofilm formation, particularly for *S. epidermidis* (Figure 19.4) and *Pseudomonas* species.
- Hypoxia may increase bacterial binding, compromise corneal integrity and impair wound healing along with stagnation of the tear film behind the CLs with reduced resistance of the cornea to infection, all factors contributing to development of contact lens-related microbial keratitis (CMIK),

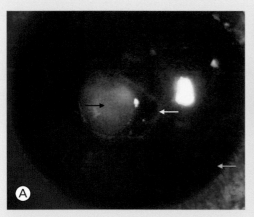 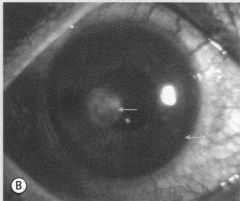

Figure 19.3 Slit lamp photograph of a 26-year-old female patient with contact lens-related microbial keratitis (A) showing a well-circumscribed corneal ulcer (black arrow) with a 5×3.5 mm corneal epithelial defect (white arrow) and circumcorneal congestion with increased vascularity suggestive of active inflammation (green arrow). On follow-up after four weeks (B), a 2×2 mm residual nebulo-macular corneal opacity (yellow arrow) with regressed circumcorneal vessels (green arrow) was seen.

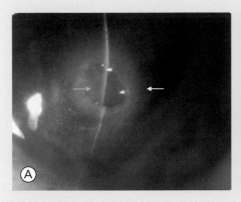
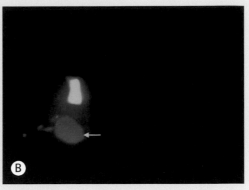

Figure 19.4 Slit lamp photograph of a young male with a history of overnight use of contact lens with resultant infective keratitis showing (A) slit illumination of the ulcer with punched out epithelial defect of 4×3 mm (yellow arrow) and surrounding infiltrates (white arrow) with central thinning. The fluorescein-stained image shows (B) a well-defined epithelial defect (yellow arrow) under cobalt blue filter.

which usually presents as paracentral, small and localised lesions without any surrounding corneal oedema in early stages of the infection (Figure 19.5).

■ Prosthetic CLs used for providing cosmesis in cases of leucomatous corneal opacities with no visual potential are also associated with risks of developing corneal ulcers and infections, usually due to poor fitting and impaired tear exchange, that leads to collection of mucopurulent discharge and debris which leads to the frequent occurrence of bacterial conjunctivitis (Figure 19.6) in these cases.

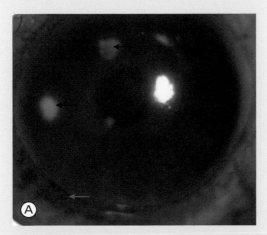
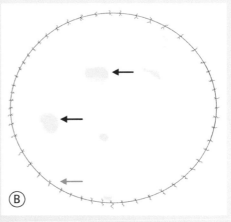

Figure 19.5 Slit lamp photograph of a patient with a recent onset of microbial keratitis following use of soft monthly disposable contact lens showing (A) paracentral, small and localised corneal infiltrates (black arrows) with diffuse limbal injection (blue arrow). The corresponding schematic diagram (B) shows the same findings.

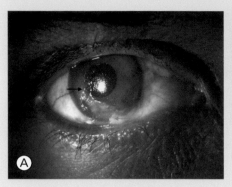
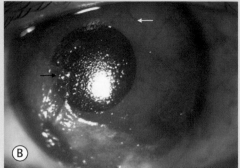

Figure 19.6 Slit lamp photograph of a patient wearing a prosthetic coloured contact lens to provide cosmesis for leucomatous corneal opacity showing (A) well-fitted contact lens with lens deposits near the pupil (black arrow) and mucopurulent discharge (blue arrow). The magnified image (B) reveals the vascularised corneal opacity beneath the prosthetic contact lens (white arrow) with lens deposits (black arrow) and mucopurulent discharge (blue arrow).

CASE 19.3

CLINICAL FEATURES

A 25-year-old male patient presented to the ophthalmic emergency department with complaints of pain, redness and watering for the past three days. He gave a history of CL usage for the past eight years and an accidental overnight usage of daily disposable CL prior to the onset of the symptoms. His clinical examination findings at presentation and follow-up are shown in Figure 19.7.

KEY POINTS

Diagnosis:
- The above scenario describes a case of CLPU.

Investigation:
- Corneal scraping specimen sent for microbiological evaluation did not reveal growth of any organism.

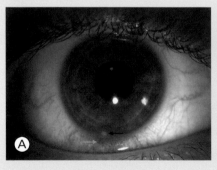
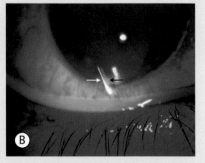

Figure 19.7 Slit lamp photograph of a male patient with history of extended use of daily disposable contact lens showing (A) circular peripheral infiltrate of approximately 1 mm in size (black arrow) with a surrounding area of conjunctival congestion (green arrow) suggestive of active inflammation. Examination under cobalt blue filter after fluorescein staining shows (B) intact overlying epithelium (white arrow) with associated anterior stromal infiltrate (black arrow) typical of contact lens-associated peripheral ulceration (CLPU).

- The CL was sent for microbiological examination for bacterial and fungal culture and sensitivity. Growth of *S. epidermidis* was noted after five days of inoculation into the blood agar culture plate. The bacterial strain isolated was reported to be sensitive to moxifloxacin, gatifloxacin, tobramycin and ofloxacin.

Treatment:
- The patient was started on moxifloxacin 0.5% drops six times a day, tobramycin 0.3% drops six times a day, homatropine 2% drops thrice a day and gatifloxacin 0.3% ointment for overnight application.

Outcome:
- The infiltrate reduced in size and depth within three days of treatment and totally disappeared by the sixteenth day after presentation.

Supplementary Information and Additional Tips
- CLPU usually presents as sterile circular epithelial lesions associated with anterior stromal infiltrates which is believed to represent an immunological reaction due to release of endotoxins by the bacteria with *Staphylococcus* species being implicated in most of the situations.

CASE 19.4

CLINICAL FEATURES

A 26-year-old male, wearing scleral CL, was maintaining a good follow-up regimen until he presented to the CL clinic with acute red eye with mild irritation and ocular discomfort. The patient was asked about the history of CL wear and it was noted that the patient had worn the lens in the right eye for 23 hours and took small naps in between, as he was unable to remove the lens in view of poor hygienic conditions while travelling on a train. The patient's visual acuity was noted to be 6/6 in both eyes. Intraocular pressure was recorded to be 19 mm Hg in the right eye and 17 mm Hg in the left eye. The examination findings and slit lamp appearance are shown in Figure 19.8.

KEY POINTS

Diagnosis:
- This was noted to be a case of CLARE with toxicity to the CL solution.

Investigations:
- Sodium fluorescein dye was instilled and the ocular surface was stained to evaluate corneal integrity for any epithelial disruption. The tear film broke up instantly, suggesting that the ocular surface health was compromised. There was no evidence of corneal infiltrates or any epithelial breakdown.
- Anterior segment optical coherence tomography (ASOCT) revealed a corneal thickness of 522 microns ruling out the presence of any corneal oedema.

Treatment:
- The patient was advised not to wear CL until the inflammation subsided and ocular surface health improved. He was advised to use spectacles for refractive correction.
- Medical management included topical loteprednol etabonate 0.5% for five days, moxifloxacin hydrochloride 0.5% thrice a day for five days, carboxymethylcellulose six times a day and hydroxypropyl methyl cellulose ophthalmic gel 0.3% at bedtime.

Outcome:
- Ocular inflammation settled and the corneal surface showed improvement with therapy.
- He was advised to wait for two weeks before resuming CL wear. Advice was given to use preservative-free saline drops to fill the scleral bowl and replenish it after every six hours while

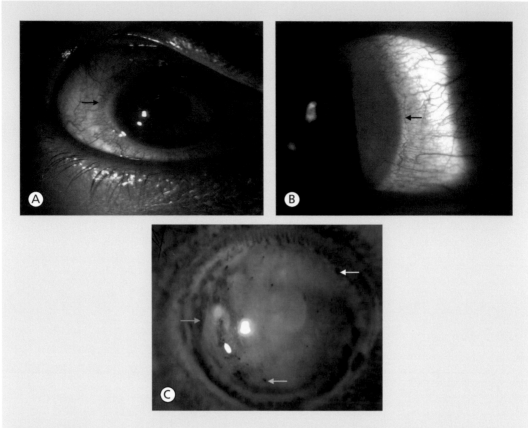

Figure 19.8 Slit lamp photograph of a patient with CLARE (contact lens-related red eye) showing (A) inflammatory reaction and profuse limbal injection (black arrow) seen as a result of prolonged wear of CL for 23 hours. Corneal infiltrates were characteristically absent. The magnified image of the limbal area (B) shows increased redness with neovascularisation (black arrow) at the limbus after removal of the scleral contact lens due to the tight mid-peripheral edge of the lens. The ocular surface was stained with fluorescein dye and it revealed (C) that the tear film broke instantly (green arrow) with mild staining noted at limbal (white arrow) and scleral tissues along with superficial punctate staining (yellow arrow) suggestive of dry eye and mild solution toxicity due to prolonged CL wear.

using CL. Strict instructions were given to refrain from sleeping with lenses.

Supplementary Information and Additional Tips

- CLARE is also referred to as tight lens syndrome.
- Various underlying reasons for CLARE include over-wearing CLs, sleeping in CLs when not indicated for that use, irritation from ill-fitting lenses, Gram-negative bacteria in

conjunction with CL overwear, reaction to bacterial toxins and solution hypersensitivity.
- Prolonged wear without removal of the scleral CL leads to hypoxia and toxicity that is compounded with prolonged contact of saline solution with the ocular surface along with closed eyelids during naps.
- Overwear of soft CLs can also lead to corneal hypoxia that triggers CLARE and results in the development of peripheral corneal neovascularisation (Figure 19.9).

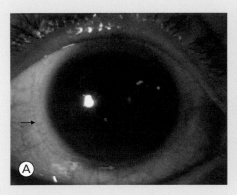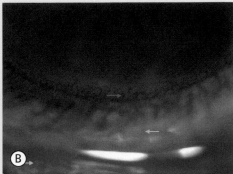

Figure 19.9 Slit lamp photograph of a patient who presented with (A) acute red eye due to overwear of conventional yearly disposable soft contact lens (black arrow) with development of peripheral corneal neovascularisation (blue arrow). The magnified image after removal of the soft contact lens reveals (B) profuse congestion of the bulbar and palpebral conjunctiva (yellow arrows) along with corneal neovascularisation (blue arrow), resulting from hypoxia and inflammation.

CASE 19.5

CLINICAL FEATURES

A 30-year-old female presented with diminution of vision in both eyes with frequent changes of glasses and reported poor improvement from spherocylindrical lenses. She experienced frequent headaches with severe pain in both eyes. She was diagnosed with pellucid marginal corneal degeneration (PMCD) and was prescribed large-diameter scleral CL (ScCL) for visual rehabilitation. On follow-up, she complained of mild stinging after lens removal, photophobia and frequent blurring of vision. Examination findings and slit lamp appearance before and after CL wear are illustrated in Figure 19.10.

KEY POINTS

Diagnosis:
- The above clinical scenario describes a case of PMCD with superficial punctate keratitis with poor wettability following ten months of scleral CL wear.

Investigations:
- A detailed ocular surface examination was performed including tear film break-up time (TBUT), Schirmer's test, corneal and conjunctival staining scores, tear osmolarity and the ocular surface disease index (OSDI).
- The tear film evaluation revealed TBUT of 3 and 11 seconds, Schirmer's test of 23 mm and 15 mm, corneal staining score of 10 and 5 and conjunctival staining score of 9 and 4, tear osmolarity values of 332 and 294 mOsmol/l and OSDI of 66 and 11 in the right and left eye, respectively.

Treatment:
- The patient was advised to stop scleral lens wear for one week and was again thoroughly counselled and trained to follow a proper lens care regimen.
- She was prescribed carboxymethyl cellulose 1% four times a day, polyethylene glycol 0.4% with propylene glycol 0.3 % four times a day and D-Panthenol 5 % ointment for topical use daily for one month. She was also prescribed fluorometholone acetate 1% twice a day that was tapered after a week to one daily instillation along with moxifloxacin 0.5% four times a day. She was asked to review after four weeks of therapy.

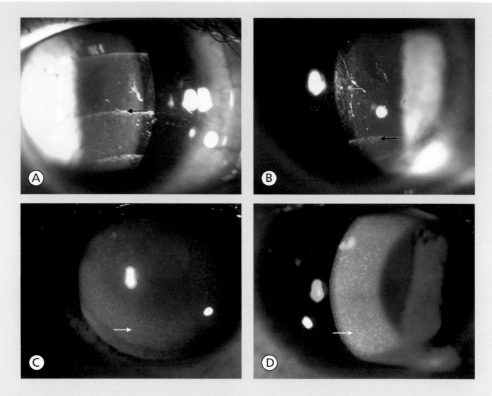

Figure 19.10 Slit lamp photograph of the patient with pellucid marginal corneal degeneration wearing scleral contact lenses (ScCL) for ten months reveals (A) debris and deposits (black arrow) on the surface of the contact lens with (B) scratches (yellow arrow) and ring-shaped lipid deposits (black arrow) affecting the surface wettability of the scleral contact lens demonstrating poor efforts at lens cleaning and hygiene. Examination after fluorescein staining under cobalt blue filter demonstrated (C) dry spots on the cornea manifesting as superficial punctate keratopathy (white arrow), more marked in the periphery on slit illumination (D) after ScCL removal.

Outcome:

- The ocular surface was evaluated after four weeks and showed an improvement in all the parameters. Corneal staining was absent with a healthy tear film.
- Visual acuity was recorded to be 6/9 and 6/6p in the right and left eye respectively.
- The scleral CL was evaluated under magnification and noted to have an optically clear surface with improved wettability.
- Subjectively, the patient was happy with the improved comfort and enhanced vision with minimal symptoms.

Supplementary Information and Additional Tips

- The lens surface of the scleral CLs can be affected by excessive and hard rubbing, taking off the special Hydra-PEG coating that provides enhanced lubrication and comfort to the eyes.
- Using rigid gas-permeable (RGP) lenses and Rose K2™ CL may lead to the development of meibomian gland dysfunction (Figure 19.11) with secretions getting deposited on the surface of the lens.
- Dry eye disease with epithelial breakdown can occur secondary to use of soft CLs (Figure 19.12).
- Superior epithelial arcuate lesion (SEAL) is an uncommon corneal complication related to CL wear that is

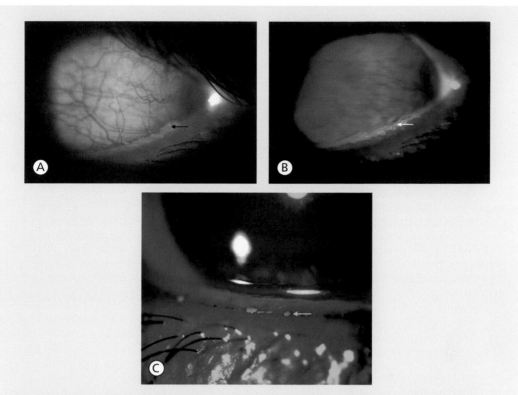

Figure 19.11 Slit lamp photograph of a patient wearing rigid gas-permeable lenses with meibomian gland dysfunction showing (A) irregular lid margin (black arrow) and foamy tear film with surfactants collected at the lid margin, that are highlighted when examined (B) under cobalt blue filter after fluorescein staining and seen as green, frothy discharge (white arrow) collected at the inferior lid margin. The magnified view reveals (C) the meibomian gland secretions (yellow arrow) plugging the gland orifices at the mucocutaneous lid junction.

also called epithelial splits or superior arcuate keratopathy. The lesions occur in the superior cornea, within about 2 mm of the superior limbus, between the limbus and the CL rim. Superficial and punctate staining is characteristic (Figure 19.13).

■ CLs alter the physiology and morphology of the epithelium and can influence corneal integrity. Signs include punctate epithelial keratopathy, epithelial abrasions (Figure 19.14), foreign body tracks, dellen, microcysts and vacuoles. The presence of epithelial defects should be monitored closely, and they may require both temporary cessation of CL wear as well as possible prophylactic antibiotic therapy, refitting of CLs, and patient education.

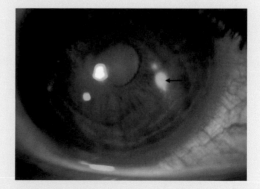

Figure 19.12 Slit lamp photograph of a patient wearing conventional soft contact lens who developed dry eye disease, manifesting as epithelial breakdown and corneal abrasion (black arrow) that was highlighted when examined under cobalt blue filter after fluorescein staining.

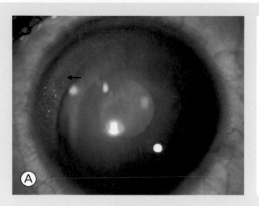 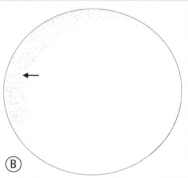

Figure 19.13 Slit lamp photograph of a patient who was prescribed a Rose K2™ contact lens for keratoconus showing (A) superior epithelial arcuate lesion (SEAL) or superior arcuate keratopathy seen in the superior cornea, between the limbus and the contact lens rim as superficial punctate staining (black arrow) when examined under cobalt blue filter after fluorescein staining. The corresponding corneal schematic diagram (B) depicts the same findings.

- The progression of keratoconus may result in flat fitting of the prescribed RGP lenses, leading to apical touch and the development of corneal abrasions and corneal stress lines (Figure 19.15) due to the tight fit of the CL.
- Corneal hypoxia may also manifest as vertical greyish-white lines called striae that appear in the posterior stroma (Figure 19.16). Upon removal of the cause, acute corneal oedema usually resolves itself within a matter of hours. To treat corneal oedema, one should select a lens material with higher oxygen permeability, decrease CL wearing time and ensure an optimal CL fit.

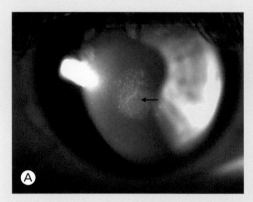 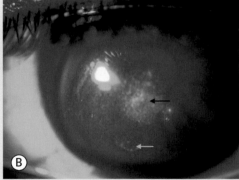

Figure 19.14 Slit lamp photograph of a patient with a corneal abrasion due to prolonged wear of a flat-fitting corneal rigid gas-permeable contact lens showing (A) central epithelial abrasion (black arrow) due to lens touch. Examination under cobalt blue filter after fluorescein staining (B) reveals a peripheral epithelial defect due to poor lens movement (yellow arrow) and highlights the central corneal abrasion (black arrow).

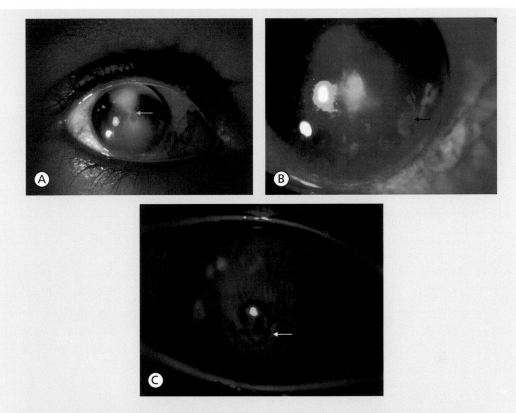

Figure 19.15 Slit lamp photograph of a patient with progressive keratoconus wearing rigid gas-permeable (RGP) corneal lenses for more than 20 months examined under cobalt blue filter after fluorescein staining showing (A) low-riding (blue arrow) and flat fitting of the RGP contact lens (yellow arrow) on the ectatic cone, leading to (B) apical touch and poor tear film exchange (black arrow) along with the development of (C) corneal abrasions (white arrow) and corneal stress lines seen on removal of the tight-fitting contact lens.

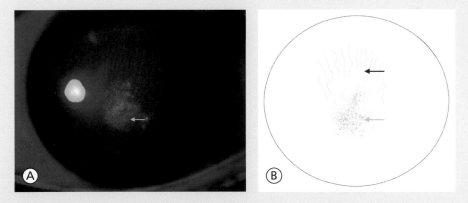

Figure 19.16 Slit lamp photograph of a patient with progressive keratoconus wearing a Rose K2™ contact lens examined under cobalt blue filter after fluorescein staining and showing (A) central corneal abrasion (yellow arrow) due to lens touch and the appearance of vertical greyish-white lines called striae or corneal stress lines (black arrow) occurring due to corneal hypoxia and flat fit of the rigid gas-permeable contact lens. The corresponding schematic diagram (B) shows the same findings.

CASE 19.6

CLINICAL FEATURES

A 30-year-old female diagnosed with advanced keratoconus (Amsler Krumeich stage IV) in both eyes with operated collagen cross-linking with riboflavin in the left eye was using ROSE K2™ CLs for keratoconus since 2014. In January 2019, she presented with a complaint of frequent dislocation and fall of lenses, with mild fluctuations in vision. As the RGP CL fitting was found to be altered with central apical touch, plasma-coated scleral CLs were prescribed for visual rehabilitation and enhanced comfort. On the annual follow-up visit, the patient complained of frequent haziness or cloudy vision after a few hours of scleral lens wear (after two to three hours) and enhanced debris in both lenses. At the end of the day after removal of the CLs, mild redness with a stinging sensation was noted and she mentioned a strong urge to rub her eyes. Examination findings and slit lamp appearance before and after CL wear are illustrated in Figures 19.17 and 19.18.

KEY POINTS

Diagnosis:

- The above case scenario represents a case of advanced keratoconus with midday fogging and post-lens tear layer debris formation due to

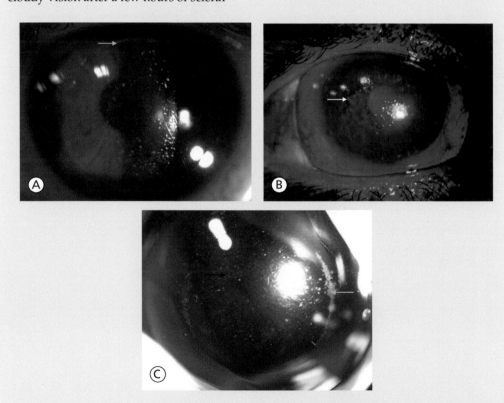

Figure 19.17 Slit lamp photograph of the patient with advanced keratoconus fitted with plasma-coated scleral lens reflects (A) debris and lipid stained front surface (black arrow) having poor wettability and severe deposits on the corneal surface mimicking the contact lens deposits (yellow arrow) with (B) heavy superficial punctate staining and dry spots on the cornea (white arrow) demonstrated on fluorescein staining under cobalt blue filter. Examination of the RGP scleral contact lens, held in the examiner's hand, after removal from the patient's eye, revealed (C) scratches, fine lipid opacities (black arrow) and ring-shaped lipid deposits (yellow arrow) over the surface of the scleral lens demonstrating poor efforts at lens cleaning and hygiene.

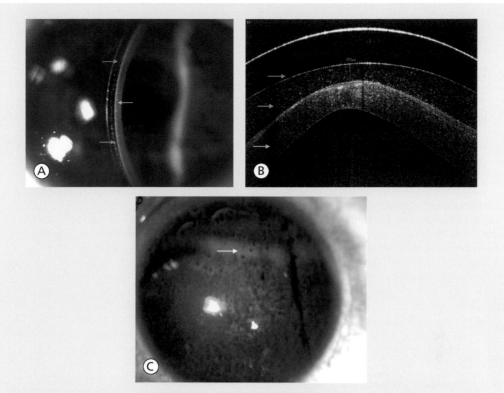

Figure 19.18 Slit lamp photograph of a patient wearing a scleral contact lens (ScCL) demonstrating (A) debris-stained tear film (green arrow) responsible for midday fogging trapped between the well-fitted scleral contact lens (blue arrow) and the ectatic cornea (yellow arrow) in keratoconus. The ASOCT imaging clearly reveals (B) the debris, seen as hyperreflective particles (green arrow) in the tear film reservoir (TFR) and the optimum ScCL vaulting (blue arrow) over steepened cornea (yellow arrow). Examination after fluorescein staining under cobalt blue filter after removal of the lens demonstrates (C) dry spots on the cornea (white arrow) manifesting as superficial punctate keratopathy and disruption of the tear film, signifying a poor ocular surface.

compromised lens hygiene and a dry ocular surface precipitated by overwear of the scleral CLs.

Investigations:
- A detailed ocular surface evaluation was performed. Tear film break-up time reflected instant break-up of the tear film, Schirmer's test demonstrated reflex tearing and increased corneal and conjunctival staining scores were noted.

Treatment:
- She was evaluated in the CL clinic and was advised to stop the use of her lenses for at least two weeks.

- She was scheduled for refitting of scleral lenses with Tangible Hydra-PEG coat lenses.
- A moist heat mask with complete usage instructions was prescribed.
- Medical therapy included azithromycin 1% eye drops three times a day for ten days, prednisolone sodium phosphate eye drops once a day for 15 days, hypromellose 0.3% eye drops four times a day and hydroxypropyl methylcellulose 0.3% eye ointment at bedtime for six weeks.
- Meanwhile, her CLs were sent to the CL laboratory for surface cleaning and polishing to remove deposits and enhance CL surface wettability.

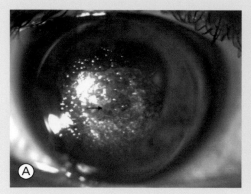
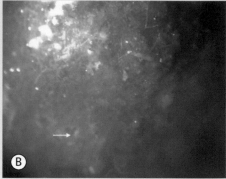

Figure 19.19 Slit lamp photograph of a patient wearing corneal RGP lenses showing (A) shiny debris (black arrow) on the surface of the CL, typically different than protein and lipid deposits, that did not get washed with a protein cleaning and disinfectant solution. The surface of the CL shows (B) yellow and green debris reflected under fluorescein (white arrow) with increase in thickness of the CL.

Outcome:
- The patient has been using the CLs successfully with no fogging or blurring of vision.

Supplementary Information and Additional Tips
- Midday fogging (MDF) occurs when there is an accumulation of debris in the post-lens tear film reservoir during scleral lens wear. Fogginess in vision disappears immediately after scleral lens reapplication, as saline is replenished. Associated ocular symptoms such as allergies, dry eye, MGD etc. must be treated

before considering lens parameter modifications.
- Factors that have been linked to scleral fogging include increased accumulation of tear debris in the lens reservoir, minimal tear exchange, increased mucin production from conjunctival tissue rubbing, accumulation of protein and lipid deposits on the front surface of the lens and corneal oedema.
- Thick lens deposits on the surface of the RGP CL can also lead to blurred vision (Figure 19.19). Guidance in an appropriate lens care regimen with maintenance of hygiene is the mainstay of therapy in these cases.

CASE 19.7

CLINICAL FEATURES

A 48-year-old female with operated radial keratotomy for moderate myopia presented to the CL clinic with complaints of reduced vision with frequent change of glasses over the last two to three years. She was considered for a ScCL trial for therapeutic use and was fitted with a 16.2 mm diameter scleral lens with edge modification to suit the contours of her eye. Visual acuity of 6/6 in the right eye and 6/6p in the left eye was achieved. The patient was comfortable with

CL wear and reported no complaints except for the mild ocular pain she felt after five to six hours of continuous lens wear with mild redness. Examination findings and slit lamp appearance before and after CL wear are illustrated in Figures 19.20 and 19.21.

KEY POINTS

Diagnosis:
- The above clinical scenario describes a case of operated radial keratotomy (RK) with conjunctival prolapse and

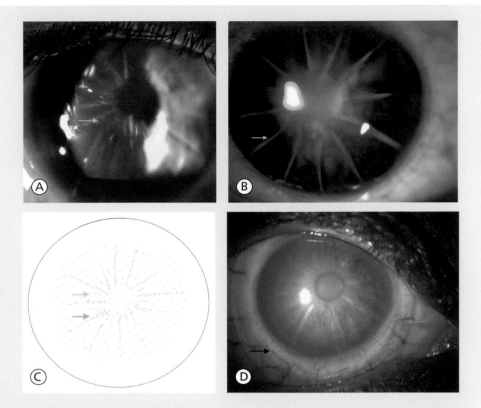

Figure 19.20 Slit lamp photograph of a patient with operated radial keratotomy for myopia depicting (A) radial and irregular pattern of cuts (yellow arrow) responsible for an irregular corneal surface along with mild corneal haze and corneal ectasia. Fluorescein-stained cornea revealed (B) instant break-up of the tear film, highlighting the surface irregularity and deficient tear film. Note the pooling of the fluorescein dye, highlighting the radial RK cuts (green arrow), that are also illustrated in (C) the schematic corneal diagram. Scleral contact lens was prescribed for visual rehabilitation and for managing the poor ocular surface, which revealed (D) adequate vaulting of ScCL but limbal hyperaemia (black arrow) with the tight edges of lens indented in the sclera (blue arrow), leading to conjunctival hooding and prolapse.

conjunctival blanching due to the steep peripheral fit of the scleral CL, precipitated by prolonged CL wear.

Investigations:
- On instillation of fluorescein dye, lens vaulting was adequate but the tight edges of the lens indented the sclera, leading to conjunctival hooding and blanching.
- An ASOCT scan was performed to assess edge details and indentation of the CL. Lens fit was thoroughly evaluated before scleral lens removal to assess the lens sinking and settling

on the eye. Conjunctival compression varied upon movement of the eye in different gazes and conjunctival flaps and folds were easily picked up on ASOCT imaging (Figure 19.22).

Treatment:
- The patient was advised to remove the CL immediately and the folds of conjunctiva disappeared.
- She was advised to wear the present lenses for shorter durations and to replace saline frequently when she received her new modified lenses.
- Total lens diameter was reduced to 16.00 mm and a better centration was

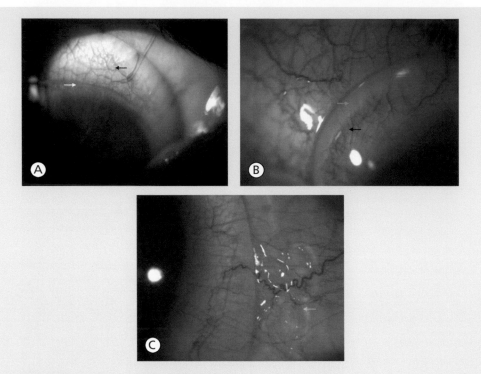

Figure 19.21 Slit lamp photograph of a patient wearing a scleral contact lens with a steep peripheral fit showing (A) conjunctival prolapse with folds (white arrow), seen as a slightly raised ridge of conjunctival tissue, that was seen underneath the superior edge of the CL due to boggy conjunctiva and pinched blood vessels underneath tight peripheral edges of the ScCL (black arrow). The magnified image revealed (B) marked compression of the blood vessels leading to blanching of the vessels (blue arrow) at the periphery of the lens (black arrow). The delamination and conjunctivochalasis (yellow arrow) were evident (C) near the superotemporal edge of the lens, probably occurring due to repeated trauma and friction of the sharp lens edge over the conjunctival tissue.

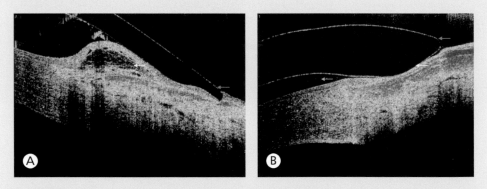

Figure 19.22 Anterior segment optical coherence tomographic scan of a patient wearing a scleral contact lens in order to assess the edge details and indentation of the lens showing (A) the peripheral edge of ScCL buried into the sclera leading to indentation of CL (blue arrow), landing of the mid-peripheral edge of ScCL compressing the conjunctiva leading to conjunctival prolapse or folds (white arrow). The lens edge was modified and on a recent follow-up visit shows (B) perfect landing of the peripheral edge (blue arrow) of the scleral contact lens on the sclera having a symbiotic relationship with the conjunctiva, without any conjunctival folds (white arrow) and adequate vault (yellow arrow) of the lens over the cornea.

achieved when the limbal curves were flattened. The recorded details with clinical images and videos were sent to the manufacturer for edge modifications and further alignment and adjustment of other parameters of the CL which may get affected by the peripheral edge modification, such as lens sag and landing of the lens.

Outcome:

■ The patient was comfortable with her new prescription of scleral lenses with 16.00 mm diameter and flattened posterior peripheral edges in both eyes. She was able to wear the new CLs for about five to six hours at a stretch without any complaints or discomfort.

Supplementary Information and Additional Tips

■ CL-related conjunctival findings include lid wiper epitheliopathy, conjunctival blanching and pinching of vessels (Figure 19.23), conjunctival

flaps, lid-parallel conjunctival folds and conjunctival indentation that are seen as scleral indentation rings with altered tear film on the cornea due to poor movement of the lens with altered tear film exchange and impaired tear dynamics (Figure 19.24).

■ Lens compression marks and corneal staining can also be seen as multicurve circular marks on the corneal surface with use of Rose K2™ RGP CLs due to impaired tear dynamics and poor movement of the CL, in spite of proper fitting (Figure 19.25).

■ Conjunctival prolapse occurs when loose perilimbal conjunctival tissue is pulled between the scleral lens and the corneal limbus, often adhering to the corneal epithelium. A prolapse positioned over the corneal limbus could reduce the nutrients available to the cornea. Conjunctival flaps resolve spontaneously with discontinuation of lens wear. Conjunctival staining may occur at the region of conjunctival folds and prolapse after removal of the scleral CL (Figure 19.26).

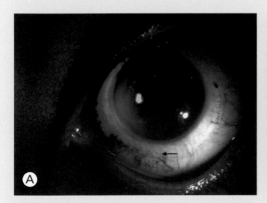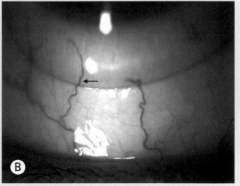

Figure 19.23 Slit lamp photograph of a patient with advanced keratoconus who was intolerant to corneal RGP lenses due to marked progression of the disease, showing (A) circumferential blanching of the blood vessels around the lens edge pinching the conjunctival blood vessels (black arrow) around the limbus, where the lens edge is causing compression on the sclera. On refitting of the scleral lens with edge modifications, smooth landing of the scleral contact lens is observed (B) with no distortion or blanching of the blood vessels (black arrow).

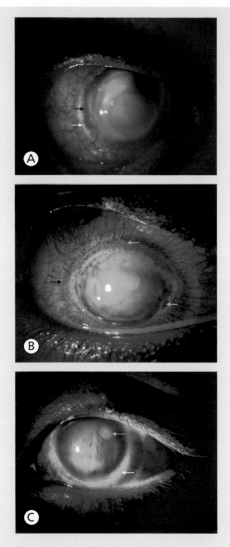

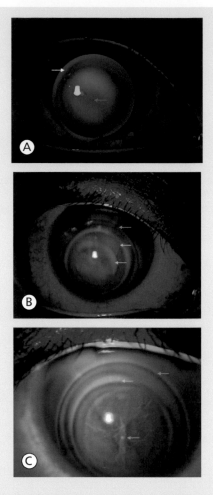

Figure 19.24 Slit lamp photograph showing contact lens-related conjunctival findings in the form of (A) scleral indentation rings (white arrow) with altered tear film due to poor movement of the lens with altered tear film exchange and impaired tear dynamics. Compressed blood vessels (black arrow) leading to limbal redness due to tight mid-periphery of CL can be seen. Examination under the cobalt blue filter highlights (B) the diffuse staining caused around the limbus due to the tight mid-periphery of ScCL (yellow arrow) and the induced limbal hyperaemia (black arrow). A circular, shiny lens indentation ring (white arrow) can be seen (C) with altered tear film (green arrow) with severely compressed conjunctival tissue due to the tight-fitting scleral contact lens.

Figure 19.25 Slit lamp photograph under cobalt blue filter after fluorescein staining of a 24-year-old female who was prescribed a Rose K2™ contact lens for visual rehabilitation, presented with altered lens fitting after nine months to reveal (A) central apical touch (blue arrow), pooling at the peripheral edge of corneal RGP lens (white arrow) and a low-riding lens (black arrow) on the cornea, denoting a poor edge-eyelid relationship with minimal tear exchange. On removal of the contact lens (B), outer (grey arrow) and inner (yellow arrows) CL compression rings over the cornea were noted, depicting the multicurve design of these lenses. On magnified view (C), the lens showed the concentric marks of the outer (grey arrow) and inner rings (yellow arrow) due to the restricted movement of the CL on blinking leading to minimal tear exchange resulting in bounding of the lens to the cornea with mild apical scarring (green arrow) caused by the CL landing on the conical apex.

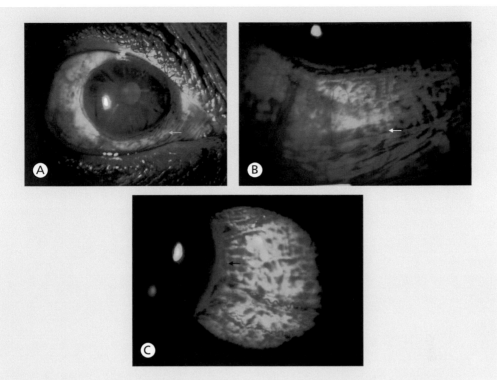

Figure 19.26 Slit lamp photograph of a patient who showed conjunctival staining on removal of ScCL, wherein the cobalt blue filter examination after fluorescein staining revealed (A) circumferential staining marks and fluorescein patches on the sclera with boggy conjunctiva near the medial canthus (yellow arrow). The conjunctival surface shows (B) fluorescein staining around the limbal area (black arrow) with marking of the tight mid-periphery of the CL along with peripheral staining of the conjunctiva due to the tight peripheral edge (white arrow) of the CL. The temporal conjunctiva (C) is also stained with marking of the tight mid-periphery of CL at the limbal area (black arrow).

CASE 19.8

CLINICAL FEATURES

A 27-year-old female using conventional one-year disposable soft CLs presented to the outpatient department with complaints of itching with ocular discomfort and reduced tolerance to CLs over a period of time. She had been using the disposable soft CLs for the past four years. She had mild mucoid discharge but no watering. She was slightly photophobic on slit lamp examination. Best corrected visual acuity in both eyes was 6/9. Examination findings and slit lamp appearance before and after CL wear are illustrated in Figures 19.27 and 19.28.

KEY POINTS

Diagnosis:
- The above clinical scenario describes a case of CLPC.

Investigations:
- Ocular surface was stained with fluorescein dye to demarcate papillae and to note other ocular details. Tear film break-up time was reduced (6 seconds) and corneal staining in the inferior quadrant of the cornea was noted.

Treatment:
- She was advised to discontinue using the CLs.

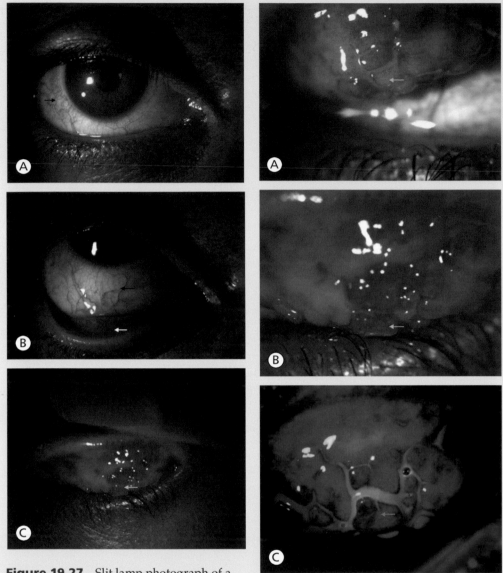

Figure 19.27 Slit lamp photograph of a patient with CLPC (contact lens-induced papillary conjunctivitis) showing (A) diffuse bulbar hyperaemia (black arrow) due to soft contact lens wear with (B) tortuous conjunctival vessels and hyperaemia (black arrow) noted in the inferior bulbar conjunctiva. The lower palpebral conjunctiva also shows marked congestion (white arrow) due to inflammation induced by the CL. On eversion of the upper lid (C) a cobblestone appearance with the presence of giant papillae (yellow arrow) was noted causing ocular discomfort and poor tolerance to CL.

Figure 19.28 Slit lamp photograph of a patient with papillary conjunctivitis due to chronic contact lens wear showing giant papillae (yellow arrow) with palpebral hyperaemia and mucus debris on eversion of the upper lids of right (A) and left eye (B). On fluorescein staining (C) multiple giant papillae (orange arrow) of more than 1 mm in size could be seen.

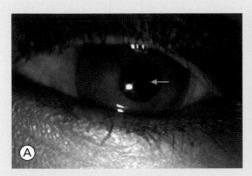
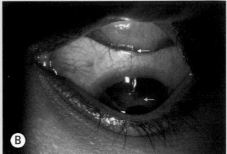

Figure 19.29   Slit lamp photograph of a patient wearing dark-pupil type of prosthetic soft contact lens (green arrow) showing (A) diffuse conjunctival congestion. On eversion of the upper lid (B), allergic response to the contact lens is seen as diffuse upper tarsal congestion along with pigment deposits (white arrow). Note the faded area of the prosthetic CL (yellow arrow), where the pigment has worn off.

- Medical therapy in the form of cold compresses thrice a day, oral cetirizine 10 mg at night for five days, topical naphazoline four times a day, topical bepotastine besilate 1.5% twice a day and carboxy methylcellulose 1% six times a day was prescribed.
- The patient was shifted to use daily disposable hydrogel CLs after the conjunctival papillae subsided with medical therapy after three months. This had the additional advantage of avoiding use of any CL solution.

Outcome:

- The patient was happy using daily disposable CLs. Her CL care regimen improved and she was advised to take all precautions to safeguard her eyes as per recommended guidelines.

Supplementary Information and Additional Tips

- CL-induced papillary conjunctivitis is a non-sight threatening and reversible condition which includes itching, ocular discomfort and leads to poor tolerance to CL and discontinuation of CL wear.
- CLPC is common in soft CLs as compared to rigid lenses and occurs in silicone hydrogel as well as hydrogel lens wearers. It can also occur with use of prosthetic CLs when pigment from the CL is deposited in the upper tarsal conjunctiva with prolonged use (Figure 19.29).

REFERENCES

1. Barr JT, Mack CJ. Contact lenses yesterday, today, and the best yet to come. Contact Lens Spectr. 2011; 26:14–15.
2. Walker M, Bergmanson JP, Marsack JD, et al. Complications and fitting challenges associated with scleral contact lenses: a review. Contact Lens Anterior Eye. 2016; 39(2):88–96.
3. Barnett M, Johns LK, eds. Contemporary Scleral Lenses: Theory and Application. Sharjah, UAE: Bentham Science Publishers; 2017; 326–34.
4. Fadela D, Kramer E. Potential contraindications to scleral lens wear. Contact Lens and Anterior Eye. 2019; 42:92–103.
5. Lim CHL, Stapleton F, Mehta JS. Review of contact lens-related complications. Eye Contact Lens. 2018; 44 Suppl. 2: S1–S10.

20 Post-Traumatic Corneal Infection and Inflammation

Nimmy Raj, Alisha Kishore, T Monikha, Neiwete Lomi, Noopur Gupta

INTRODUCTION

Ocular trauma is an significant cause of preventable monocular blindness in the world. Contusions, lamellar or full-thickness laceration of the ocular coats and posterior segment afflictions are the major clinical manifestations.[1] Ocular trauma represents the main risk factor for infectious keratitis. Work safety guidelines, vigilance in initiating treatment and education by front-line physicians should be reinforced.[2]

Post-traumatic microbial keratitis also adds to the extent of ocular morbidity. A high degree of suspicion and treatment of each case of possible infection with broad-spectrum antibiotics (while keeping in mind the chances of Gram-negative or polymicrobial aetiology) is important in reducing the incidence of post-traumatic blindness.[3]

CASE 20.1

CLINICAL FEATURES

A 25-year-old male presented with decrease in vision, watering and discomfort in the right eye following trauma to the right eye with a wooden stick one day earlier. On examination, the vision in the right eye was 6/36. The intraocular pressure was within normal limits. Slit lamp findings are illustrated in Figure 20.1.

KEY POINTS

Diagnosis:
- The above clinical scenario describes a case of post-traumatic self-sealed corneal perforation.

Investigations:
- The diagnosis is made on clinical history and examination.
- A pressure Seidel test should be done to rule out full-thickness corneal perforation which was negative in this case. Ultrasound B-scan of the right eye to rule out any posterior segment pathology was done and was found to be anechoic.

Treatment:
- The patient was managed on topical antibiotic (moxifloxacin 0.5% four times a day for two weeks) and lubricant (carboxymethylcellulose 0.5% six times a day for two weeks).

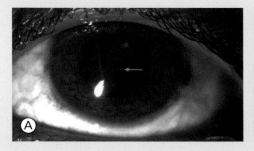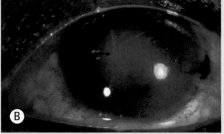

Figure 20.1 Slit lamp photograph of a patient with a post-traumatic, self-sealed corneal perforation showing (A) a vertical, linear self-sealed corneal perforation of about 6 mm (black arrow) with surrounding Descemet's folds (grey arrow). Examination under a cobalt blue filter (B) after instilling fluorescein dye demonstrated a negative pressure Seidel test (black arrow).

Moxifloxacin ointment was prescribed at night.

Outcome:
- There was a fine, vertical, linear nebular scar in the area of corneal perforation. The surrounding Descemet's folds were resolved with treatment. The vision was documented to be 6/12.

Supplementary Information and Additional Tips
- The need for intervention in cases of self-sealed perforation should be assessed on a case-to-case basis. In cases where the anatomy of the eye is conserved (i.e. the iris and lens are in their normal position) with no aqueous leak, the patient can be managed conservatively on antibiotics and lubricants and kept on close follow-up.

CASE 20.2

CLINICAL FEATURES

A 5-day-old female child was presented by the parents with complaints of redness and whitish opacity in the right eye since birth. The child was born at full term by forceps assisted normal vaginal delivery. The examination of the child was performed under anaesthesia and the findings are as shown in Figure 20.2.

KEY POINTS

Diagnosis:
- The above clinical scenario describes a case of post-traumatic (forceps induced) corneal abrasion.

Investigations:
- The diagnosis is based on clinical history and examination.

Treatment:
- The child was given prophylactic antibiotic treatment (topical moxifloxacin 0.5% four times a day for one week) with lubricant drops (carboxymethylcellulose 0.5% four times a day for one week).

Outcome:
- The corneal abrasion and subconjunctival haemorrhage with microtear resolved with the treatment within a week.

Supplementary Information and Additional Tips
- An examination under anaesthesia is always necessary to make a definitive diagnosis in a case of an infant or neonate with whitish opacity since birth with associated redness and watering. Primary congenital glaucoma and infective keratitis are important differential diagnoses.

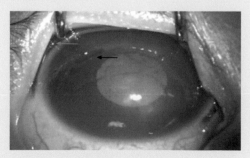

Figure 20.2 Clinical photograph of a newborn child with post-traumatic (forceps delivery) corneal abrasion showing superior subconjunctival haemorrhage (green arrow) and corneal abrasion of around 5 mm temporally (black arrow).

CASE 20.3

CLINICAL FEATURES

A 35-year-old male presented with decrease in vision, pain, watering and photophobia in the right eye following trauma with a bull horn one week earlier. Visual acuity at presentation was 6/24. Examination and slit lamp examination findings are shown in Figure 20.3.

KEY POINTS

Diagnosis:

- The above clinical scenario describes a case of post-traumatic corneal perforation with uveal tissue prolapse.

Investigations:

- The diagnosis is based on clinical history and examination. Ultrasound B-scan can be performed to rule out any posterior segment pathology in case fundus evaluation is not possible.

Treatment:

- A corneal patch graft was done in this case since the perforation was around 5 mm size.
- Postoperatively, topical antibiotic (moxifloxacin 0.5% four times a day for two weeks), cycloplegic (homatropine 2% twice daily for two weeks), topical steroids (four times a day tapered gradually over four weeks) and lubricants were given. Antibiotic ointment was administered at night.

Outcome:

- The patient was followed at one week. The postoperative vision was 5/60. Close follow-up was advised for the patient.

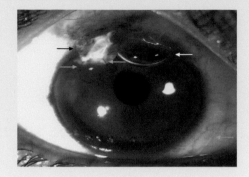

Figure 20.4 Slit lamp photograph of a patient with post-traumatic peripheral corneal perforation showing an operated tenon's patch graft (black arrow) sutured with 10-0 monofilament nylon sutures (yellow arrows) and surrounding conjunctival congestion (grey arrow). Note the bandage contact lens in place (green arrow) and well-formed anterior chamber with an air bubble (white arrow) superiorly near the wound site.

Supplementary Information and Additional Tips

- Linear corneal perforations can be sutured to seal the defect, but for bigger corneal tissue defects suturing will not suffice. A defect of up to 3 mm can be treated with cyanoacrylate glue and a bandage contact lens.
- In corneal tissue defects up to 3–5 mm, a corneal patch graft can be done; bigger defects require penetrating keratoplasty. A tenon's patch graft with or without a tissue adhesive can also be used to close defects if corneal tissue is unavailable (Figure 20.4).

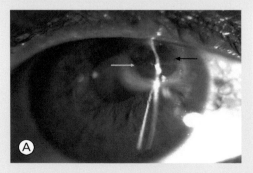

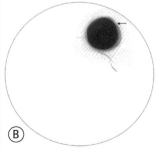

Figure 20.3 Slit lamp photograph of a 35-year-old patient showing (A) post-traumatic corneal perforation (bull horn injury) measuring 5×4 mm (green arrow) with uveal tissue prolapse (black arrow). The corresponding schematic diagram (B) depicts the same findings.

CASE 20.4

CLINICAL FEATURES

A 40-year-old male presented with decrease of vision, watering, redness and pain in the right eye for the previous day following trauma with a knife. He had a history of operated radial keratotomy for myopia in both eyes 15 years ago. Examination findings and slit lamp appearance are shown in Figure 20.5.

KEY POINTS

Diagnosis:
- The above clinical scenario describes a case of both-eyes operated radial keratotomy (RK) for myopia with right eye post-traumatic corneal perforation.

Investigations:
- The diagnosis is based on clinical history and examination.
- An ultrasound B-scan was performed to rule out any posterior segment pathology and was found to be anechoic.

Treatment:
- A corneal perforation repair was done under general anaesthesia.
- Continuous sutures were applied. It is important to assess all the RK incision scar sites for any gaping at the completion of surgery.
- Suturing of gaping RK cuts was needed at four scar sites in this case.

Outcome:
- Postoperatively, the perforation site and all the incision site were sealed with the anterior chamber well formed at one week follow-up.

Supplementary Information and Additional Tips

- Any previous corneal surgery including RK, laser in situ keratomileusis (LASIK) treatment or penetrating keratoplasty affects the tensile strength of the cornea and creates weak areas in the cornea which can easily give way following any blunt or penetrating injury.

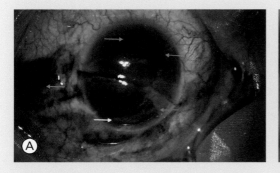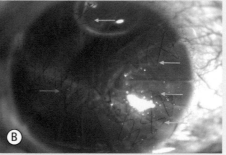

Figure 20.5 Clinical photograph of a patient with operated radial keratotomy presenting with post-traumatic corneal perforation (A) showing subconjunctival haemorrhage (green arrow) with linear, limbus to limbus corneal perforation (black arrow) with radial keratotomy incision scar marks (grey arrows) and hyphaema (white arrow). Postoperative slit lamp examination (B) demonstrates a continuous suturing technique performed at the corneal perforation site (blue arrow) along with repaired ruptures at the radial keratotomy incision sites (yellow arrows) to secure globe integrity.

CASE 20.5

CLINICAL FEATURES

A 44-year-old male presented with sudden loss of vision, watering, redness and pain in the left eye for the past day following trauma with a fist during a fight. He had a history of left-eye operated keratoplasty for healed keratitis four months prior. His visual acuity was positive perception of light with inaccurate projection of rays in two quadrants. The examination and slit lamp findings are shown in Figure 20.6.

KEY POINTS

Diagnosis:
- The above clinical scenario describes a case of post-traumatic graft dehiscence with uveal tissue prolapse.

Investigations:
- The diagnosis is based on clinical history and examination. Ultrasound to rule out any posterior segment pathology was done and was found to be anechoic.

Treatment:
- Graft dehiscence repair along with iris tissue abscission was done under general anaesthesia and interrupted 10-0 nylon sutures were applied.
- Postoperatively, topical antibiotic (moxifloxacin 0.5% four times a day), steroids (prednisolone every two hours in tapering doses) and lubricants were given.

Outcome:
- Following graft dehiscence repair, the graft-host junction was well apposed with an oedematous graft at the one week follow-up. The patient was kept on close follow-up.

Supplementary Information and Additional Tips

- A patient who has undergone a penetrating keratoplasty is at high risk of a graft dehiscence following even minor trauma due to the weak graft-host junction which can easily give way.
- There is a very high chance of graft failure following post-traumatic graft dehiscence (Figure 20.7).

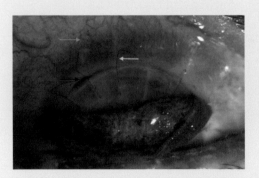

Figure 20.6 Slit lamp examination of a patient with post-traumatic graft dehiscence showing conjunctival congestion with superficial vascularisation (green arrow) with graft dehiscence of six clock hours extending from 9–3 o'clock (black arrow) with broken sutures (yellow arrow) and uveal tissue prolapse (grey arrow).

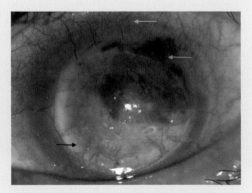

Figure 20.7 Slit lamp examination in a patient presenting with post-traumatic graft dehiscence showing conjunctival congestion with 360 degrees of superficial vascularisation (yellow arrow) with graft dehiscence of four clock hours extending from 11–3 o'clock with uveal tissue prolapse (green arrow) resulting in opacified and failed graft (black arrow).

CASE 20.6

CLINICAL FEATURES

A 10-year-old male was brought by his parents to the eye casualty department with complaints of watering, redness and whitish opacity in the right eye with associated diminution of vision for the past 25 days. The child had a history of fingernail injury to his eye from his elder brother. Examination findings and clinical appearance are shown in Figure 20.8.

KEY POINTS

Diagnosis:
- A diagnosis of post-fingernail trauma infective keratitis with perforation was made.

Investigations:
- Diagnosis was made based on history and clinical examination.

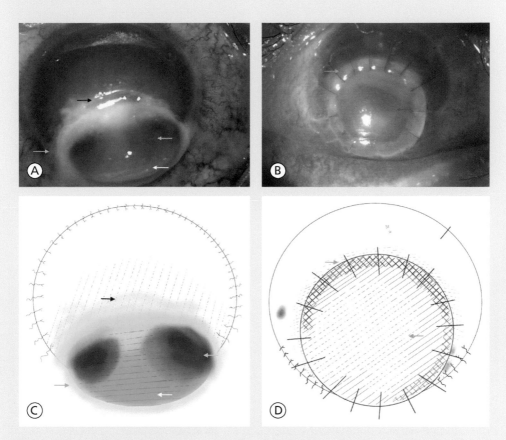

Figure 20.8 Slit lamp examination of a patient with post-fingernail trauma infective keratitis showing (A) conjunctival congestion with inferior corneal melt measuring 9×10 mm in size (green arrow) with surrounding corneal infiltrates and oedema (black arrow) with pseudocornea formation (white arrow) and iris tissue prolapse visible through the defect (yellow arrow). Postoperative slit lamp photograph of the patient reveals (B) corneal patch graft (blue arrow) with well-apposed graft-host junction and intact sutures (grey arrow) and well-formed anterior chamber. The corresponding preoperative (C) and postoperative (D) schematic diagrams illustrate the same findings.

- Bacterial culture of the corneal scrapings was suggestive of Gram-negative bacilli.
- An ultrasound B-scan was done preoperatively to rule out associated posterior segment pathology and was found to be anechoic.

Treatment:
- The patient was taken for a therapeutic patch graft under guarded visual prognosis under general anaesthesia.
- Postoperative treatment in the form of broad-spectrum fortified antibiotics (concentrated vancomycin 5% drops and concentrated tobramycin 1.3% drops were given six times a day) with topical antiglaucoma medication. Systemic antibiotics for seven days and vitamin C capsules were also given along with analgesics to the child.

Outcome:
- Postoperatively, the graft-host junction was seen to be healthy and well apposed with impaired graft clarity due to corneal oedema. Globe integrity was restored. The patient was kept on frequent follow-up visits. The host button was sent for bacterial culture and was reported to be sterile.

Supplementary Information and Additional Tips

- Any case of fingernail trauma should be managed carefully especially if the injury occurred in the setting of playing in soil or a field because of the increased chance of fingernails being contaminated.
- Fingernail injuries can also occur in adults and present as peripheral keratitis (Figure 20.9).
- Keep in mind the chance of anaerobic or Gram-negative infection, which can progress quickly with resulting ulceration and perforation if not properly managed.
- Techniques like sutureless corneal patch graft can be used in cases of perforations of 3–5 mm size with the help of tissue adhesives like fibrin–aprotinin complex along with a bandage contact lens (Figure 20.10).

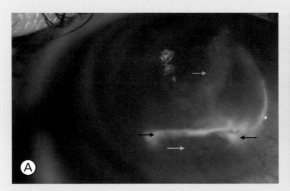
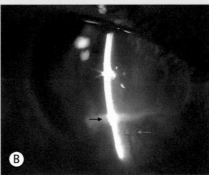

Figure 20.9 Slit lamp photograph of a patient with post-fingernail trauma with healed infective keratitis showing (A) a curvilinear leucomatous corneal scar of 7 mm (black arrows) with cojunctivalisation (yellow arrow) and macular corneal opacity (green arrow). Slit view of the same eye reveals (B) full-thickness corneal involvement (black arrow).

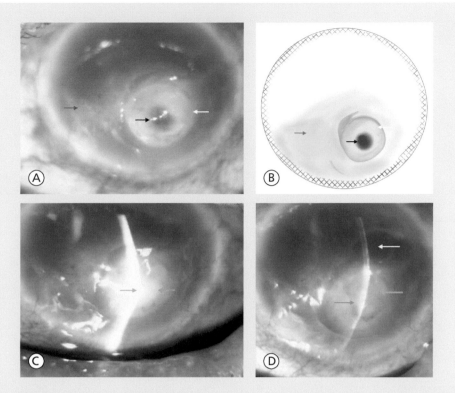

Figure 20.10 Slit lamp photograph of a case of post-traumatic infective keratitis following trauma to the eye with vegetative matter showing (A) defect of approximately 4×4 mm size with infiltrates (white arrow) and surrounding corneal oedema (blue arrow) with descemetocele formation (black arrow). The clinical findings are depicted in (B) a schematic corneal diagram. The patient was treated with (C) a sutureless corneal patch graft (green arrow) to provide tectonic support. The patch graft was held in place with the help of tissue adhesive (fibrin–aprotinin) and a bandage contact lens (grey arrow). The corneal patch (green arrow) was well adhered (D) two weeks after surgery and the resolution of infiltrates with the formation of corneal opacity (yellow arrow) and a well-formed anterior chamber (white arrow) was observed.

CASE 20.7

CLINICAL FEATURES

A 50-year-old female patient came to the emergency department with complaints of pain, redness and watering associated with diminution in vision which started a week prior when she sustained trauma to her eye from the twig of a plant while working in an agricultural field. After sustaining the trauma, she rubbed her eyes and splashed water into them but with no improvement in irritation and redness. Recorded visual acuity was 2/60 with accurate projection of rays. The examination findings and slit lamp appearance are shown in Figure 20.11.

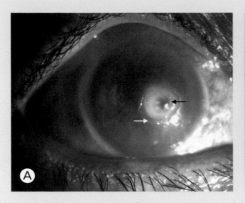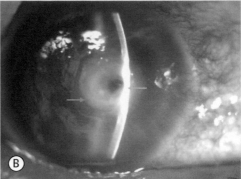

Figure 20.11   Slit lamp photograph of a patient with post-traumatic infective keratitis showing (A) corneal ulcer of size 4×3.5 mm (black arrow) with surrounding infiltrates (white arrow) and oedema with central thinning (yellow arrow). Slit illumination of the same patient (B) better shows the appreciable corneal thinning (yellow arrow) and shallow anterior chamber with surrounding corneal oedema (green arrow).

KEY POINTS

Diagnosis:

- The above scenario describes a case of left-eye post-traumatic infective keratitis.

Investigations:

- Corneal scraping was sent for both Gramstain and KOH smear examination as well as bacterial culture and sensitivity and fungal culture. The KOH smear showed the presence of hyphae and septate branching filaments under the microscope. As the patient had difficulty in cooperating for indirect ophthalmoscopic examination, an ultrasonography B-scan was done for posterior segment examination and was found to be anechoic.

Treatment:

- The patient was started on topical antifungal treatment with natamycin 5% and voriconazole 1% drops with antibiotic cover (moxifloxacin 0.5%) with antiglaucoma and cycloplegic medications. Oral vitamin C was prescribed to promote collagen synthesis and healing.

Outcome:

- Resolution of symptoms was reported with the healing of the epithelial defect along with a decrease in infiltration resulting in a leucomatous corneal opacity after four weeks of therapy. Eventual visual acuity was 6/24 in the left eye.

Supplementary Information and Additional Tips

- Proper primary management by the general practitioner with a broad-spectrum antibiotic, avoidance of topical steroids and urgent referral to an ophthalmologist should be sought in all such cases.
- Trauma to the eye with small insects is a common history obtained in some cases of corneal ulcers and needs to be treated effectively, keeping in mind the anaphylactic reaction to and additional chemical insult from the insect (Figure 20.12).

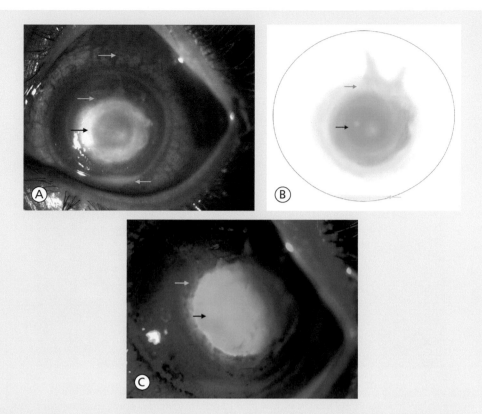

Figure 20.12 Slit lamp photograph of a case of post-traumatic (insect falling into the eye) infective keratitis in an 8-year-old male showing (A) conjunctival hyperaemia (green arrow) corneal ulcer measuring 6×5 mm (black arrow) with surrounding infiltrate of 7×6.5 mm size (grey arrow) and a hypopyon measuring 1 mm in height (yellow arrow). The corresponding schematic diagram (B) shows the same findings. On examination under cobalt blue filter (C) the epithelial defect (black arrow) with a surrounding area of infiltrates (grey arrow) is seen better after staining with fluorescein dye.

CASE 20.8

CLINICAL FEATURES

A 33-year-old male, a carpenter by profession, presented to the emergency department with a history of trauma to the eye while carving wood with complaints of pain, redness, watering and associated blurring of vision in his left eye. Examination findings and slit lamp appearance are illustrated in Figure 20.13.

KEY POINTS

Diagnosis:

■ The above clinical scenario describes a case of post-traumatic intrastromal corneal foreign body (wooden stick) with secondary infection.

Investigation:

■ Ultrasonography was done to rule out any associated posterior segment pathology and was found to be anechoic with no intraocular foreign body.

■ An X-ray orbit antero-posterior (AP) and lateral view was done to rule out any intraocular or intraorbital foreign body and none could be detected.

■ The retrieved foreign body was sent for microbiological analysis.

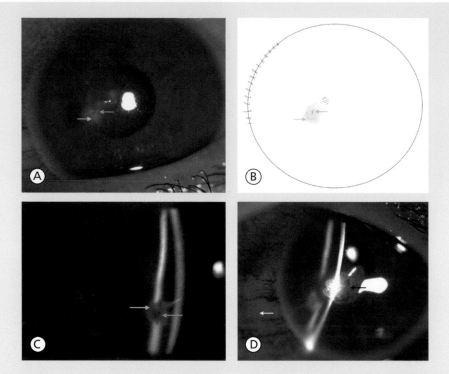

Figure 20.13 Slit lamp imagery of a patient with intrastromal corneal foreign body showing (A) a wooden foreign body embedded in anterior stroma (green arrow) along with associated nebulo-macular corneal opacity and infiltrates (yellow arrow); the same findings being depicted in a colour coded schematic diagram (B). Slit illumination clearly exhibits (C) the foreign body (green arrow) with surrounding infiltrates (yellow arrow). The foreign body was removed from the corneal stroma, leaving a site of leak due to resulting tissue defect that was sealed (D) with the help of cyanoacrylate glue (black arrow) with application of a bandage contact lens (white arrow); note the well-formed anterior chamber.

Treatment:
- Foreign body removal was done under topical anaesthesia taking all aseptic precautions with the help of an operating microscope. As there was an aqueous leak following the removal of the foreign body, the defect was sealed using a tissue adhesive (cyanoacrylate glue) with bandage contact lens (BCL) application.

Outcome:
- The patient was symptomatically better following the procedure and fared well after the removal of the BCL after two weeks.

Supplementary Information and Additional Tips

- Corneal foreign bodies are an important cause of ocular morbidity and a common workplace-related injury. Workers should be counselled on the importance of wearing protective eye gear while doing high-risk activities.
- Anterior segment optical coherence tomography imaging helps to assess the depth of penetration of a foreign body and aids in planning management. A corneal foreign body may get lodged near the corneal limbus and serve as a nidus of infection (Figure 20.14).
- Farmers are also prone to trauma to their eye with vegetative matter which lead to abrasions, but occasionally large corneal foreign bodies like a sugar cane twig may cause penetrating injury to the eye and necessitate suturing to maintain globe integrity (Figure 20.15).

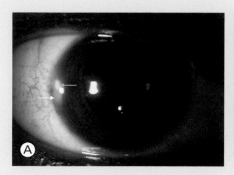

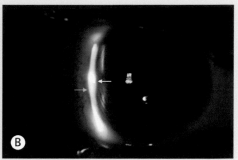

Figure 20.14 Slit lamp photograph of a patient with post-traumatic intrastromal corneal foreign body showing (A) wooden foreign body in situ (yellow arrow) with associated corneal macular opacity (white arrow). Slit illumination picture of the same patient demonstrates (B) increased reflectivity in the area of foreign body (green arrow) with macular corneal opacity (white arrow).

■ Lipid keratopathy can infrequently occur secondary to those penetrating injuries that are self-sealing in nature, so that the patient presents late to the health-care setup. Corneal thinning and vascularisation may be seen in these long-standing cases (Figure 20.16).

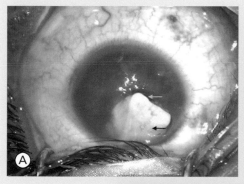

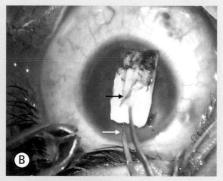

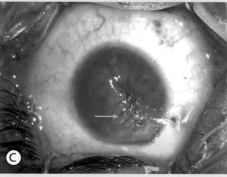

Figure 20.15 Clinical photograph of a patient who sustained agricultural trauma showing (A) sugar cane stick piercing the cornea and reaching the anterior chamber (black arrow) causing a full-thickness corneal perforation with surrounding corneal oedema (yellow arrow). The foreign body (B) was removed with forceps (white arrow) and a relatively large foreign body with iris tissue pigment (black arrow) was observed. Corneal perforation (C) was repaired with 10-0 monofilament nylon sutures (green arrow).

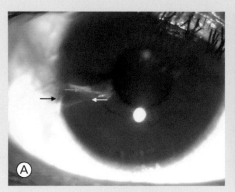
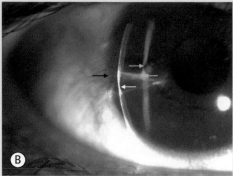

Figure 20.16 Slit lamp biomicroscopic image of post-traumatic lipid keratopathy showing (A) lipid deposits in the corneal stroma (green arrow) with associated corneal thinning (white arrow) and an area of superficial vascularisation seen near the limbal area (black arrow). Slit illumination of the same patient shows (B) corneal thinning (white arrow) which is better seen with the slit, whitish intrastromal lipid deposits (green arrow), anterior synechiae (yellow arrow) and an adjacent area of conjunctivalisation (black arrow).

CASE 20.9

CLINICAL FEATURES

A 70-year-old female patient who had undergone cataract surgery with intra ocular lens (IOL) implantation five years ago presented with a history of penetrating trauma to the eye with a cow's horn followed by the lens extruding from the eye and associated loss of vision in her left eye of one day's duration. Examination findings and clinical appearance are shown in Figure 20.17.

KEY POINTS

Diagnosis:
- The above clinical scenario describes a case of post-traumatic zone 1 open-globe injury perforating type with uveal tissue and IOL prolapse with infection.

Investigation:
- A gentle ultrasonography B-scan examination was done which showed

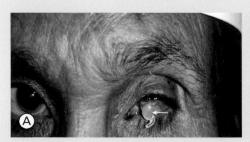
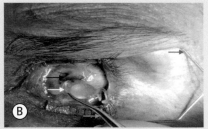

Figure 20.17 Clinical photograph of a case of a post-traumatic penetrating type of open-globe injury (cow's horn) showing (A) intra ocular lens (IOL) extrusion (white arrow). A magnified view reveals (B) the prolapsed IOL (white arrow) being removed with a pair of forceps (green arrow) and a corneal perforation with uveal tissue prolapse (black arrow) with oedematous opaque corneal tissue (yellow arrow). A wire speculum can also be seen (blue arrow) in the image which is used to keep the eyes widely open during the procedure.

mild-to-moderate amplitude spikes in the vitreous cavity suggestive of vitreous haemorrhage/vitreous exudates.

Treatment:
- The protruding IOL was removed using a pair of forceps, the corneal perforation was repaired under general anaesthesia under guarded visual prognosis and intravitreal antibiotics were administered.
- Postoperatively, broad-spectrum fortified antibiotics (concentrated vancomycin 5% drops and

concentrated tobramycin 1.3% drops) were given six times a day; cycloplegic (homatropine 2%) twice daily for two weeks, topical steroids four times a day tapered gradually over four weeks and lubricants were given.

Outcome:
- The patient was put on close follow-up and conservative management was done for the associated vitreous haemorrhage. The eye was salvaged but the vision could not be restored due to extensive damage to the ocular structures with retinal detachment.

CASE 20.10

CLINICAL FEATURES

A 30-year-old male patient presented with history of shotgun injury to his right forehead which happened four days before with complaints of diminution in vision in the right eye associated with photophobia, foreign body sensation and watering from the eye. Examination findings and slit lamp appearance are shown in Figure 20.18.

KEY POINTS

Diagnosis:
- The above scenario describes a case of shotgun injury with multiple corneal

and conjunctival pellets with corneal decompensation.

Investigations:
- Ultrasonography B-scan to rule out intraocular pellets and associated posterior segment involvement were done and found to anechoic. Non-contrast computed tomography (NCCT) head and orbit was already done from the outside and showed multiple superficial radio opaque circular foreign bodies in the scalp and forehead region.

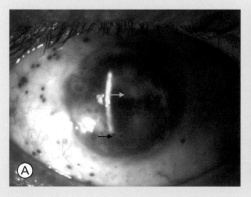 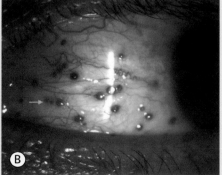

Figure 20.18 Slit lamp image in a case of shotgun injury with multiple pellet foreign body in situ showing (A) deeply embedded corneal pellets (black arrow) with associated nebulo-macular corneal opacity (yellow arrow). A magnified image (B) reveals multiple superficial conjunctival foreign bodies (grey arrow) along with deeper sub-conjunctival pellets (green arrow).

Treatment:
- The foreign bodies over the conjunctival surface and that present in the sub-conjunctival space were removed with the help of an operating microscope. The corneal pellets were embedded more deeply and could not be removed. Poor visual prognosis was explained.
- Penetrating keratoplasty was planned when the episode of acute inflammation was controlled.

Outcome:
- The patient had vision of 4/60 on follow-up visit and a definitive corneal surgery was planned.

Supplementary Information and Additional Tips
- Ocular injuries are occasionally seen with facial and cranial gunshot wound injuries that may result in permanent visual dysfunction.
- Limbal stem cell deficiency, corneal decompensation and corneal scarring may also be seen in cases of bomb-blast injury (Figure 20.19).

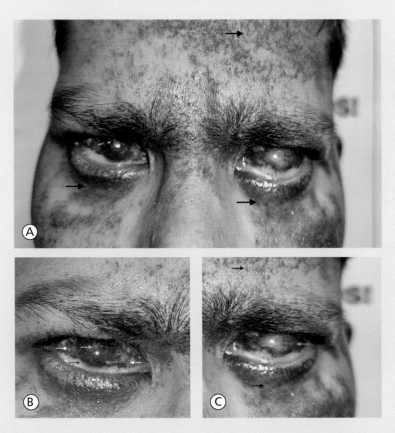

Figure 20.19 Clinical photograph of a patient who sustained a bomb-blast injury showing (A) dispersed gunpowder seen in both the palpebral apertures and in the skin over the adnexal areas and face (black arrows). The right eye shows (B) diffuse pigmentation with gunpowder deposition over the conjunctiva (white arrow) and cornea with areas of macular corneal opacity (yellow arrow) with associated limbal ischaemia (blue arrow). The left eye is more adversely affected showing (C) leucomatous corneal opacity (yellow arrow) with limbal stem cell deficiency (blue arrow) and charring of the palpebral aperture (grey arrow).

CASE 20.11

CLINICAL FEATURES

A 30-year-old male patient was brought to the emergency department with complaints of bleeding, watering and redness associated with diminution of vision in his right eye following a car-tire blast injury which happened one day prior to the presentation. There was a history of expulsion of intra ocular contents. Corneal perforation repair was done under general anaesthesia with the administration of prophylactic intravitreal antibiotic injections. Examination findings and slit lamp appearance are illustrated in (Figure 20.20).

KEY POINTS

Diagnosis:
- Post-traumatic zone 1 open-globe injury perforating type with infective keratitis.

Investigations:
- A postoperative ultrasound examination was done to rule out associated posterior segment afflictions like vitreous haemorrhage and retinal detachment.

- An X-ray orbit AP and lateral view was done to rule out the presence of an intraocular foreign body.
- Microbiological investigations were performed from corneal scrapings and vitreous tap: Gram stain, Giemsa stain, calcofluor white stain, KOH mount, bacterial culture on blood agar, fungal culture on Sabouraud dextrose agar and thioglycollate broth, and drug sensitivity testing.

Treatment:
- The patient was started on fortified antibiotics (concentrated vancomycin 5% drops and concentrated tobramycin 1.3% drops were given six times a day) with topical antiglaucoma medication. Systemic antibiotics for seven days and vitamin C 500 mg thrice a day were also given.
- Topical steroids were not started in view of a suspicion of infective keratitis.

Outcome:
- The ulcer healed with formation of a leucomatous corneal opacity after four weeks of therapy. Eventual visual

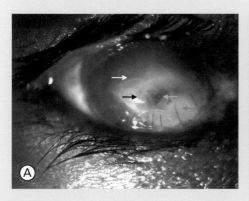
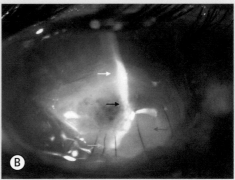

Figure 20.20 Slit lamp photograph of a patient who underwent repair of corneal perforation that resulted from a car-tyre blast injury demonstrating (A) corneal ulcer of size 6×5 mm (black arrow) with associated infiltrate measuring 7×7 mm (white arrow) with an area of abscess formation with haemorrhage in the centre (green arrow) along with repaired corneal perforation (blue arrow). Note the loose sutures (yellow arrow) that were sent for microbiological analysis. Parellopiped illumination of the same patient showing (B) area of thinning (black arrow) with associated full-thickness corneal infiltrate with surrounding corneal oedema (white arrow) and repaired corneal perforation (blue arrow) with loose sutures (yellow arrow).

acuity was finger counting close to face with accurate projection of rays.

Supplementary Information and Additional Tips

■ In such cases, when the trauma is from a highly contaminated source or a chemical injury is suspected (Figure 20.21), a polymicrobial aetiology (Gram-negative organisms like *Pseudomonas aeruginosa* and rare organisms like *Bacillus cereus*) should be kept in mind and an empirical treatment with topical broad-spectrum fortified antibiotics should be started.

■ Topical steroids should be withheld in such cases of perforation with infective keratitis after the perforation repair.

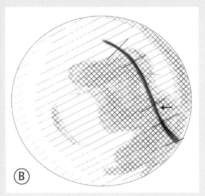

Figure 20.21 Slit lamp photograph of a patient with a post-traumatic acid injury (inverter battery blast) repaired corneoscleral perforation with healed keratitis showing (A) linear corneal perforation of 8 mm size (green arrow) repaired with 10-0 monofilament nylon (black arrow) with associated scleral perforation (yellow arrow) and leucomatous corneal opacity (grey arrow). The corresponding schematic diagram (B) depicts the same findings.

CASE 20.12

CLINICAL FEATURES

A 48-year-old female patient was brought to the emergency department with left eye pain, watering and redness associated with increase in diminution of her vision in the left eye for the past month. She gave a history of penetrating injury to both her eyes (scissor injury) three years back following which her right eye was enucleated and also gave a history of multiple lid reconstruction procedures performed in her left eye. The clinical appearance and the examination findings are shown in Figure 20.22.

KEY POINTS

Diagnosis:
■ The above clinical scenario describes a case of post-open-globe penetrating injury with right eye anophthalmos and left-eye operated lid reconstruction surgery with upper and lower lid entropion with lagophthalmos with exposure keratopathy and secondary infectious keratitis.

Investigations:
■ An ultrasound examination of the posterior segment was done to rule out associated endophthalmitis and was found to be grossly anechoic.

Treatment:
■ The patient was initially planned for corrective lid surgery to correct entropion and lagophthalmos with concurrent medical management of infective keratitis.

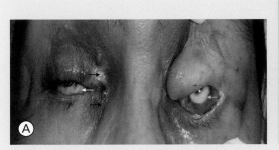
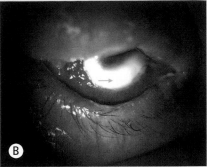

Figure 20.22 Clinical photograph of a case of bilateral penetrating injury to the eyes with the blades of a pair of scissors showing (A) scarred lids on the right side (black arrow) with an anophthalmic socket (white arrow) and the left eye of the patient shows a deformed upper lid (blue arrow) following multiple lid reconstruction procedures with loss of cilia, along with exposure keratopathy and inferior infective keratitis (yellow arrow). Slit lamp photograph of the left eye reveals (B) thickened lid margins, boggy and drooping eye lids (grey arrow), lagophthalmos, exposure keratopathy with dense corneal infiltrates (green arrow).

Outcome:

- The keratitis resolved with treatment and the patient is planned for optical keratoplasty following corrective lid surgeries by the oculoplastic surgeon.

Supplementary Information and Additional Tips

- Associated lid injuries are commonly seen in cases of polytrauma and

appropriate management of these conditions are paramount for effective management and avoidance of complications. Residual lid abnormalities like entropion, ectropion and scarring with associated lagophthalmos can lead to secondary ocular surface diseases like exposure keratopathy and infectious keratitis.

REFERENCES

1. Lin YB, Gardiner MF. Fingernail-induced corneal abrasions: case series from an ophthalmology emergency department. Cornea. 2014; 33(7):691–5.

2. Wong TY, Klein BE, Klein R. The prevalence and 5-year incidence of ocular trauma. The beaver dam eye study. Ophthalmology. 2000; 107(12):2196–202.

3. Lim BX, Koh VTC, Ray M. Microbial characteristics of post-traumatic infective keratitis. Eur J Ophthalmol. 2018; 28(1):13–8.

21 Chemical Injury

Saumya Yadav, T Monikha, Alisha Kishore, Neiwete Lomi, Radhika Tandon

INTRODUCTION

Ocular chemical burns constitute an important ophthalmic emergency which can permanently damage visual function. Alkali injuries are more frequent and cause more severe damage than acid injuries. Most cases of chemical or thermochemical injuries are seen in children and young adults and the accidents happen mainly at home, workplace or as criminal assault. Extensive damage to the ocular surface and intraocular structures caused by these injuries cause significant ocular morbidity and may require long-term care and multiple interventions for visual rehabilitation.[1] Prompt assessment of the nature and grade of injury and initiation of treatment to control corneal inflammation and infection serves as the cornerstone in determining final visual outcome in these cases.[2,3]

CASE 21.1

CLINICAL FEATURES

A 5-year-old male, accompanied by his parents, presented to the eye emergency with complaints of sudden onset of diminution of vision, watering, pain and whitish opacity in his left eye for one day. As per the parents, the child had sustained an eye injury while playing with a packet of edible 'chuna' (calcium hydroxide) paste that had burst open. Visual acuity at presentation was perception of light with accurate projection of rays in left eye and 6/6 in the right eye. Intraocular pressures were normal on digital assessment. The examination findings are shown in Figure 21.1.

KEY POINTS

Diagnosis:
- The relevant history and examination findings were consistent with the diagnosis of a case of acute grade V chemical ('chuna' particle) injury to the left eye with total limbal ischaemia.

Investigations:
- As the child was highly uncooperative for detailed ocular examination, an examination under anaesthesia (EUA) was performed. On EUA there were no signs of chemical injury in the right eye. In the left eye, inflamed conjunctiva with opaque cornea and 360° limbal ischaemia were noted.

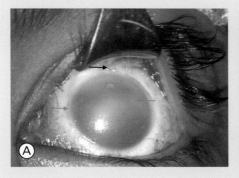 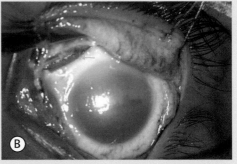

Figure 21.1 Clinical photograph of a case of acute chemical injury ('chuna' particle) showing (A) total corneal opacification (green arrow) with 360° limbal ischaemia (grey arrow), conjunctival inflammation (yellow arrow) and early symblepharon (black arrow). On double eversion of the upper lid using a Desmarres retractor (B), retained 'chuna' particles (blue arrow) can be seen in the upper fornix.

- On double eversion of the upper lid, using a Desmarres retractor, impacted 'chuna' particles were seen in the fornices.
- B-scan ultrasonography for evaluation of the posterior segment was done and was found to be anechoic.

Treatment:
- Under EUA, copious irrigation of the eye and fornices (with double eversion) with normal saline was done to remove any residual chemical and was continued till forniceal pH as measured using pH strips was normal.
- For removing impacted 'chuna' particles in the superior fornix a localised peritomy was performed and the retained particles were removed using forceps.
- The patient was managed medically using topical steroids (prednisolone acetate 1% four times a day for seven days), cycloplegic (homatropine 2% twice a day for two weeks), antibiotic (moxifloxacin 0.5% four times a day for two weeks), lubricants (carboxymethylcellulose 0.5% every two hours tapered to six times a day after a week), antiglaucoma treatment (betaxolol 0.5% twice a day), sodium citrate 10% and sodium ascorbate 10% (four times a day for one week). Oral vitamin C (250 mg twice a day for four weeks) was also given.
- Weekly sweeping of the conjunctival fornices using a moistened cotton tip applicator was advised to the parents to prevent symblepharon formation.

Outcome:
- Acute inflammation was controlled within two weeks and vision improved to 4/60. Limbal stem cell deficiency and corneal haziness were still present. Patient has been kept on close follow-up for further intervention and long-term visual rehabilitation.

Supplementary Information and Additional Tips

- The aim of treatment in a case of acute chemical injury is to reduce inflammation, promote surface epithelialisation and healing, maintain normal intraocular pressures and prevent secondary infections.

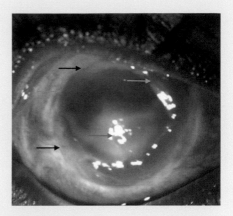

Figure 21.2 Slit lamp photograph of a 14-year-old child with grade V alkali (powdered lime) injury showing more than nine clock hours of limbal stem cell deficiency (black arrows) with a patch of healthy limbal stem cells (grey arrow), pannus (yellow arrow) and a persistent corneal epithelial defect (green arrow).

- 'Chuna' (calcium hydroxide) is an important cause of chemical injury in the paediatric age group and causes severe alkali burns to the eye with corneal melting and opacification (Figure 21.2).
- Depending upon the force of impact and form of 'chuna' (liquid/paste/ powder), 'chuna' particles often get impacted in the sub-conjunctival space forming a depot, resulting in persistent inflammation and continued damage (Figure 21.3).

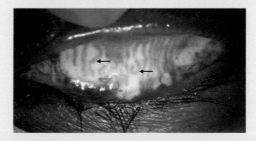

Figure 21.3 External photograph of a case of 'chuna' particle injury with impacted 'chuna' (green arrows) in the superior sub-conjunctival space with overlying conjunctival blanching resulting in visualisation of the meibomian gland ducts (black arrows).

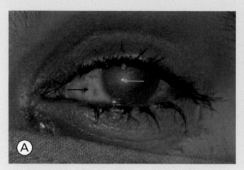 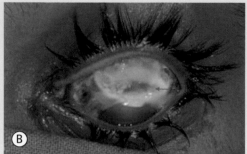

Figure 21.4 External photograph of a case of acute alkali ('chuna' particle) injury showing (A) diffuse conjunctival congestion (black arrow), 360° limbal ischaemia and total corneal haze (yellow arrow). On downgaze (B), impacted 'chuna' particle (green arrow) can be seen in the superior fornix.

- It is important to double evert the lids using a Desmarres retractor to look for any retained 'chuna' particles in the fornices as found in this case.
- Lime particles may also get impacted in the sclera and in some cases the posterior limit of the impacted material may not be seen on routine examination (Figure 21.4), hence surgical EUA is recommended.

CASE 21.2

CLINICAL FEATURES

A 24-year-old male presented to the eye emergency with complaints of sudden onset pain, redness, diminution of vision and burning sensation in his right eye of two days duration. He gave a history of an accidental fall of household cleaning agent into his right eye two days previously. Visual acuity of 6/36 in his right eye was recorded and on examination conjunctival congestion with epithelial defect was noted with no associated limbal ischaemia (Figure 21.5).

KEY POINTS

Diagnosis:
- The above clinical presentation is consistent with the diagnosis of a case of acute, grade III chemical injury.

Investigations:
- No additional investigations were performed.

Treatment:
- An immediate, thorough saline wash was given to remove any residual chemical from the eye.
- Patient was managed medically with topical steroids (prednisolone acetate 1% four times a day for seven days), cycloplegic (homatropine 2% twice a day for two weeks), antibiotic (moxifloxacin 0.5% four times a day for two weeks), antiglaucoma medication (timolol 0.5% twice a day) lubricants (carboxymethylcellulose 0.5% six times a day), sodium citrate 10% and sodium ascorbate 10% (four times a day for one week).

Outcome:
- The epithelial defect healed with residual nebular corneal opacity within one month and the patient attained best corrected visual acuity of 6/12.

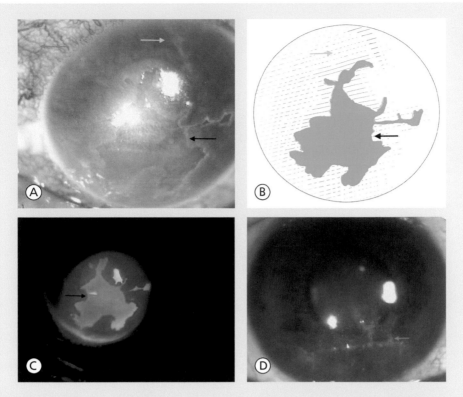

Figure 21.5 Slit lamp photograph of a case of acute chemical injury showing (A) conjunctival congestion (green arrow) with corneal epithelial defect (black arrow) and surrounding corneal haze (yellow arrow). The schematic corneal diagram (B) depicts the same findings of acute chemical injury. The epithelial defect is delineated on viewing (C) under a cobalt blue filter after staining with sodium fluorescein dye (black arrow). The epithelial defect healed (D) with residual mild nebular corneal opacity within one month of medical management (grey arrow).

Supplementary Information and Additional Tips

- Mild cases of chemical injury, especially if not complicated by limbal ischaemia, usually heal completely without causing significant damage to visual function, especially with timely and adequate management.

CASE 21.3

CLINICAL FEATURES

A 28-year-old male presented to the ophthalmic outpatient department 12 days after sustaining injury with battery acid to his left eye while working. Prior to presentation he had been receiving treatment at a different hospital. His visual acuity in the left eye was 6/24. Slit lamp appearance and examination findings are demonstrated in Figure 21.6.

KEY POINTS

Diagnosis:

- The clinical scenario is that of a partially treated grade IV chemical injury with partial limbal ischaemia.

Investigations:

- No additional investigations were performed.

321

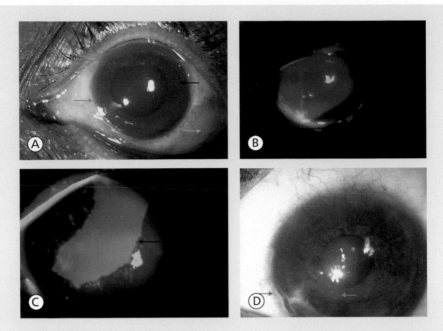

Figure 21.6 Slit lamp photograph depicting (A) conjunctival congestion (yellow arrow), corneal epithelial defect (black arrow) and limbal ischaemia (green arrow) in a case of acute chemical injury. Epithelial defect can be seen clearly under (B) cobalt blue filter after staining with sodium fluorescein dye (black arrow). A decrease in size of the epithelial defect (C) is noted after five days of medical management. Following four months of medical management, the inflammatory process resolved completely (D) with residual mild nebular corneal opacity (grey arrow) and partial limbal stem cell deficiency (green arrow).

Treatment:
- Patient was medically managed with topical steroids (prednisolone acetate 1% four times a day for seven days), cycloplegic (homatropine 2% twice a day for two weeks), antibiotic (moxifloxacin 0.5% four times a day for two weeks), lubricants (carboxymethylcellulose 0.5% six times a day) and antiglaucoma medication (timolol 0.5% and brimonidine 0.2% twice a day). Sodium citrate 10% and sodium ascorbate 10% (four times a day for one week) were started along with oral vitamin C (500 mg thrice a day for four weeks).

Outcome:
- After four months of medical management, the epithelial defect resolved completely, leaving behind a mild nebular corneal opacity. Partial limbal stem cell deficiency ensued in two quadrants. Patient attained best corrected visual acuity of 6/12.

CASE 21.4

CLINICAL FEATURES

A 30-year-old male, an industrial worker by occupation, presented with sudden onset redness, decrease of vision, watering and pain in the left eye following an accidental injury to the left eye with hot molten aluminium at his workplace on the previous day. On examination, the vision in the left eye was perception of light with accurate projection of rays. Examination findings and slit lamp appearance are illustrated in Figure 21.7.

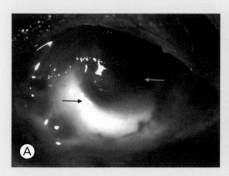 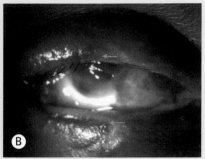

Figure 21.7 Slit lamp photograph of a case of acute thermochemical injury (molten aluminium) demonstrating (A) diffuse conjunctival congestion and chemosis (grey arrow) with inferior limbal ischaemia (black arrow) and corresponding inferior corneal epithelial defect (green arrow). Note (B) the superior and inferior lid burns and singed eyelashes (yellow arrows).

KEY POINTS

Diagnosis:

- The clinical scenario describes a case of acute thermochemical injury with localised limbal ischaemia due to a workplace accident.

Investigations:

- The clinical diagnosis was based on history and examination.
- B-scan ultrasonography to rule out any posterior segment pathology was done and found to be anechoic.

Treatment:

- Copious irrigation with isotonic saline was done before starting topical medications.
- Topical steroids (prednisolone acetate 1% four times a day for seven days), cycloplegic (homatropine 2% twice a day for two weeks), antibiotic (moxifloxacin 0.5% four times a day for two weeks), lubricants (carboxymethylcellulose 0.5% every two hours and vitamin A-carbomer ointment at night), antiglaucoma therapy (timolol 0.5% and brimonidine 0.2% twice a day) and sodium citrate 10% and sodium ascorbate 10% (four times a day for one week) were started along with oral vitamin C (500 mg thrice a day for four weeks) and oral doxycycline (100 mg twice a day for two weeks).
- An amniotic membrane transplantation was performed after a week of medical management.

Outcome:

- The inflammation was controlled in two weeks with complete healing of the corneal epithelial defect. Visual acuity improved to 5/60. Patient has been kept on close follow-up for further management of limbal stem cell deficiency.

Supplementary Information and Additional Tips

- Workplace chemical burns (industrial chemicals and molten metals) can cause severe damage to ocular structures due to a combination of chemical injury, thermal assault and mechanical trauma and may lead to eyelid burns, corneal and/or scleral melt with uveal tissue prolapse (Figure 21.8) and

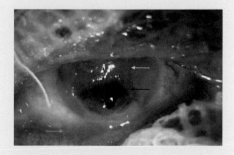

Figure 21.8 Slit lamp photograph of a case of acute thermochemical injury showing diffuse conjunctival congestion and chemosis (green arrow) with inferior corneal melt and exposure of underlying uveal tissue (black arrow) with surrounding oedematous cornea (yellow arrow).

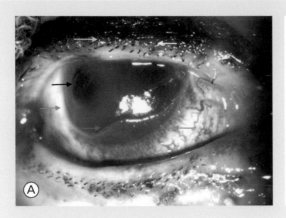
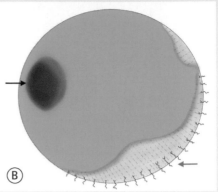

Figure 21.9 Slit lamp photograph of a case of acute thermochemical injury with molten metal showing (A) superficial lid burns (yellow arrow), ciliary congestion (blue arrow), near total epithelial defect (green arrow), corneal thinning (black arrow), nasal area of limbal ischaemia (grey arrow) and trimmed eyelashes (white arrow). The corresponding schematic diagram (B) demonstrates the same findings.

non-healing epithelial defects with corneal thinning and descemetocele formation (Figure 21.9).

- The compromised ocular surface in patients with ocular chemical injuries is prone to secondary infection due to direct invasion of microbes with contaminated chemicals (Figure 21.10) or due to associated eyelid abnormalities and trichiasis in these cases (Figure 21.11), worsening the prognosis.

- Chemical injuries may result in corneal melting and perforations with infective keratitis. Techniques like sutureless corneal patch graft can be used in cases of descemetocele or perforations of 3–5 mm size with the help of tissue adhesives like fibrin-aprotinin complex along with a bandage contact lens. The graft provides tectonic support and promotes healing eventually resulting in a vascularised corneal scar (Figure 21.12).

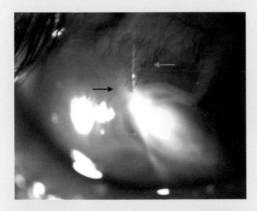

Figure 21.10 Slit lamp photograph of a case of infective keratitis that developed in a patient following acute thermochemical injury showing superficial corneal vascularisation (grey arrow), corneal infiltrates with associated corneal thinning (yellow arrow) and surrounding corneal opacification (black arrow).

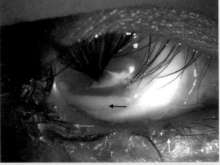

Figure 21.11 Slit lamp photograph of a patient with secondary infective keratitis following injury to his right eye with a liquid disinfecting agent (phenyl). Mild inferior lid burns with singeing of eyelashes (white arrow), crusting and matting of eyelashes (yellow arrow), upper lid trichiasis, corneal infiltrates (grey arrow) with diffuse haze along with a hypopyon (black arrow) can be seen.

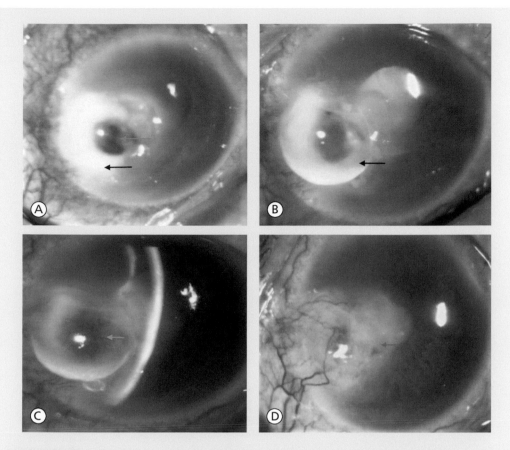

Figure 21.12 Slit lamp photograph of a patient with secondary infective keratitis following alkali injury showing (A) corneal infiltrates (black arrow) with perforation (grey arrow). A sutureless corneal patch graft (B) secured with fibrin glue was performed to promote healing and provide tectonic support (black arrow). At 1.5 months of follow-up (C), a significant reduction in infiltrates and the formation of a frond of vessels (yellow arrow) with a well-formed anterior chamber, seen on slit view, were noted. The corneal ulcer healed completely (D) with formation of a vascularised, leucomatous corneal opacity (green arrow) that was seen three months after the surgery.

CASE 21.5

CLINICAL FEATURES

A 21-year-old male painter presented to the eye casualty department with complaints of sudden onset pain, diminution of vision and redness in his left eye for five days. He gave a history of a fall of whitewash solution into his left eye five days prior for which he had received irrigation and topical treatment at another hospital. On presentation his visual acuity was 5/60. Examination findings and slit lamp appearance are illustrated in Figure 21.13.

KEY POINTS

Diagnosis:
- The clinical scenario describes a case of acute grade IV chemical injury caused by an alkaline agent.

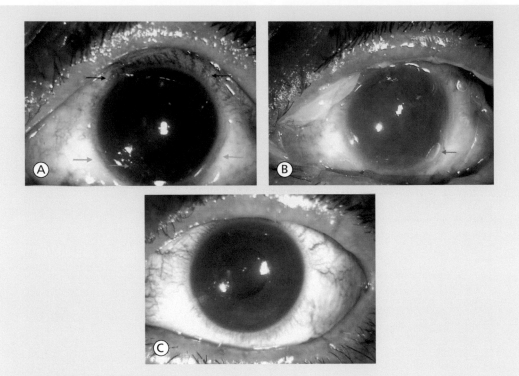

Figure 21.13 Slit lamp photograph of the left eye of a patient with chemical injury showing (A) circumcorneal congestion (black arrows), epithelial defect (grey arrow) and limbal ischaemia in inferonasal and inferotemporal quadrants (yellow arrows). An amniotic membrane graft (B) can be seen in situ (green arrow), which led to (C) complete healing of the epithelial defect one month following the injury.

Investigations:
- Forniceal pH was assessed using pH strips and was found to be within normal range. No further investigations were performed.

Treatment:
- The patient was initially started on topical steroids (prednisolone acetate 1% four times a day for seven days), cycloplegic (homatropine 2% twice a day for two weeks), antibiotic (moxifloxacin 0.5% four times a day for two weeks), lubricants (carboxymethylcellulose 0.5% six times a day), antiglaucoma therapy (timolol 0.5% and brimonidine 0.2% twice a day), sodium citrate 10% and sodium ascorbate 10% (four times a day for one week) along with oral vitamin C (500 mg thrice a day for four weeks) and carbomer ointment at night.
- Due to a non-healing epithelial defect, an amniotic membrane

transplantation (AMT) was performed on the eighth day after presentation.

Outcome:
- Following one month of the AMT, the epithelial defect healed completely and the patient achieved a best corrected visual acuity of 6/9.

Supplementary Information and Additional Tips

- An amniotic membrane graft (AMG) acts as a therapeutic bandage in the management of acute chemical injuries. It reduces the severity of inflammation and promotes re-epithelisation (Figure 21.14). Rarely, a secondary infection following AMT may occur resulting in severe infective keratitis with dense vascularisation, resulting in poor visual outcome (Figure 21.15).

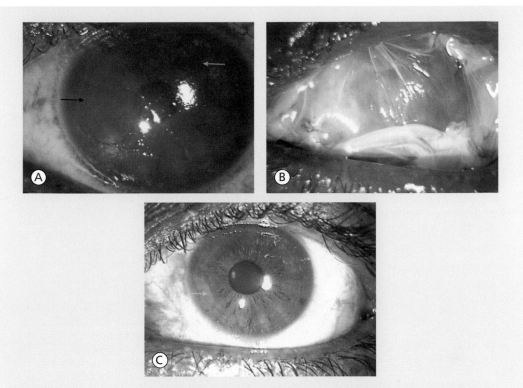

Figure 21.14 Slit lamp photograph of a case of chemical injury showing (A) conjunctival congestion (green arrow) with corneal epithelial defect (black arrow) and surrounding corneal oedema (grey arrow). (B) Amniotic membrane transplantation (yellow arrow) was done for the non-healing epithelial defect. The epithelial defect (C) had healed completely after one month with minimal residual scarring (blue arrow).

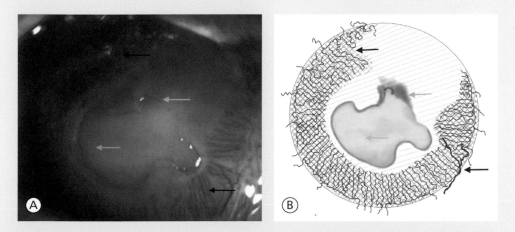

Figure 21.15 Slit lamp photograph of a case of secondary infective keratitis following amniotic membrane transplantation for acute chemical injury, showing (A) a large epithelial defect with amniotic graft melt (green arrow), corneal infiltrates (yellow arrow) and intense superficial vascularisation (black arrows). The corresponding schematic diagram (B) shows the same findings.

CASE 21.6

CLINICAL FEATURES

A 58-year-old male presented with complaints of sudden onset diminution of vision in both eyes following an accidental splash of chemical at his workplace. On examination, his vision was 2/60 in the right eye and 1/60 in the left eye. The examination findings and slit lamp appearance are described in Figure 21.16.

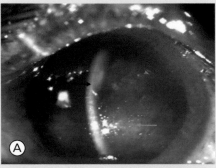

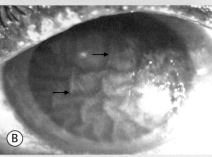

Figure 21.16 Slit lamp photographs of a patient with bilateral chemical injury with toxic endotheliitis depicting (A) total epithelial defect with moderate corneal oedema (yellow arrow) and several Descemet's folds (black arrow) in the right eye and (B) total epithelial defect and cobblestone keratopathy with marked Descemet's membrane folds due to endothelial decompensation (black arrows) in the left eye.

KEY POINTS

Diagnosis:
- The clinical scenario describes a case of bilateral chemical injury presenting as toxic endotheliitis with corneal oedema.

Investigations:
- A B-scan ultrasound was done to look for any posterior segment pathology and was found to be anechoic.

Treatment:
- An immediate bilateral copious irrigation of the eye was done to remove any residual chemical.
- The patient was started on bilateral topical steroids (prednisolone acetate 1% four times a day for seven days), cycloplegic (homatropine 2% twice a day for two weeks), antibiotic (moxifloxacin 0.5% four times a day for two weeks), lubricants (carboxymethylcellulose 0.5% six times a day), antiglaucoma therapy (timolol 0.5% and brimonidine 0.2% twice a day), sodium citrate 10% and sodium ascorbate 10% (four times a day for one week) along with oral vitamin C (500 mg thrice a day for four weeks) and oral doxycycline (100 mg twice a day for two weeks).

Outcome:
- The corneal oedema resolved completely in the right eye and complete epithelialisation was achieved after four weeks.
- The left eye sustained irreversible endothelial injury resulting in long-term endothelial decompensation. Hence, the patient was scheduled for endothelial keratoplasty for visual rehabilitation.

CASE 21.7

CLINICAL FEATURES

An 11-year-old male presented to the ocular emergency with complaints of sudden onset pain, redness and diminution of vision. He gave a history of sustaining a firecracker injury the previous day. On presentation, his visual acuity was 6/60 in the right eye and 6/9 in the left eye. Dilated fundus examination did not reveal any associated fundus pathology. Examination findings and slit lamp appearance are illustrated in Figure 21.17.

KEY POINTS

Diagnosis:
- The clinical scenario describes a case of post-firecracker (thermochemical) injury with facial burns and focal endothelial oedema.

Investigations:
- The diagnosis was established on the basis of history and clinical examination.
- No additional investigations were performed.

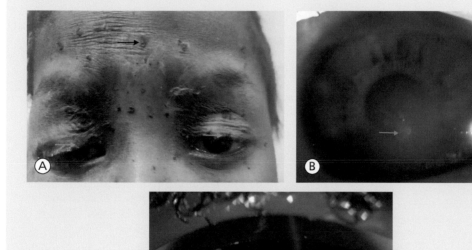

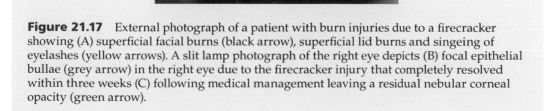

Figure 21.17 External photograph of a patient with burn injuries due to a firecracker showing (A) superficial facial burns (black arrow), superficial lid burns and singeing of eyelashes (yellow arrows). A slit lamp photograph of the right eye depicts (B) focal epithelial bullae (grey arrow) in the right eye due to the firecracker injury that completely resolved within three weeks (C) following medical management leaving a residual nebular corneal opacity (green arrow).

Treatment:

- Immediate copious irrigation of the eye with normal saline was done.
- Medical management was started with topical steroids (prednisolone acetate 1% four times a day for seven days), cycloplegic (homatropine 2% twice a day for two weeks), antibiotic (moxifloxacin 0.5% four times a day for two weeks), lubricants (carboxymethylcellulose 0.5% six times a day), antiglaucoma therapy (timolol 0.5% and brimonidine 0.2% twice a day), sodium citrate 10% and sodium ascorbate 10% (four times a day for one week). In view of the focal endothelial oedema, topical hypertonic saline (5% four times a day and 6% ointment at night) was prescribed to the patient.

Outcome:

- The focal endothelial oedema resolved completely within three weeks without any residual scarring and the patient attained a best corrected visual acuity of 6/6.

Supplementary Information and Additional Tips

- Firecrackers can result in mechanical, chemical and thermal injuries to the eye. These injuries are very common among children and cause significant morbidity. Secondary infection may occur in repaired corneoscleral perforations resulting from the sudden force and mechanical impact of firecracker injuries (Figure 21.18), that are associated with a poor prognosis.

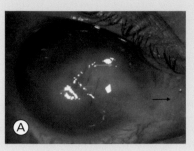

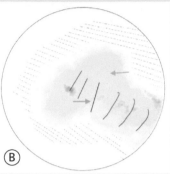

Figure 21.18 Slit lamp photograph of a case of a post-firecracker injury repaired corneoscleral perforation that presented with secondary infection. The clinical picture reveals (A) corneal infiltrates (yellow arrow) with corneal (green arrow) and scleral sutures (black arrow) to seal the perforation occurring due to the impact of the injury. The corresponding schematic corneal diagram (B) depicts the same findings.

- Firecracker injuries may also result in unusual presentations such as corneal cyst with endothelial involvement and Descemet's folds (Figure 21.19) due to the focal, high impact nature of firecracker injuries.

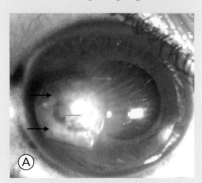

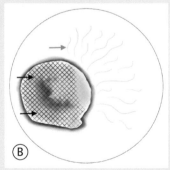

Figure 21.19 Slit lamp photograph (A) and corresponding schematic diagram (B) of a patient with a firecracker (thermochemical) injury showing corneal cyst (black arrows) with overlying pigmentation (yellow arrow) and Descemet's membrane folds (grey arrow).

CASE 21.8

CLINICAL FEATURES

A 56-year-old male patient presented to the outpatient department with complaints of pain and diminution of vision in both eyes following accidental trauma with molten metal at his workplace seven days ago. He gave a prior history of undergoing AMT and lid laceration repair in his right eye at another hospital. His visual acuity at presentation was hand movements close to face with accurate projection of rays in the right eye and 6/24 in the left eye. Examination findings and slit lamp appearance of his right eye are illustrated in Figure 21.20.

KEY POINTS

Diagnosis:
- The clinical scenario describes a case of bilateral thermochemical injury with right eye sutured AMG with corneoscleral thinning.

Investigations:
- Posterior segment assessment with B-scan ultrasound did not reveal any pathology.

Treatment:
- Emergency tectonic sclero-keratoplasty was performed due to significant thinning of the cornea, limbal ischaemia and thinned out friable scleral tissue.

- The postoperative regimen included topical steroids (prednisolone acetate 1% four times a day), antibiotic (moxifloxacin 0.5% four times a day), lubricants (carboxymethylcellulose 0.5% six times a day), cycloplegic (homatropine 2% twice a day for two weeks), antiglaucoma therapy (timolol 0.5% and brimonidine 0.2% twice a day), along with systemic corticosteroids and oral antibiotic therapy.

Outcome:
- At the two-month follow-up the patient achieved best corrected visual acuity of 3/60 and is currently under close follow-up for further intervention and long-term visual rehabilitation.

Supplementary Information and Additional Tips

- Acute chemical/thermochemical injuries can often lead to significant corneal thinning (Figure 21.21), which, depending upon the severity, is managed by increased topical lubrication, autologous serum drops, therapeutic bandage contact lenses, multi-layered AMT, lamellar corneal patch graft or tectonic keratoplasty.

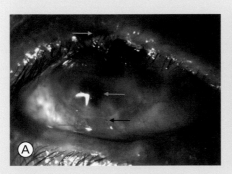 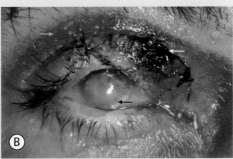

Figure 21.20 Slit lamp photograph of a patient with acute thermochemical (molten metal) injury with (A) sutured amniotic membrane graft (black arrow). Singed eyelashes (yellow arrow), inferior corneal (grey arrow) and scleral (green arrow) thinning can be seen. Slit lamp photograph (B) on the first postoperative day following eccentric tectonic sclero-keratoplasty demonstrates a well-sutured corneal graft (black arrow) with amniotic membrane overlay, appreciated better on the lower eyelid (green arrow). Charred eyelid (white arrow), singed eyelashes (yellow arrow) and periorbital ecchymosis (blue arrow) can also be seen.

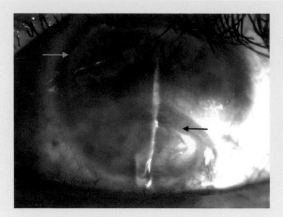

Figure 21.21 Slit lamp photograph of a patient of acute acid injury showing diffuse conjunctival congestion, inferior corneal thinning (black arrow) and an inferiorly decentred bandage contact lens (grey arrow), placed unsuccessfully to provide tectonic support.

CASE 21.9

CLINICAL FEATURES

A 25-year-old male presented with sudden decrease of vision, watering, redness and pain in the left eye after enduring a blast injury at his workplace five days previously. He also gave a history of undergoing penetrating keratoplasty for a corneal scar due to healed keratitis two years ago. The patient's records showed that he had good vision in both eyes prior to injury. On examination, his best corrected vision in the right eye was 6/12 and perception of light with accurate projection of rays in the left eye. Examination findings and clinical appearance are illustrated in Figure 21.22.

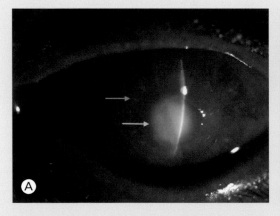
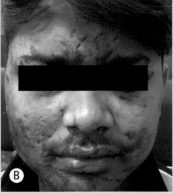

Figure 21.22 Slit lamp photograph of a patient with a thermochemical (blast) injury (A) who developed infective keratitis in a previously operated full-thickness graft; note the diffuse conjunctival congestion (black arrow) with a 7×6 mm corneal ulcer and surrounding infiltrates (yellow arrow). The graft-host junction and suture marks (green arrow) can also be seen. External face photograph of the patient (B) shows multiple abrasions and lacerations due to the blast injury (grey arrows).

KEY POINTS

Diagnosis:
- The clinical scenario describes a case of acute thermochemical (blast) injury with infective keratitis in a patient with operated penetrating keratoplasty.

Investigations:
- Corneal scraping samples were sent for Gram and KOH stains and for bacterial and fungal cultures but no specific organism was isolated.
- B-scan ultrasound revealed no coexisting posterior segment pathology.

Treatment:
- The patient was managed medically with topical concentrated antibiotics (vancomycin 5% every hour and tobramycin 1.3% every hour tapered gradually over four weeks according to clinical response), cycloplegic (homatropine 2% four times a day for two weeks) and preservative-free lubricants (carboxymethylcellulose 0.5% six times a day).
- In addition, oral doxycycline (100 mg twice a day) and vitamin C (500 mg QID) were also prescribed.

Outcome:
- The patient showed a good response to medical management within the first week; fortified antibiotics were accordingly tapered.
- The ulcer healed in about four weeks leaving behind a residual leucomatous corneal opacity.

CASE 21.10

CLINICAL FEATURES

A 14-year-old female presented to the cornea clinic of a tertiary eye care hospital with complaints of pain, poor vision and foreign body sensation. She gave a history of sustaining bilateral chemical injury two years ago following which she had undergone right-eye, full-thickness tectonic keratoplasty. At presentation her visual acuity in the right eye was hand movements close to face with accurate projection of rays and perception of light with inaccurate projection of light in the left eye. Examination findings and slit lamp appearance are illustrated in Figure 21.23.

KEY POINTS

Diagnosis:
- The clinical scenario describes a case of bilateral post-chemical-injury sequelae with 360° limbal stem cell deficiency with right eye operated tectonic keratoplasty and graft melt.

Investigations:
- Diagnosis was based on the history and clinical examination.
- Posterior segment assessment on B-scan ultrasonography was normal in the right eye while it revealed optic nerve head cupping in the left eye.

Treatment:
- An emergency tectonic keratoplasty was performed in the right eye.
- Postoperative regimen of topical steroids (prednisolone acetate 1% four times a day), antibiotic (moxifloxacin 0.5% four times a day), cycloplegic (homatropine 2% four times a day for two weeks) and lubricants (carboxymethylcellulose 0.5% six times a day) was started.
- Antiglaucoma therapy was started in the left eye. No surgical intervention was planned in the left eye due to poor visual potential.

Outcome:
- On follow-up, successful anatomic restoration was achieved with best corrected visual acuity of 2/60 in the right eye.

Supplementary Information and Additional Tips
- Healthy limbal stem cells are a prerequisite for early epithelialisation

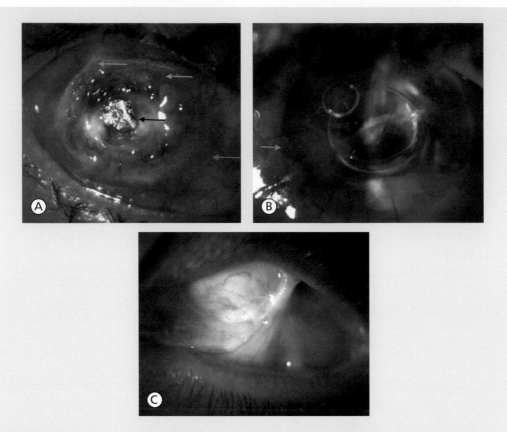

Figure 21.23 Slit lamp photograph of a case of post-chemical-injury sequelae showing (A) operated tectonic penetrating keratoplasty with 360° limbal stem cell deficiency with graft melt (black arrow). Sutures of keratoplasty (yellow arrows) and ciliary congestion (green arrow) can be seen. An emergency full-thickness tectonic keratoplasty (grey arrow) (B) was performed. Examination of the left eye shows (C) features of post-chemical-injury sequelae with inferior large symblepharon (blue arrow).

and hence, success of the corneal grafts. Limbal stem cell deficiency is often an unavoidable complication of chemical injury. Other late complications include corneal scarring, dry eyes, symblepharon formation (Figure 21.24), ankyloblepharon, glaucoma and lid abnormalities.

■ Rarely, a neurotrophic ulcer may develop following ocular chemical trauma (Figure 21.25) and is managed with topical preservative-free artificial tears, soft bandage contact lenses/ patching, topical autologous serum or umbilical cord serum and AMG in non-responding cases.

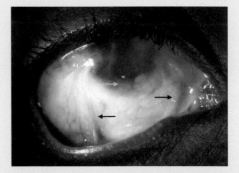

Figure 21.24 Slit lamp photograph of a patient with post-chemical-injury sequelae showing inferior and nasal symblepharon (black arrows) with at least 270° limbal stem cell deficiency (green arrow).

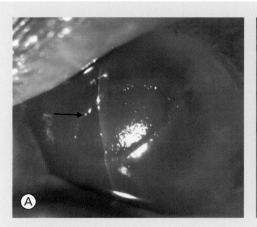 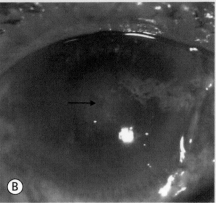

Figure 21.25 Slit lamp photograph of a case of post-alkali injury demonstrating (A) central neurotrophic ulcer (black arrow) with heaped-up margins. The ulcer (B) significantly decreased in size (black arrow) within three weeks of treatment with topical autologous serum.

REFERENCES

1. Singh P, Tyagi M, Kumar Y, Gupta KK, Sharma PD. Ocular chemical injuries and their management. Oman J Ophthalmol. 2013 May; 6(2):83–6.
2. Eslani M, Baradaran-Rafii A, Movahedan A, Djalilian AR. The ocular surface chemical burns. J Ophthalmol. 2014; 2014:196827.
3. McGhee CNJ, Crawford AZ, Meyer JJ, Patel DV. Chapter 94. Chemical and Thermal Injuries of the Eye. In: Cornea; Volume 1 – Fundamentals, Diagnosis and Management. 4th ed. USA: Elsevier; 2017; 1106–19.

22 Crystalline Keratopathy

Aishwarya Rathod, Ritika Mukhija, Radhika Tandon

INTRODUCTION

Crystalline keratopathy is an important clinical entity in which crystalline deposits are noted in the cornea; it can occur secondary to a variety of causes including infections, systemic diseases and even topical medications. Infectious crystalline keratopathy (ICK), the commonest variant, is a rare, indolent corneal infection that results in greyish-white and branching stromal opacities with minimal anterior chamber or corneal inflammation. The most common risk factors for ICK include a history of penetrating keratoplasty and the associated use of topical steroids. ICK has also been reported with the use of contact lens wear and topical anaesthetic, and following lamellar keratoplasty, corneal relaxing incisions, laser in situ keratomileusis (LASIK) and cataract surgery.[1,2]

CASE 22.1

CLINICAL FEATURES

A 52-year-old male with a prior history of sclerokeratitis in the left eye presented with pain, photophobia, watering and diminution of vision for the last ten days. There was no history of any ocular trauma or use of contact lens. Examination findings and slit lamp appearance are illustrated in Figure 22.1.

KEY POINTS

Diagnosis:
- The above clinical scenario describes a case of ICK in a patient with healed sclerokeratitis.

Investigations:
- The mainstay of investigations includes corneal scrape sampling for Gram stain, KOH mount and microbiological culture with drug sensitivity.
- In vivo confocal microscopy (IVCM) and polymerase chain reaction (PCR) can be done as useful adjuncts.

Treatment:
- The patient was empirically treated with topical fortified cefazolin (5%) six times a day, topical fortified tobramycin (1.3%) six times a day, cycloplegic (homatropine hydrobromide 2% four times a day), and lubricants (preservative-free carboxymethylcellulose 0.5% six times a day). After a negative fungal culture report, topical fluorometholone drops were also administered from the fifth day.

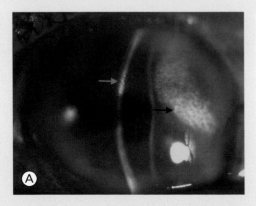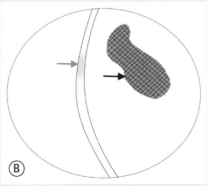

Figure 22.1 Slit lamp photograph of the left eye (A) and corresponding corneal diagram (B) of a patient with infectious crystalline keratopathy showing crystalline branching opacity (black arrow) and stromal deposition of the crystals in the overlying slit (grey arrow).

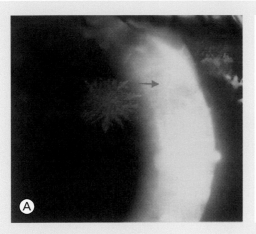
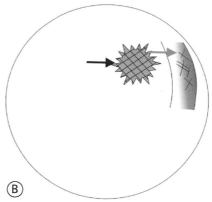

Figure 22.2 Slit lamp photograph of a patient (A) and corresponding corneal diagram (B) of a patient with infectious crystalline keratopathy showing arborising, needle-like branching with a characteristic snowflake pattern (black arrow) along with white-grey crystalline deposits in the anterior to middle stroma (grey arrow).

Outcome:

- The stromal infiltrate cleared within two weeks and the keratopathy resolved with treatment within a month following which the topical antibiotics were stopped and steroids gradually tapered.

Supplementary Information and Additional Tips

- The most common risk factors for ICK include a history of penetrating keratoplasty and the associated use of topical steroids; peripheral crystalline keratopathy, as in this case, is a rare sequel of sclerokeratitis.[3]
- Typical cases may reveal the presence of an arborising, needle-like branching with a characteristic snowflake pattern (Figure 22.2).
- The clinical response to pharmacological treatment can be poor and may require prolonged application of antibiotic therapies with refractive/contact lens correction or lamellar/penetrating keratoplasty for management.

CASE 22.2

CLINICAL FEATURES

A 7-year-old male was referred to our outpatient department with severe photophobia and decreased visual acuity in both eyes for the past week. He had been diagnosed with nephropathic cystinosis at the age of 4 years and was on systemic treatment for the same. Examination findings, slit lamp appearance and confocal imaging scans are illustrated in Figures 22.3.

KEY POINTS

Diagnosis:

- The above clinical scenario describes a case of bilateral crystalline keratopathy with conjunctival crystalline deposits in a patient with nephropathic cystinosis.

Investigations:

- IVCM was performed (Figure 22.4), which revealed numerous, discrete, hyperreflective, needle-like crystals in the corneal stroma.

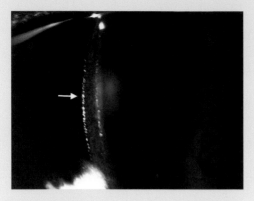

Figure 22.3 Slit lamp photograph of the right eye of a patient with nephropathic cystinosis and crystalline keratopathy showing anterior- to mid-stromal crystalline deposits diffusely present in the slit section with an overlying intact epithelium (white arrow).

- Apart from IVCM, a multitude of investigations can aid in the diagnosis including anterior segment optical coherence tomography (ASOCT), transmission electron microscopy (TEM) and light microscopy (following keratoplasty).

- A gene analysis can also be done to identify the mutation.

Treatment:
- The patient was managed with topical cysteamine bitartarate drops six times a day and lubricants along with ongoing course of oral cysteamine for the systemic disease.

Outcome:
- The patient responded to treatment and had a significant reduction in photophobia with gradual disappearance of the crystals from the cornea and conjunctiva.

Supplementary Information and Additional Tips

- The cystine crystals are polychromatic and demonstrate maximum density in the peripheral cornea but are usually present throughout the anterior stroma.[4]
- The amount of these crystals does not correlate with the symptoms of the disease.
- Ocular cystinosis may be the first presenting feature of this disease and it is imperative to refer the patient to a primary care physician for definitive management.

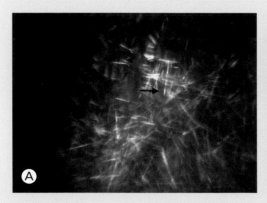
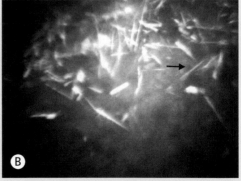

Figure 22.4 Confocal microscopy images of the right and left eye (A and B) of the above patient demonstrating multiple, needle-like, thin, linear and hyperreflective objects (black arrows) in anterior- and mid-stroma crisscrossing each other at all levels.

CASE 22.3

CLINICAL FEATURES

A 42-year-old male presented to our emergency department with a history of diminution of vision, watering and photophobia in his right eye for the past four days. The patient also gave a history of an ocular trauma to the right eye with an iron particle while welding at the factory five days prior. The patient was prescribed topical fortified antibiotics, lubricants and oral non-steroidal anti-inflammatory drugs by a local ophthalmologist. Examination findings and slit lamp appearance are illustrated in Figure 22.5.

KEY POINTS

Diagnosis:
- The above clinical scenario describes a case of right eye intrastromal foreign body with crystalline keratopathy. Diagnosis is based on clinical features vis-à-vis presence of a foreign body lodged in the cornea along with surrounding crystalline deposits.

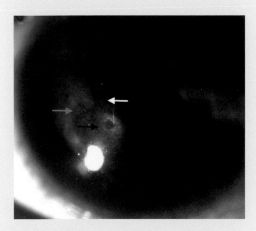

Figure 22.5 Slit lamp photograph of a patient showing a corneal foreign body with surrounding crystalline keratopathy. A small circular foreign body (black arrow) has been embedded in the inferotemporal quadrant with surrounding crystalline deposits (white arrow) with sparse brownish-black pigmentation (grey arrow).

Investigations:
- The depth of the dislodged foreign body was documented with ASOCT imaging.
- Corneal scrapings for microbiological cultures were also sent after discontinuing the antibiotics for 12 hours.
- A thorough posterior segment examination with indirect ophthalmoscopy and/or ultrasound is important to rule out any retained intraocular foreign body.

Treatment:
- The treatment of this foreign body-induced crystalline keratopathy mainly includes removing the foreign body either at the slit lamp itself or in the operating room depending on how deep it has been embedded. Here, the iron particle was embedded in the anterior corneal stroma, hence it was removed using a 26 G needle under topical anaesthesia at the slit lamp.
- The patient was additionally treated with topical steroids (fluorometholone 0.1%) and the ongoing topical antibiotics and lubricants were continued.

Outcome:
- The lesions resolved almost completely with approximately four weeks of treatment; steroids and antibiotics were gradually tapered, while lubricants were continued for three months.

Supplementary Information and Additional Tips

- It is recommended to send corneal scrapings even after the topical antibiotics have already been prescribed after discontinuing them for 12–24 hours. Diagnostic testing such as Gram stain, KOH mount and bacterial and fungal cultures as well as acid-fast stain and mycobacterial cultures should be done if indicated. However, the culture yield for ICK is generally low.

■ Unless the corneal foreign body is evidently superficial, removal should not be attempted without confirming its depth on ASOCT or ultrasound biomicroscopy (UBM).

■ Even after the removal of the foreign body, the patient might develop crystalline keratopathy diffusely involving the stroma with minimal stromal infiltrates and no anterior chamber inflammation (Figure 22.6).

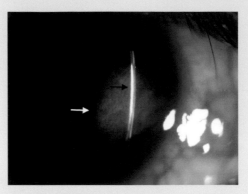

Figure 22.6 Slit lamp photograph demonstrating a well-circumscribed patch of crystalline keratopathy with very minimal surrounding stromal infiltrates (white arrow); overlying slit helps to show that the crystals are diffusely deposited in the stroma (black arrow).

CASE 22.4

CLINICAL FEATURES

A 66-year-old female presented to our outpatient department with recurrent episodes of pain, watering, glare, photophobia and diminution of vision in her left eye. She had a history of bone pain for two years and had been diagnosed with multiple myeloma, for which she was on chemotherapy. Examination findings and slit lamp appearance are illustrated in Figure 22.7.

KEY POINTS

Diagnosis:
■ The above clinical scenario describes a case of left eye crystalline keratopathy associated with lymphoproliferative disorder with a central ring of ferritin deposits.

Treatment:
■ The patient was initially treated with tear substitutes for four weeks but due to lack of any significant response, she was additionally prescribed hydroxyl propyl methyl cellulose (HPMC) gel

four times a day following which she reported symptomatic relief.
■ Refractive correction with anti-glare coating was prescribed.
■ A trial of a short course of low-potency steroids was also given for two weeks to reduce the inflammation but with no significant benefit.

Outcome:
■ There was no change in the lesion even after two months of treatment but the patient was relieved of the debilitating symptoms.

Supplementary Information and Additional Tips

■ Crystalline keratopathy associated with lymphoproliferative disorders can present with variable ocular symptoms and usually does not demonstrate a typical clinical picture.
■ The role of the ophthalmologist in treating such patients is mainly to provide symptomatic care.

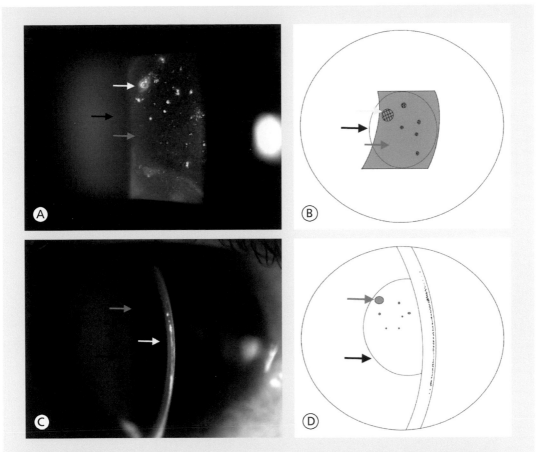

Figure 22.7 Slit lamp photograph of the right eye of a patient with lymphoproliferative disorder (A) and corresponding corneal diagram (B) showing a few central circular corneal opacities (grey arrow) with a circle of deposition of brownish iron deposits centrally (black arrow) and deposition of the crystals of varied sizes (white arrow). Slit lamp photograph of the other eye (C) and corresponding corneal diagram (D) showing similar but relatively subtle findings; note the central mid-stromal corneal deposits (white arrow) with surrounding diffuse mild stromal haze (grey arrow) along with a faint ring of iron deposits (black arrow).

REFERENCES

1. Kaufman HE, Barron BA, McDonald MD, eds. The Cornea. 2nd ed. Boston: Butterworth-Heinemann; 1998.
2. Weisenthal RW, Afshari NA, Bouchard CS, Colby KA, Rootman DS, Tu EY, de Freitas D. BCSC External Disease and Cornea, Section 8. San Francisco: American Academy of Ophthalmology; 2019-2020:533-553.
3. Gupta N, Ganger A, Bhartiya S, Verma M, Tandon R. In vivo confocal microscopic characteristics of crystalline keratopathy in patients with sclerokeratitis. Ocul Immunol Inflamm. 2018; 26(5):700–5.
4. Gahl WA, Kuehl EM, Iwata F, et al. Corneal crystals in nephropathic cystinosis: natural history and treatment with cysteamine eyedrops. Mol Genet Metab. 2000; 71:100–20.

23 Corneal Hydrops

Aishwarya Rathod, Ritika Mukhija, Noopur Gupta

INTRODUCTION

Acute corneal hydrops describes an abnormal accumulation of fluid in the corneal stroma caused by the acute disruption of Descemet's membrane in the background of corneal ectasia. Although majority of the cases are associated with keratoconus, it has also been seen with pellucid marginal degeneration (PMD), keratoglobus, Terrien's marginal degeneration (TMD), laser in situ keratomileusis (LASIK)-associated keratectasia, keratectasia after radial keratotomy (RK) deep anterior lamellar keratoplasty (DALK) and penetrating keratoplasty (PKP).[1,2] Most of the cases are seen in the second or the third decade with a preponderance for the male gender, often with a preceding history of vigorous eye-rubbing.[2,3]

CASE 23.1

CLINICAL FEATURES

A 23-year-old male presented to our outpatient department with history of painful diminution of vision and severe photophobia in his left eye for the last six days. The patient was a known case of bilateral keratoconus and was using rigid gas-permeable (RGP) lenses routinely. He had stopped using them since the onset of symptoms. The patient was already on topical antibiotics (moxifloxacin), topical hypertonic saline (5%), cycloplegic and lubricants prescribed by a local ophthalmologist; however, there was no significant improvement. Examination findings and slit lamp appearance are illustrated in Figure 23.1.

KEY POINTS

Diagnosis:
- With the given clinical scenario, the patient was diagnosed as a case of left eye acute corneal hydrops associated with keratoconus.

Investigations:
- Anterior segment optical coherence tomography (AS-OCT) was performed to quantify the extent and location of corneal oedema and thickness and the extent of the break in Descemet's membrane.
- Corneal Scheimpflug tomography was performed to assess the other eye and no significant progression was noted.

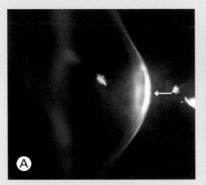 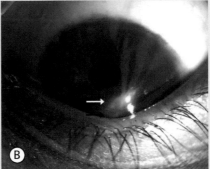

Figure 23.1 Slit lamp photograph of a patient with keratoconus showing (A) central corneal oedema (black arrow) and the slit view shows the conical protrusion of the cornea and the increased thickness depicts the magnitude of corneal oedema (white arrow). On downgaze (B), the central area of corneal oedema (white arrow) along with a V-shaped indentation of the lower eyelid in inferior gaze (black arrow), commonly known as Munson's sign, can be appreciated.

Treatment:

- In addition to the above medications, topical steroids (prednisolone acetate 1% four times a day) and antiglaucoma (timolol maleate 0.5% twice a day) were also added.
- Pneumatic descemetopexy using sulphur hexafluoride (SF6) was performed and a bandage contact lens (BCL) was placed on the cornea at the end of the procedure to provide temporary symptomatic relief.

Outcome:

- The stromal oedema settled and the patient reported relief in his symptoms; at four weeks follow-up, the BCL was removed. Steroids were tapered and stopped and the lubricants were continued.

- The hydrops healed with a macular corneal opacity and the patient was asked to continue the use of RGP and follow-up regularly.

Supplementary Information and Additional Tips

- Although the use of topical steroids is controversial, they are often employed to reduce the inflammation and subsequent neovascularisation that can accompany these episodes.
- Hydrops often resolves with para-central scarring as the cone usually does not involve the central cornea and can even cause flattening of the cone in some cases (Figure 23.2); hence visual acuity and lens-fitting may show improvement after healing.

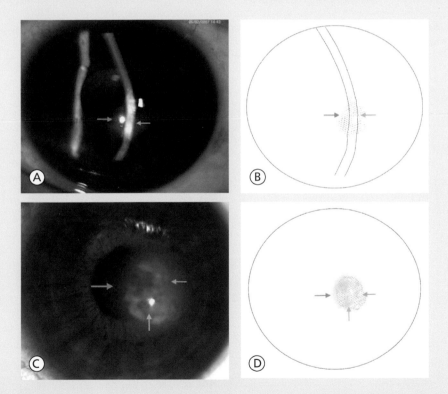

Figure 23.2 Slit lamp photograph of a patient with keratoconus showing (A) a central nebulo-macular opacity with healed hydrops (grey arrow) and absence of inflammation. Note the corneal ectasia and steepening along with flattening (yellow arrow) at the site of healed hydrops due to corneal scarring. The corresponding schematic diagram (B) depicts the same findings. Slit lamp photograph (C) and corresponding schematic corneal diagram (D) of another patient with keratoconus demonstrating localised corneal hydrops (grey arrow) showing signs of resolution with decrease in corneal oedema, scarring (green arrow) and appearance of clear areas (yellow arrow).

■ In some cases with severe and long-standing corneal hydrops, partial or delayed response may be observed, with corneal oedema taking days or months to subside even after pneumo-descemetopexy (Figure 23.3).

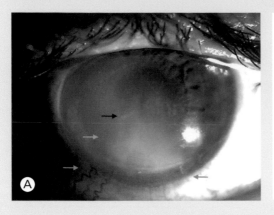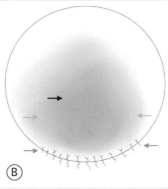

Figure 23.3 Slit lamp photograph of a patient with keratoconus demonstrating (A) features of resolving corneal hydrops after three days of pneumodescemetopexy. Note Descemet's membrane folds (black arrow) and corneal oedema (yellow arrows) with circumcorneal congestion (grey arrows), a sign of active inflammation. The corresponding schematic diagram (B) illustrates the same clinical findings.

CASE 23.2

CLINICAL FEATURES

A 36-year-old female presented to our outpatient department with an episode of sudden pain, watering, photophobia and diminution of vision in her right eye following rigorous itching. She was a known case of bilateral PMD diagnosed a year ago and was using spectacles for refractive correction. There was no history of any ocular trauma or contact lens wear over the past year. Examination findings and slit lamp appearance along with management of the case are illustrated in Figures 23.4 and 23.5.

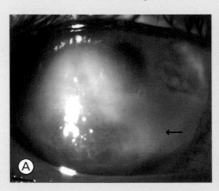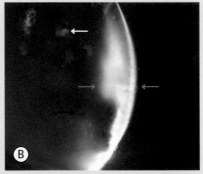

Figure 23.4 Slit lamp photograph of a patient with pellucid marginal corneal degeneration showing (A) inferior ectatic cornea with extensive central and inferior corneal oedema (black arrow) with circumcorneal congestion. Magnified slit view (B) reveals microcystic oedema (black arrow), corneal opacities of varied sizes superiorly (white arrow) and thickened cornea with severe oedema (grey arrows).

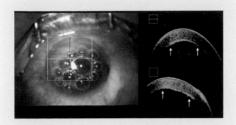

Figure 23.5 Intraoperative photograph of the patient with PMD and acute hydrops showing presence of the gas (sulphur hexafluoride) that had been injected inside the anterior chamber with its corresponding ASOCT on the right half of the image, demonstrating the attached hyper-reflective Descemet's membrane (white arrows), a sign of successful descemetopexy. The upper image depicts the horizontal cut section and the lower image depicts the vertical cut section as illustrated by blue and pink arrows.

KEY POINTS

Diagnosis:
- The above clinical scenario describes a case of right eye acute corneal hydrops associated with PMD.

Investigations:
- On Scheimpflug imaging, the classic topographic pattern of inferior steepening with superior flattening, described as a 'crab-claw' or 'lobster-claw' pattern, was seen in the left eye; AS-OCT was also performed to quantify the extent of corneal oedema in the right eye.

Treatment:
- The patient was started on preservative-free lubricants, topical hypertonic saline (5%), topical antibiotics (moxifloxacin 0.5%), antiglaucoma (timolol 0.5%) and cycloplegic (homatropine 2%). Oral acetazolamide 250 mg thrice a day was administered orally and intermittent patching was advised.
- The patient was subsequently managed by intracameral SF6 gas injection along with corneal stromal punctures performed under the guidance of intraoperative optical coherence tomography (iOCT); BCL was placed at the end of the procedure.

Outcome:
- The best corrected visual acuity significantly improved and was restored to 20/40 in the right eye at three months follow-up.
- Patient was continued on lubricating eye drops and counselled against eye-rubbing.

Supplementary Information and Additional Tips

- Large disruptions of Descemet's membrane are associated with prolonged resolution of the stromal oedema (Figure 23.6) resulting in

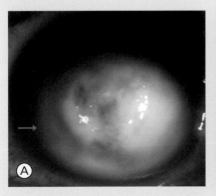
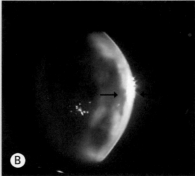

Figure 23.6 Slit lamp photograph of a patient with corneal ectasia and long-standing hydrops showing (A) non-resolving, chronic corneal oedema involving the visual axis with a large, circular maculo-leucomatous opacity (grey arrow). The corresponding slit image (B) reveals a thickened cornea with stromal opacification and presence of oedema (black arrows) and microcysts.

impaired corneal clarity because of scarring and surface irregularity, and a higher risk of neovascularisation, necessitating the need for corneal transplantation for visual rehabilitation.

- Excessive rubbing of the eyes in ectatic corneal disorders causes microtrauma and may result in Descemet's membrane rupture and eventual manifestation of acute corneal hydrops.
- Similar manifestations of acute corneal hydrops may rarely be seen in cases with post-LASIK ectasia (Figure 23.7).

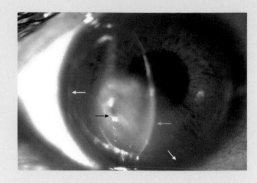

Figure 23.7 Slit lamp photograph of a patient with post-LASIK (laser in situ keratomileusis) ectasia presenting with focal oedema (yellow arrow) with areas of corneal thinning (black arrow); the peripheral edges of the LASIK flap (white arrows) are also faintly visible.

REFERENCES

1. Tuift SJ, Gregory WM, Buckley RJ. Acute corneal hydrops in keratoconus. Ophthalmology. 1994; 101:1738–44.
2. Grewal S, Laibson PR, Cohen EJ, Rapuano CJ. Acute hydrops in the corneal ectasias: Associated factors and outcomes. Trans Am Ophthalmol Soc. 1999; 97:187–203.
3. Feder RS, Neems LC. Chapter 72. Noninflammatory Ectatic Disorders. In Krachmer JH, Mannis MJ, Holland EJ (eds) Cornea. 4th edition. USA: Mosby Publishers. 2017; 820–44.

Index

Note: Locators in *italics* represent figures and **bold** indicate tables in the text.